Technology Driven
LIVESTOCK FARMING

THE EDITOR

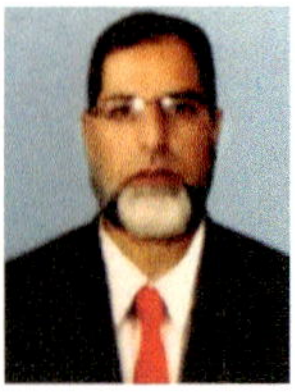

Dr. Zahoor A. Pampori Professor and Head, Division of Veterinary Physiology, Faculty of Veterinary Sciences, SKUAST-Kashmir, Srinagar. Has graduated in veterinary sciences from Ranchi Veterinary College in 1989 and did doctorate in Animal Physiology from National Dairy Research Institute, Karnal, Haryana. The editor has 32 years of service career and has served the State Animal Husbandry Department for 13 years and is discharging his duties in the Faculty of Veterinary Sciences, SKUAST-Kashmir for last 22 years in different capacities. He has over 60 publications in international and national journals and authored four books. He has organized several national & international workshops and training programmes.

Technology Driven
LIVESTOCK FARMING

— *Editor* —

Zahoor A. Pampori

2023

Daya Publishing House®
A Division of
Astral International Pvt. Ltd.
New Delhi – 110 002

ISBN: 978-93-5222-166-0 (HB)

Published by : **Daya Publishing House®**
A Division of
Astral International Pvt. Ltd.
– ISO 9001:2015 Certified Company –
4736/23, Ansari Road, Darya Ganj
New Delhi-110 002
Ph. 011-43549197, 23278134
E-mail: info@astralint.com
Website: www.astralint.com

Printed at : Replika Press Pvt. Ltd.

Sher-e-Kashmir
University of Agricultural Sciences & Technology of Kashmir
www.skuastkashmir.ac.in

Prof. Nazir A. Ganai
Vice-Chancellor

FOREWORD

The most significant increase in the world's population since the 1950s, is mainly attributed to medical advancement and increase in agricultural productivity. The food production per unit land has also increased several folds, mainly due to genetically improved varieties, mechanised agriculture practices and use of chemical fertilizers. However, intensive cultivation, grazing, soil mineralization, overuse of chemical fertilizers, deforestation, climate change and environmental degradation is not sustaining the food production for the growing global population. In such a scenario any form of intervention that could sustain the food production and nutritional security of the hug global population while respecting conservation of nature resource & environmental concern will be boon humanity.

There is dire need to look beyond existing farming systems and bring in the new innovative sophisticated technologies of robotics, sensors, aerial imaging, artificial intelligence, machine learning, digitization, automation in farming system to make livestock industry more profitable, efficient, safe, environmental friendly and more importantly sustainable.

The present book on *"Technology Driven Livestock Farming"* contains different chapters, dealing with challenges and solutions in livestock farming for future smart, efficient and precision farming. The chapters are lucid, vivid and encompass various strategies, policies, means and methods to increase the global food production, through use of emerging technologies of biotechnology, reproduction, bioinformatics, robotics, biosensors, IoT, machine learning and artificial intelligence. The contributions made by various international and national experts of repute in this book have made this book a policy document for planners and researchers. I am confident that this book, with strong science and policy commitment, will serve a guiding torch for researchers, academicians, policy makers and students to pursue the goal of technology driven livestock farming in future.

Place: Shalimar, Srinagar

Dated: 10.04.2023

(Nazir Ahmad Ganai)

Shalimar, Srinagar-190025, J&K India
Phone: (Office) 0194-246-1028; Fax: 0194-2461160(Resid.) 0194-2463655, 2461543

Preface

The first technology revolution in agriculture made impressive strides between 1961 to 2004 with tremendous increase in cereal production through use of mechanized farm practices, development of more productive varieties, use of chemical fertilizers and pesticides. However, efficiency gains are tumbling and the challenges are mounting owing to the exhausting natural resources, enormous increase in the expected food demand and simultaneously coping with climate change. Human population growth curve illustrates a spike and we have global human population of 7.2 billion in 2021that is projected to be 9.6 billion by 2050. The demand for agriculture products is expected to increase by 70% by 2050. The demand for meat and milk in 2050 is projected to grow by 73 and 58 percent, respectively especially in developing countries and emerging economies. Livestock is an important sector in global food security and globally accounts for 40% of global agricultural gross domestic product, and provides over 33% of the world's protein intake and 7% of global kilo calorie consumption. Livestock provides protein and nutritional security and can play a vital role in improving the lives of millions by providing the sufficient and reliable supplies of meat, milk, eggs and dairy products. Livestock is an important sector in agriculture food systems, diversifying food basket with animal-source foods; helping to generate income and creating employment, strengthening the rural household assets, improving the livelihood and supporting sustainable economic growth. The urbanization, improved incomes and dietary changes has increased the demand for foods of animal origin. Since livestock production has to get increased owing to increasing demands but cannot afford to produce it in a traditional farming system without protecting natural resources and respecting environment. We need to rethink on the conservation and judicial use of natural resources, efficient use of inputs, processing, value addition & availability of livestock products and conversion of animal waste into wealth to have future sustainable production system. There is dire need to look beyond existing farming systems and bring in the new innovative sophisticated technologies of robotics, sensors, aerial imaging, artificial intelligence, machine learning, digitization, automation in farming system to make livestock industry more profitable, efficient, safe, environmental friendly and more importantly sustainable. Future livestock farming must be smart and technology driven with efficient use of inputs for maximum output. It is with this intention that the book has been engraved and contains chapters from reputed experts from the field of animal physiology, reproduction, biotechnology, bioengineering and livestock management. The book is dealing with the challenges associated with livestock farming and solutions to transition away from the dominant industrial agriculture paradigm designed for massive production & self-sufficiency to one of sustainable agriculture that conserves natural resources & animal genetic resources via use of emerging appropriate technologies for economically viable and socially acceptable livestock food production. It contains 22 chapters on different topics relevant to title of the book.

I am confident and of firm belief that this book will serve as a guide for livestock scientists, managers, academicians and farmers in building their capacity, skills and technologies, besides a policy document for government functionaries to plan and design the policies related to technology driven livestock food production. In this noble mission I thankfully acknowledge the support rendered by the authors of this book. I also do thankfully acknowledge the help provided by Dr. Aasif A Sheikh, Dr. M. Rayees Dar, Dr. Dilruba Hasin, Dr. Ovais Aarif, Dr. Fozia Shah, Ms. Aroos Ali, Ms. Sumiera Shafi and Ms. Nowsheen Amin. I would like to acknowledge and appreciate Astral International Pvt Ltd, New Delhi for their support and responsibility of disseminating the knowledge/ science through publishing & printing of this manuscript.

(Zahoor A. Pampori)

Contents

List of Contributors

A. A. Sheikh
Division of Veterinary Physiology, Sher-e-Kashmir University of Agricultural Sciences and Technology, Srinagar, India

A. Nowsheen
Division of Veterinary Sciences & AH, SKUAST-Kashmir, Shuaham, Alusteng-190006, JK, India

A. Uroos
Division of Veterinary Sciences & AH, SKUAST-Kashmir, Shuaham, Alusteng-190006, JK, India

Aasif Ahmad Sheikh
Division of Veterinary Physiology, Faculty of Veterinary Sciences and Animal Husbandry, Sher-e-Kashmir University of Agricultural Sciences and Technology of Kashmir, Srinagar, Jammu & Kashmir
e-mail: aasifvet1@gmail.com

Abrar Malik
Cloning & Transgenic Laboratory, Division of Animal Biotechnology, SKUAST-K, Shuhama
e-mail: abrarmalik33@gmail.com

Abrar O. Ismail
Biomedical Sciences, Clinical Embryology and Reproductive Biology, College of Medicine, Alfaisal University, Riyadh, Saudi Arabia.

Amit Kumar
ICAR-Indian Veterinary Research Institute, Izatnagar,
Bareilly 243122, Uttar Pradesh, India
e-mail: amit.kumar@icar.gov.in, amitkat791@gmail.com

Anamika Pandey
Physiology & Climatology Division
ICAR-Indian Veterinary Research Institute, Izatnagar-243122
e-mail: anamikabulbul1396@gmail.com

Anjali
Physiology & Climatology Division
ICAR-Indian Veterinary Research Institute, Izatnagar-243122
e-mail: anjalibramhane@gmail.com

Ankita Bhatt
Chemical Biology Lab, Department of Biological Sciences and Bioengineering
Indian Institute of Technology Roorkee, Roorkee, Uttarakhand, India 247667"
e-mail: ankita_b@ah.iitr.ac.in

Ashok Kumar
Department of Biological Sciences and Bioengineering, Indian Institute of Technology Kanpur, Kanpur, U.P., India
e-mail: ashokkum@iitk.ac.in

Ashok Kumar Balhara
CAR-Central Institute for Research on Buffaloes, Hisar-125001
e-mail: balharaak@gmail.com

Azmat Alam Khan
Sher-e-Kashmir University of Agricultural Sciences and Technology of Kashmir, Srinagar,\ Jammu and Kashmir
e-mail: azmatalamkhan@gmail.com

C. Devaraj
Centre for Climate resilient Animal Adaptation Studies, ICAR-National Institute of Animal Nutrition and Physiology, Adugodi, Hosur Road, Bangalore-560030
e-mail: drcdeva@gmail.com

C.G. Shashank
Centre for Climate resilient Animal Adaptation Studies, ICAR-National Institute of Animal Nutrition and Physiology, Adugodi, Hosur Road, Bangalore-560030
e-mail: shanko009@gmail.com

Celus C.S.
ICAR-Indian Veterinary Research Institute, Izatnagar, Bareilly 243122, Uttar Pradesh, India
e-mail: cdlmcelus@gmail.com

Chandrasekhar B.
Dairy Microbiology Department, Warner College of Dairy Technology, SHUAT, Prayagraj, UP, India
e-mail: chandrundri93@gmail.com

D Hasin
Division of Veterinary Physiology, Faculty of Veterinary Sciences and Animal Husbandry, Sher-e-Kashmir University of Agricultural Sciences and Technology of Kashmir, Srinagar, Jammu & Kashmir

Dharmendra Kumar
Animal Physiology and Reproduction Division, ICAR-Central Institute for Research on Buffaloes, Hisar-125001, Haryana, India
e-mail: dkumarbt@gmail.com

Dilruba Hasin
Division of Veterinary Physiology, Faculty of Veterinary Sciences & Animal Husbandry, Shuhama, SKUAST-Kashmir
e-mail: dhasin7@gmail.com

Dr. Mahendra Singh
Division of Animal Physiology, ICAR-National Dairy Research Institute, Karnal-132001,
e-mail: chhokar.ms@gmail.com

Fozia Shah
Division of Veterinary Physiology, Faculty of Veterinary Sciences and Animal Husbandry, Sher-e-Kashmir University of Agricultural Sciences and Technology of Kashmir, Srinagar, Jammu & Kashmir
e-mail: drfozia_vet@rediffmail.com

G. Girish Varma
Vice Chairman, Bioengine Synergies Industries Private Ltd. & Former Faculty Dean (Dairy Science), Faculty
e-email: girish@kvasu.ac.in

Gyanendra Kumar Gaur
ICAR-Indian Veterinary Research Institute, Izatnagar, Bareilly 243122, Uttar Pradesh, India
e-mail: gyanendrakg@gmail.com

Gyanendra Singh
Physiology & Climatology Division ICAR-Indian Veterinary Research Institute, Izatnagar-243122
e-mail: gyansidd@gmail.com

Henna Hamadani
Sher-e-Kashmir University of Agricultural Sciences and Technology of Kashmir, Srinagar, Jammu and Kashmir
e-mail: hamadani.hh@gmail.co

Iqbal Hyder
Department of Physiology & Biochemistry, College of Veterinary Science, Garividi, A.P. - 535 101.
e-mail: iqbvet@gmail.com

Ishfaq A. Sheikh
Reproductive Biology Laboratory, King Fahd Medical Research Center, King Abdulaziz University, Jeddah, Saudi Arabia
e-mail: iasheikh@kau.edu.sa

Jonali Devi
Division of Veterinary Physiology & Biochemistry
e-mail: drjonali2011@gmail.com

K. Raji
Assistant Professor, Kerala Veterinary & Animal Sciences University
e-mail: raji@kvasu.ac.in

Kajal Sankar Roy
Principal Scientist, ICAR-National Institute of Animal Nutrition and Physiology, Adugodi, Bangalore- 560 030, Karnataka, India
e-mail: ksroy123star@gmail.com

Kamal Sarma
Division of Veterinary Anatomy Faculty of Veterinary Sciences & Animal Husbandry, SKUAST-Jammu, R. S. Pura (UT of J & K)
e-mail: kamalsarma73@gmail.com

Kawardeep Kour
Division of Veterinary Physiology & Biochemistry
email: vet26kawar@gmail.com

M. R. Dar
Division of Veterinary Physiology, Faculty of Veterinary Sciences and Animal Husbandry, Sher-e-Kashmir University of Agricultural Sciences and Technology of Kashmir, Srinagar, Jammu & Kashmir

M. Rayees
Division of Veterinary Sciences & AH, SKUAST-Kashmir, Shuaham, Alusteng-190006, JK, India

M.V.Silpa
Institute of Animal Breeding and Genetics, Justus-Liebig-Universität Gießen, Gießen, Germany
e-mail: mv.silpa@gmail.com

Mohammad Rayees Dar
Division of Veterinary Physiology, Faculty of Veterinary Sciences & Animal Husbandry, Shuhama, SKUAST-Kashmir
e-mail: rayeesr21@gmail.com

Mohan Mondal
Reproductive Physiology Laboratory, ICAR-National Dairy Research Institute, Eastern Regional Station, Kalyani, Nadia, West Bengal-741235, INDIA
e-mail: drmmondal@gmail.com

Mohd A. Beg
Reproductive Biology Laboratory, King Fahd Medical Research Center, King Abdulaziz University, Jeddah, Saudi Arabia
e-mail: mabeg51@gmail.com

Muneer Dar
Cloning & Transgenic Laboratory, Division of Animal Biotechnology, SKUAST-K, Shuhama" e-mail: darmuneer9858@gmail.com

N Amin
Division of Veterinary Physiology, Sher-e-Kashmir University of Agricultural Sciences and Technology, Srinagar, India

Naveen Kumar Navani
Chemical Biology Lab, Department of Biological Sciences and Bioengineering, Indian Institute of Technology Roorkee, Roorkee, Uttarakhand, India 247667"
e-mail: naveen.navani@bt.iitr.ac.in

Nida Handoo *Cloning & Transgenic Laboratory, Division of Animal Biotechnology, SKUAST-K, Shuhama e-mail: nidahandoo@gmail.com*

Nowsheen Amin
Division of Veterinary Physiology, Faculty of Veterinary Sciences and Animal Husbandry, Sher-e-Kashmir University of Agricultural Sciences and Technology of Kashmir, Srinagar, Jammu & Kashmir
e-mail: nowsheenamin7@gmail.com

Nukula Ramesh
Department of Veterinary Extension, College of Veterinary Science, Rajendranagar, Hyderabad, P. V. Narasimha Rao Telangana Veterinary University, Telangana, India
e-mail: ramesh.vet80@gmail.com

O. Aarif
Division of Veterinary Physiology, Faculty of Veterinary Sciences and Animal Husbandry, Sher-e-Kashmir University of Agricultural Sciences and Technology of Kashmir, Srinagar, Jammu & Kashmir
e-mail: ovaisaarif@gmail.com

P S Yadav
Animal Physiology and Reproduction Division, ICAR-Central Institute for Research on Buffaloes, Hisar-125001, Haryana, India
e-mail: psycirb@gmail.com

Pavan Kumar Pesingi
Department of Veterinary Public Health and Epidemiology, Faculty of Veterinary and Animal Sciences, Institute of Agricultural Sciences, Rajiv Gandhi South Campus, Banaras Hindu University, Barkachha, Mirzapur, Uttar Pradesh, India
e-mail: pavanpesingi@gmail.com

R. Bhatta
Centre for Climate resilient Animal Adaptation Studies, ICAR-National Institute of Animal Nutrition and Physiology, Adugodi, Hosur Road, Bangalore-560030
e-mail: directornianp@gmail.com

Riaz Shah
Cloning & Transgenic Laboratory, Division of Animal Biotechnology, SKUAST-K, Shuhama
e-mail: drriazshah@gmail.com

S Shafi
Division of Veterinary Physiology, Sher-e-Kashmir University of Agricultural Sciences and Technology, Srinagar, India

S. Sumeira
Division of Veterinary Sciences & AH, SKUAST-Kashmir, Shuaham, Alusteng-190006, JK, India

Saba Nazir
Cloning & Transgenic Laboratory, Division of Animal Biotechnology, SKUAST-K, Shuhama
e-mail: sabanazir389@gmail.com

Safia Zahoor
Division of Veterinary Physiology, Faculty of Veterinary Sciences & Animal Husbandry, Shuhama, SKUAST-Kashmir
e-mail: safiakawoosa530@gmail.com

Sakshi Vaishnav
ICAR-Indian Veterinary Research Institute, Izatnagar, Bareilly-243122, Uttar Pradesh, India
e-mail: sakshivaishnav1996@gmail.com

Sandhya S Chaudhary
Department of Veterinary Physiology and Biochemistry College of Veterinary Science and A.H., Kamdhenu University, Navsari (Gujarat)
e-mail: sandhyachaudhary6@gmail.com

Sheikh Firdous Ahmad
ICAR-Indian Veterinary Research Institute, Izatnagar, Bareilly 243122, Uttar Pradesh, India
e-mail: sheikh.ahmad@icar.gov.in

Shubham Jain
Chemical Biology Lab, Department of Biological Sciences and Bioengineering, Indian Institute of Technology Roorkee, Roorkee, Uttarakhand, India 247667
e-mail: jainshubham167@gmail.com

Sohan Vir Singh
Animal Physiology Division
ICAR-National Dairy Research Institute, Karnal, India
e-mail: sohanvir2004@yahoo.com

Subodh Kumar
ICAR-Indian Veterinary Research Institute, Izatnagar,
Bareilly 243122, Uttar Pradesh, India
e-mail : subkum@gmail.com

Suhail A. Khan
Division of Veterinary Physiology, Faculty of Veterinary Sciences & Animal Husbandry, Shuhama,
SKUAST-Kashmir e-mail: suhailkhann4321@gmail.com

Suhail Magray
Cloning & Transgenic Laboratory, Division of Animal Biotechnology, SKUAST-K, Shuhama
e-mail: suhailmagray@gmail.com

Suman Sangwan
CAR-Central Institute for Research on Buffaloes, Hisar-125001

Sumeira Shafi
Division of Veterinary Physiology, Faculty of Veterinary Sciences and Animal Husbandry, Sher-e-Kashmir University of Agricultural Sciences and Technology of Kashmir, Srinagar,
Jammu & Kashmir
e-mail: sumeirashafi@gmail.com

Swati Thakur
Animal Physiology and Reproduction Division, ICAR-Central Institute for Research on Buffaloes,
Hisar-125001, Haryana, India

Syed Hilal
Cloning & Transgenic Laboratory, Division of Animal Biotechnology, SKUAST-K, Shuhama
e-mail: hilalyaqoob3@gmail.com

Thulasiraman Parkunan
Department of Veterinary Physiology and Biochemistry, Faculty of Veterinary and Animal Sciences, Institute of Agricultural Sciences, Rajiv Gandhi South Campus, Banaras Hindu
e-mail: dr.thula89@gmail.com

Triveni Dutt
ICAR-Indian Veterinary Research Institute, Izatnagar,
Bareilly 243122, Uttar Pradesh, India
e-mail: director.ivri@icar.gov.in

Uroos Ali
Division of Veterinary Physiology, Faculty of Veterinary Sciences and Animal Husbandry, Sher-e-Kashmir University of Agricultural Sciences and Technology of Kashmir,
Srinagar, Jammu & Kashmir
e-mail: uroosali786@gmail.com

V. Sejian
Centre for Climate resilient Animal Adaptation Studies, ICAR-National Institute of Animal Nutrition and Physiology, Adugodi, Hosur Road, Bangalore-560030
e-mail: drsejian@gmail.com

Varshetha Muthukumar
Department of Public Health, School of Health, Bioscience and Sport, University of East London, UK
e-mail: varshetham@gmail.com

Virendra Kumar Singh
Department of Veterinary Physiology and Biochemistry College of Veterinary Science and A.H., Kamdhenu University, Navsari (Gujarat)
e-mail: drvksingh1981@gmail.com

VP Maurya
Physiology & Climatology Division ICAR-Indian Veterinary Research Institute, Izatnagar-243122
e-mail: vijaipmaurya@gmail.com

Wilfried Kues
Department of Biotechnology, FLI-Institute of Farm Animal Genetics, Neustadt, Germany - 31535
e-mail: wilfried.kues@fli.de

Younis Farooq
Cloning & Transgenic Laboratory, Division of Animal Biotechnology,SKUAST-K, Shuhama
e-mail: younisfarooqwani@gmail.com

Z. A. Pampori
Division of Veterinary Physiology, Faculty of Veterinary Sciences and Animal Husbandry, Sher-e-Kashmir University of Agricultural Sciences and Technology of Kashmir, Srinagar, Jammu & Kashmir
e-mail: drzap64@gmail.com

Chapter 1

Genetically Engineered Whole-cell Biosensors: From Naïve Bugs to Protean Detectives

Shubham Jain, Ankita Bhatt, Naveen Kumar Navani*
Chemical Biology Lab, Department of Biological Sciences and Bioengineering, Indian Institute of Technology Roorkee, Roorkee, Uttarakhand, India 247667
naveen.navani@bt.iitr.ac.in

INTRODUCTION

Biosensors in the current scenario are playing a pivotal role in biomedical diagnosis as well as a wide range of other areas like point-of-care devices for environmental monitoring, food security, drug discovery as well as forensics[1,2]. The first use of biosensors dates back to 1956 by Leyland C. Clark for oxygen detection[3]. Biosensor is defined as a detection entity made up of a molecular recognition element 'MRE' (which invariably is a biological moiety) linked to a transducer which converts molecular recognition into a detectable signal. MRE or biorecognition elements in biosensors range from nucleic acids, proteins, enzymes, and antibodies to entire cells. Macromolecule-based biosensors are highly specific but are usually expensive due to their downstream processing and instability in complex and extreme environments which leads to a short shelf life thus restricting their application in real-time sample analysis[4]. However, advancements in genetic engineering have led to the development of whole-cell biosensors which provide specificity, sensitivity, and stability to the biosensing platforms. As a base for whole-cell biosensors, bacterial cells have several advantages over eukaryotic cells when utilized as a biosensing element to engineer whole-cell biosensors. Some of the advantages are - their ubiquitous nature, ability to adapt and metabolize a wide range of chemical compounds, ability to thrive in adverse conditions, ability to degrade new molecules with time, and are amenable to genetic modifications. All these properties impart bacterial whole-cell biosensors a cutting edge over other biosensors. Being inexpensive, and field-deployable whole-cell biosensors can replace expensive and sophisticated analytical techniques like GC, HPLC, etc.

Whole-cell biosensors comprise of a genetic regulatory element based on mostly a transcription factor, that acts as an activator or a repressor protein; an inducible promoter as a biosensing element, and reporter proteins (such as *crtA, lux, luc, gfp,* etc.) as a transducer element[5]and wastewater-based epidemiology (WBE. Usually, the transcription factor controls the initiation of transcription, either by blocking the operator site in the case of repressor-based sensors or being unable to bind alone to transcriptional factor binding sites present in the promoter region in the case of activator-based sensors, resulting in no binding of RNA polymerase at the promoter site. However, in the presence of a cognate analyte, the repressor protein kicks off from the operator site and binds to the analyte due to better affinity, providing the site for RNA polymerase binding and generating a detection signal eventually. In the case of activator-based biosensors, the analyte act as a co-inducer allowing the activator protein to bind to TFBS and facilitating RNA polymerase binding to switch on transcription of the downstream reporter protein. The binding affinity of the transcription factor to the cognate analyte imparts specificity to the biosensor, while the sensitivity and detection limits of the biosensor are determined by the reporters or transducer elements used.

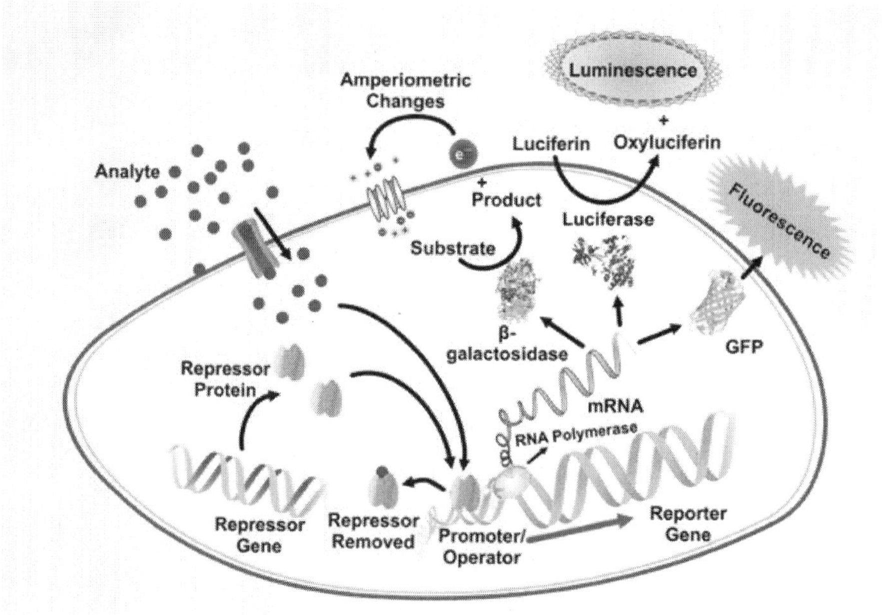

Figure 1a: Whole-cell biosensor: its principle and mechanism

CHARACTERISTICS OF WHOLE-CELL BIOSENSORS

There are certain attributes that all biosensors must possess. The optimization of these parameters is reflected in the performance of whole-cell biosensors.

1. **Selectivity:** The selectivity of a whole-cell biosensor depends on the specific interaction between the transcription factor and the analyte of interest. However, many naturally occurring transcription factors are promiscuous, so cells can respond to many similar molecules without the

requirement of a specific sensing part for each molecule. The binding of non-specific molecules can lead to false-positive results. In such cases, directed evolution is one of the strategies used to improve the selectivity of the transcription factor by altering the binding pocket. Genetic circuits build using logic gates can also be used to enhance the specificity. As, in the case of the promiscuous biosensing element, multiple sensing parts can be combined via AND gate where the signal is produced only when both the biosensing parts are activated.

2. **Sensitivity:** Another important parameter for a biosensor is its sensitivity. The sensitivity of the whole-cell biosensor depends on the minuscule quantity of analyte good enough to cross the cell membrane and interact with the transcription factor to facilitate the binding of RNA polymerase to the promoter and ultimately, produce a detectable signal. Therefore, increasing the intracellular concentration of the analyte is one way to enhance the sensitivity which could be achieved either by overexpressing the importer proteins or by the knockout of efflux pumps. Another approach would be to increase or decrease the concentration of transcription factor inside the cell depending of the fact that whether the transcription factor is an activator or repressor protein.

3. **Dynamic Range:** Dynamic range is the ratio of the leaky expression of the promoter to the maximum inducible expression of the promoter, also termed the "signal-to-noise ratio". Maximizing the dynamic range of the biosensor is one of the important attributes of a biosensor. The dynamic range of a whole-cell biosensor majorly depends on the strength of the promoter used. With strong promoters, there is a probability of more leaky expression, although weak promoters fail to give high analyte inducible expression, resulting in a low signal-to-noise ratio. Hence, the binding equilibrium between RNA polymerase and the promoter is to be determined. One of the ways to increase the translation rate is to change the RBS strength. Genetic amplifiers, like the hrpRS amplification system, can also be used to boost the response of whole-cell biosensors.

4. **Stability:** Stability is another important parameter to widen the applicability of whole-cell biosensors. Whole-cell biosensors are quite stable as compared to molecular sensors as the microbes are under a constant phase of evolution to survive extremities. Currently, lyophilization and encapsulation have been studied to enhance the shelf life of whole-cell biosensors. Another approach to increase the stability of whole-cell biosensors is to use spore-forming bacteria like *Bacillus subtilis* as biosensor chassis. These spores can be induced to reanimate the sensor activity for 12 months when refrigerated.

ADVANCEMENTS IN WHOLE-CELL BIOSENSOR ENGINEERING

With the increasing trust in the potential of whole cell biosensors to identify previously undetectable critical analytes, it quickly became a complimentary detection tool with performance either at par or better than its standard analytical detection counterparts. Improvised strategies have been able to increase the detection efficiency, molecular specificity, detection limit, and dynamic range for optimal biosensor performance. This has been made possible due to advancements in the fields of microbial genomics, microbial evolution, and bioinformatics in the past decades.

1. **Protein engineering and genetic element optimization:** The most important feature of a successful whole-cell biosensor is its ability to specifically interact with its target analyte present even in trace concentrations in complex samples. However, there still exist some concerns in the widespread usage of these biosensors as detection platforms because of their lack of specificity, variable dynamic ranges, and genetic instability of the sensing circuits. This made it imperative to optimize the detection platform with enhanced attributes to establish it as a sustainable alternative to the existing analytical methods. The most significant approaches either involve the redesigning of the regulator protein or altering the genetic elements that are critical for the regulator-operator interaction, ultimately controlling the downstream expression of the reporter gene[6]rapid, *in situ*, and real-time analytical tools for monitoring environments. The development of synthetic biology has enabled emergence of genetically engineered whole-cell microbial biosensors. This review updates the design and optimization principles for a diverse array of whole-cell biosensors based on transcription factors (TF. Such adaptations in genetic elements of whole-cell biosensors impart tunability to their sensitivity, specificity, dynamic range, and optimal detection range.
2. **Reporter element modifications:** It is established that an ideal transducing element plays a major role in determining the sensitivity of the biosensor and its subsequent success in field applications. Over decades, many reporters have been in practice to make whole-cell biosensors better than other biosensors. Amelioration of reporters has changed the common colorimetric whole-cell biosensors to several classes, like, fluorescence, luminescence, olfactory, magnetic, electrochemical, etc. These modified reporters widen the applications of whole-cell biosensors for rapid and sensitive detection of analytes in remote settings[7].
3. **Artificial Intelligence and Directed evolution:** The constant need to develop novel analyte recognition elements for expanding the application range of WCB has inspired researchers to develop advanced algorithms that can elucidate the optimal modification of both regulator and transduction domains to increase the specificity and binding affinity of a regulator protein to a certain analyte. Thus, expanding the toolbox of transcription factors that recognize new analytes is of considerable interest in many applications[8]. The development of AI-based models eventually eases the directed evolution of genetic elements by predicting the fate of the proposed evolution, thus, facilitating new endeavors of repurposing already-known whole-cell biosensors.

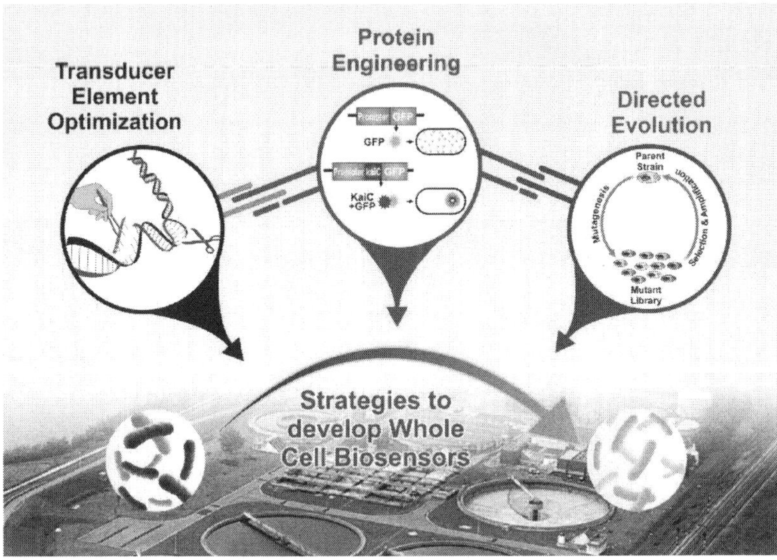

Figure : 1b. Advanced strategies to develop whole-cell biosensors for wider applicability.

APPLICATIONS OF WHOLE-CELL BIOSENSORS

1. **Food and feed toxins:** Around 48 million people suffer due to foodborne illness every year in the United States, emphasizing the quick, and sensitive detection of toxins and toxin-producing microbes in food to maintain food safety. Wu et al. generated a QscR quorum sensing system-based biosensor, which detects the Acyl Homoserine Lactones (AHLs) synthesized by *Pseudomonas aeruginosa* and *Burkholderia pseudomallei*[9]. The detection was based on colorimetric signal generation in the form of lycopene with a range of detection of about 1-100 nM. Several whole-cell biosensors for bacterial and fungal toxins are also present in the literature, playing a vital role in food security and safety.

2. **Antibiotics and their derivatives:** The screening methods for antibiotic residues starts in the early 1970 with many advances through the decades however, the scientific community is searching for more facile, efficient, and user-friendly methods. Over the past few decades, the use of various transcriptional factor-based biosensors for several antibiotics and their residues has been attempted but these bacterial sensors require genetic engineering for better performance. Ma et al. proposed a biosensing strategy based on genetically modified *E. coli* for paper-based detection of tetracycline in different environmental matrices[10]. This paper-based biosensor has a quantitative range of 75-10000 μg/L with a detection limit of 5.23 – 17.1 μg/L and could be a part of a simple, inexpensive point-of-care field kit. Another interesting biosensor for fluoroquinolone detection was engineered by Srivastava et al., which was highly specific and sensitive with a detection limit of 1 μg/mL[11].

3. **Metabolites:** Metabolites are important biomarkers for the detection of various communicable or non-communicable diseases. The abnormal accumulation or depletion of such metabolites is the result of abnormal metabolism occurring during the diseased state in the patients. Hence, clinicians require simple yet efficient point-of-care diagnostic tools for the quantitative determination of such metabolites in physiological fluids without complicated pre-treatment procedures. Dhyani et al. developed two whole-cell biosensors for the quantitative estimation of homocysteine and tryptophan to detect homocystinuria and tryptophanuria with LOD of 3.8 and 3 μM, respectively[12]and cost-effective diagnostic tools for the quantitative determination of amino acids in physiological fluids for the detection of metabolic disorder diseases. Besides, amino acids also act as biological markers for different types of cancers and cardiovascular diseases. Herein, we applied an in-silico based approach to identify potential amino acid-responsive genetic regulatory elements for the detection of metabolic disorders in humans. Identified sequences were further transcriptionally fused with GFP, thus generating an optical readout in response to their cognate targets. Screening of genetic regulatory elements led us to discover two promoter elements (pmetE::GFP and ptrpL::GFP. Both biosensors are highly specific for their cognate analytes however, the tryptophan biosensor is a turn-off type biosensor, decreasing the GFP synthesis in presence of tryptophan. Similarly, Dhyani et al. also engineered a biosensor for the rapid detection of alkaptonuria, a rare inherited disorder of amino acid metabolism[13]"ISSN":"15206882","abstract":"Clinicians require simple quantitative tools for the detection of homogentisic acid in alkaptonuria patients, a rare inherited disorder of amino acid metabolism. In this study, we report a whole-cell biosensor for homogentisic acid to detect alkaptonuria disease through the expression of green fluorescence protein. The assay system utilizes a promoter sequence (hmgA. The biosensor detects homogentisic acid to the detection limit of 3.9 μM in 4 hrs in urine samples of the patient. Thus, whole-cell biosensors are creating their recognition in the biomedical field as well.

4. **Surfactants:** Surfactants and detergents are one of the most commonly found chemicals in industrial and domestic waste. Their wide range of applications has increased their use to alarming levels. Thus, it is important to generate specific and rapid biosensors which can detect detergents in wastewater and sewage quickly and reliably. Recently, Dey et al. developed a whole-cell biosensor using *P. aeruginosa* as chassis and GFP as reporter gene having a linear range of detection 0.4-62.5 ppm of SDS in wastewater[14]agricultural operations, and industries is leading to its subsequent disposal in waterways. There is an apprehension of the adverse effect of such detergents on various living organisms. Thus, an efficient, specific, and simple detection method to monitor SDS reliably in the environment is needed. We used sdsB1 activator protein and SDS-responsive promoter of sdsA1 gene along with Green Fluorescent Protein (GFP. The LOD of the engineered biosensor is 0.1 ppm. It is the first and only WCB,

which is highly specific to SDS and has minimal interference with other detergents (SDBS), metals, and inorganic ions.

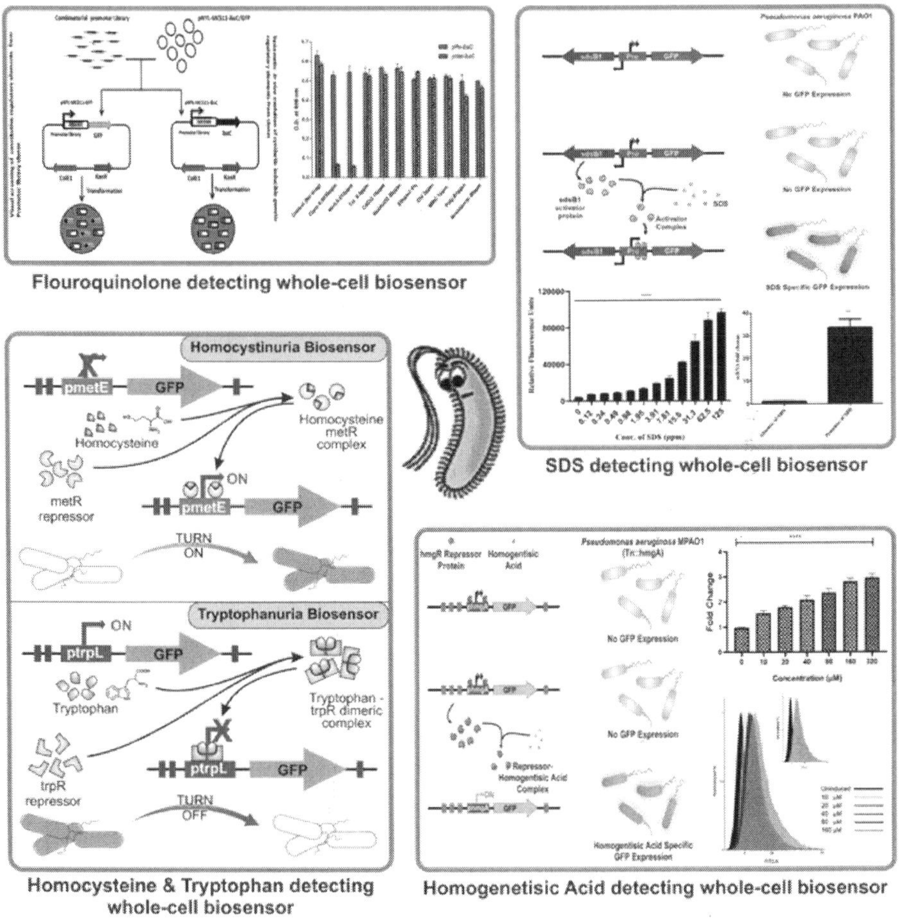

Figure : 1c. Some recently developed whole-cell biosensors for the detection of antibiotics, metabolites, and surfactants [11,12,13,14].

CONCLUSION

Over the last decade, our understanding of the prokaryotic world has increased manifold as a result researchers have taken advantage to generate whole-cell biosensors for detection of chosen targets. Furthermore, biotechnology, synthetic biology, and protein engineering have emerged as systematic approaches to rationalizing genetic modifications of the cells, leading to the generation of reliable, sensitive, and specific whole-cell biosensors. AI-based platforms have also leveraged learned knowledge to tackle specific tasks in the upliftment of whole-cell biosensors. We believe that future development of whole-cell biosensors would focus on mining sensing elements through high-throughput screening and machine learning, resolving biosafety issue of WCBs, and exploiting novel biosensors such as microbial electrochemical sensors and cell-free sensors for monitoring and treatment of a plethora of analytes ranging from simpler small molecules to complex bacterial cells. Thus, whole cell biosensors are poised to become Sherlock Holmes of the bio-future!

Acknowledgement – Research in Navani lab is generously supported by funds from DBT, ICMR and ICAR, Govt of India.

REFERENCES

Karunakaran, C., Rajkumar, R. & Bhargava, K. *Introduction to Biosensors. Biosensors and Bioelectronics* (Elsevier Inc., 2015). doi:10.1016/B978-0-12-803100-1.00001-3

Navani, N. K. & Li, Y. Nucleic acid aptamers and enzymes as sensors. *Curr. Opin. Chem. Biol.* 10, 272–281 (2006).

Heineman, W. R. & Jensen, W. B. Leland C. Clark Jr. (1918–2005). *Biosens. Bioelectron.* 21, 1403–1404 (2006).

Morales, M. A. & Halpern, J. M. Guide to Selecting a Biorecognition Element for Biosensors. *Bioconjug. Chem.* 29, 3231–3239 (2018).

Mao, K., Zhang, H., Pan, Y. & Yang, Z. Biosensors for wastewater-based epidemiology for monitoring public health. *Water Res.* 191, (2021).

Liu, C. et al. Engineering whole-cell microbial biosensors: Design principles and applications in monitoring and treatment of heavy metals and organic pollutants. *Biotechnol. Adv.* 60, 108019 (2022).

Polat, E. O. et al. Transducer Technologies for Biosensors and Their Wearable Applications. *Biosensors* 12, (2022).

Andon, J. S., Lee, B. & Wang, T. Enzyme directed evolution using genetically encodable biosensors. *Org. Biomol. Chem.* 20, 5891–5906 (2022).

Wu, Y., Wang, C. W., Wang, D. & Wei, N. A Whole-Cell Biosensor for Point-of-Care Detection of Waterborne Bacterial Pathogens. *ACS Synth. Biol.* 10, 333–344 (2021).

Ma, Z., Liu, J., Sallach, J. B., Hu, X. & Gao, Y. Whole-cell paper strip biosensors to semi-quantify tetracycline antibiotics in environmental matrices. *Biosens. Bioelectron.* 168, 112528 (2020).

Srivastava, S. K. et al. Isolation of a non-genomic origin fluoroquinolone responsive regulatory element using a combinatorial bioengineering approach. *Nucleic Acids Res.* 44, 2451–2461 (2016).

Dhyani, R., Jain, S., Bhatt, A., Kumar, P. & Navani, N. K. Genetic regulatory element based whole-cell biosensors for the detection of metabolic disorders. *Biosens. Bioelectron.* 199, 113869 (2022).

Dhyani, R. et al. Homogentisic acid-based whole-cell biosensor for detection of alkaptonuria disease. *Anal. Chem.* 93, 4521–4527 (2021).

Dey, S., Baba, S. A., Bhatt, A., Dhyani, R. & Navani, N. K. Transcription factor based whole-cell biosensor for specific and sensitive detection of sodium dodecyl sulfate. *Biosens. Bioelectron.* 170, 112659 (2020).

Chapter 2

Gene Editing Technologies for Livestock Improvement in India: Present Scenario and Future Prospects

Riaz Shah*, Abrar Malik, Nida Handoo, Younis Farooq, Syed Hilal, Suhail Magray, Muneer Dar, Saba Nazir

Cloning & Transgenic Laboratory, Division of Animal Biotechnology, SKUAST-K, Shuhama

**Email: drriazshah@gmail.com*

INTRODUCTION

Advancements in genetic manipulation have propelled the field of biotechnology into an exciting era. High-throughput DNA sequencing and genome editing have revolutionized research on model organisms, evolutionary studies, food organisms, and medical applications. These innovative technologies are game-changing tools for the scientific community and have opened up new possibilities.

The field of genetic modifications in mammals has significantly progressed over the years, from insertional transgenesis to advanced techniques like gene targeting and editing. Most recently, base and prime editing have emerged as powerful tools that utilize CRISPR-derived systems to enhance precision and efficiency in gene editing (Kalds *et al.*, 2020). These techniques offer permanent and cumulative results that can be accomplished in a relatively short ramp-up period (Doudna and Charpentier, 2014).

Since its first application in the mammalian genome (Cong *et al.*, 2013), CRISPR technology has been extended to a broad range of cell lines and mammalian species, including livestock. The advent of CRISPR/Cas9-based genome editing tools has brought about a significant breakthrough in this field, enabling efficient and easy modifications to be made in livestock genomes (Urnov *et al.*, 2010; Joung and Sander,

2013; Laible *et al.*, 2015; Lillico *et al.*, 2016; Georges *et al.*, 2019). This technology has opened up avenues for introducing modifications that can enhance livestock production traits, improve animal health and welfare, generate more refined large animal models of human diseases, produce pharmaceutical proteins, and study gene function.

GENOME EDITING PLATFORMS

Gene editing has been revolutionized by the development and successful use of several nucleases, such as Zinc Finger Nuclease (ZFN), Transcription Activator-Like Effector Nuclease (TALEN), and the Clustered Regularly Interspaced Short Palindromic Repeat (CRISPR) and RISPR-associated (Cas) protein 9 system. All of these platforms arose from investigations into natural biological processes and not from intentions to find genome editing reagents. Compared to conventional gene targeting based on homologous recombination (HR), these nuclease-based gene editing tools offer significant advantages in terms of targeted genome engineering, including higher efficiency, lower cost, and greater simplicity. This has ushered in a new era of genetic modifications, particularly in large animals, facilitating biological and biomedical investigations. '

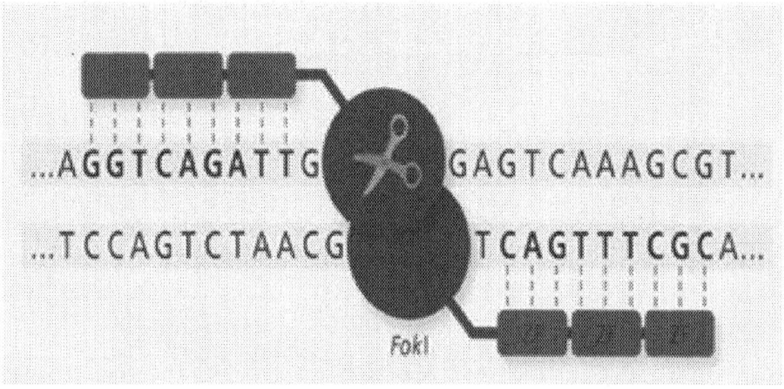

Figure 1: Zinc-finger nucleases (ZFNs)

a. The first synthetic genome editing agents were Zinc Finger Nucleases (ZFNs), (Figure 1) which consist of a zinc finger protein (ZFP) binding module and the Flavobacterium okeanokoites endonuclease (FokI) as a restriction enzyme domain. To induce double-strand breaks (DSBs) during genome editing, a pair of ZFPs must bind flanking regions of the target locus and form a FokI dimer.

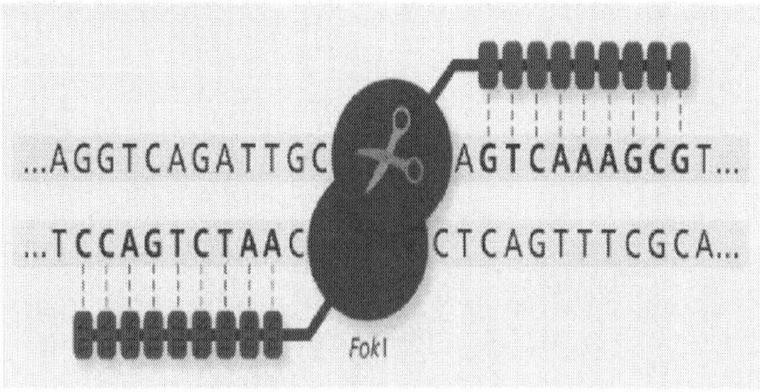

Figure 2: Transcription activator-like effector nucleases (TALENs)

b. Transcription activator-like effector nucleases (TALENs) (Figure 2) are also modular proteins containing a customizable DNA-binding domain (TALE) and a FokI nuclease domain. Like ZFNs, TALENs generate DSBs through FokI dimerization by cutting TALE-binding DNA sequences. TALEN-mediated gene editing was recognized as one of the top 10 scientific breakthroughs of 2012, and both ZFNs and TALENs have been used to generate genetically modified large animals. However, their extensive protein-DNA contacts and highly repetitive nature made it challenging to target different sites in the genome without re-engineering a new set of proteins. This, along with the difficulty in cloning and protein engineering, has limited their adoption by the scientific community. Since 2013, the CRISPR system has dominated the genome editing field due to its efficiency and ease of use. Compared to ZFNs and TALENs, CRISPR is simpler, more flexible, and has fewer technical barriers, making it a more accessible tool for the scientific community (Table 1).

Table-1: Comparison between ZFNs, TALENs, and CRRISR/Cas systems for genome editing.

Features of Gene ZFNs editing tools	ZFNs	TALENs	CRISPR/Cas9
Target DNA recognition Key components Function mode	Protein-DNA ZF-Fok I fusion protein ZF proteins recognize target DNA sequences R dimerization of Fok I nucleases induces DSBs of DNA RDSBs are repaired by NHEJ or HDR	Protein-DNA TALE-Fok I fusion protein TALE proteins recognize target DNA sequences R dimerization of Fok I nucleases induces DSBs of DNA R BSDs are repaired by NHEJ or HDR Highly efficient and specific	RNA-DNA Guide RNA and Cas9 protein Guide RNA recognizes target DNA sequence next to a NGG motifRCas9 induces DSBs of DNARDSBs are repaired by NHEJ or HDR
Advantages	Highly efficient and specific	Highly efficient and specific	Highly efficient, easy to be constructed, and capable of editing multiple sites simultaneously
Disadvantages	Large-scale screening, time-consuming, expensive to be constructed	Tedious and time consuming to be constructed	Pam motif next to target sequence required
DSB=Double-strand break, NHEJ=Non-homologous end joining,HDR=Homology-direct repair, ZFNs=Zinc finger nucleases, Talens =Transcription activator-like effector nuclease, CRISPR/ Cas9=Clustered regularly interspaced short palindromic repeats			

c. In 2007, CRISPR (Figure 3) was discovered as a defense mechanism utilized by bacteria to defend against viruses. In 2012, the CAS protein was found to have the ability to cleave specific DNA sequences guided by short synthetic pieces of RNA in vitro. Subsequently, in 2013, the power of CRISPR-mediated genome modification was demonstrated in mammalian cells by various laboratories. The CRISPR/Cas system has revolutionized the life sciences with its scalability, affordability, and engineering flexibility, allowing for efficient and versatile genetic modifications such as deletions, knock-ins, RNA regulation, and chromatin modification of targeted gene loci.

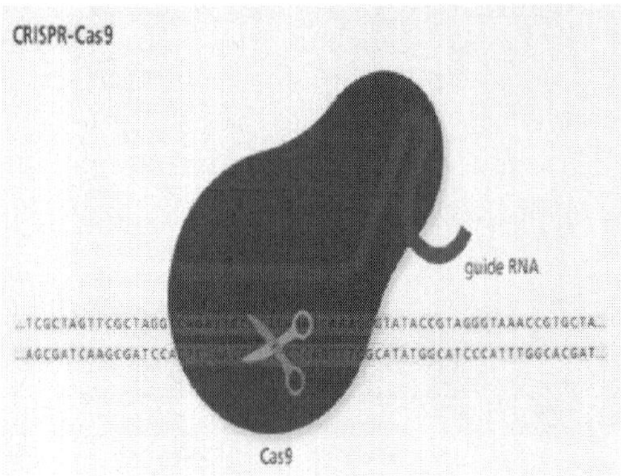

Figure 3

CRISPR/CAS MECHANISM

CRISPR/Cas-9 genome editing involves three main steps: recognition, cleavage, and repair (Figure 4). The process is initiated when the designed sgRNA guides the Cas-9 protein to the target sequence in the gene of interest by recognizing it through its 5 crRNA complementary base pair component. In the absence of sgRNA, the Cas-9 protein remains inactive. Once the Cas-9 protein finds the target site, it makes a double-stranded break (DSB) at a site 3 base pair upstream to PAM, which is a short conserved DNA sequence downstream to the cut site.

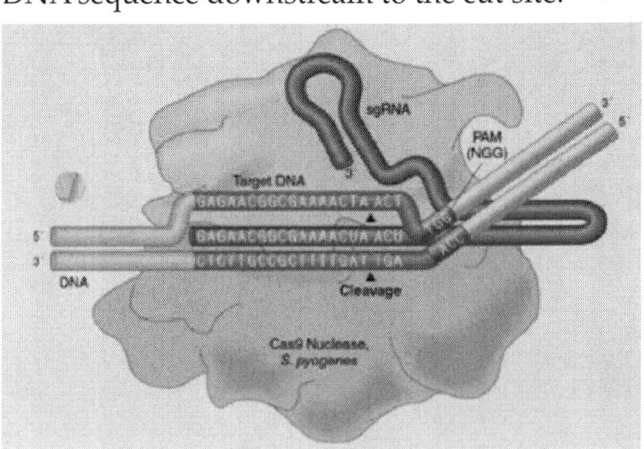

Figure 4

The PAM sequence varies in size depending on the bacterial species, and the Cas-9 protein recognizes the PAM sequence at 5-NGG-3 (N can be any nucleotide base). After finding the appropriate PAM, Cas-9 triggers local DNA melting followed by the formation of RNA-DNA hybrid (Figure 5).

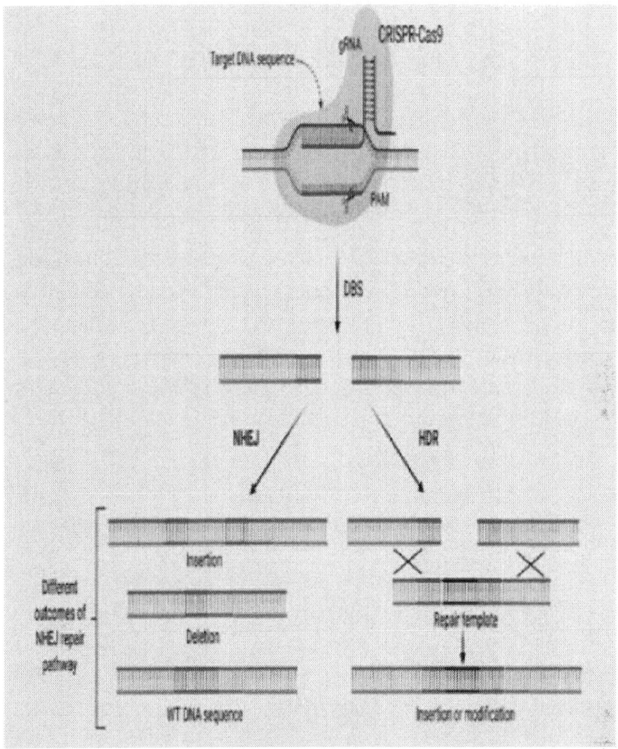

Figure 5

The mechanism by which Cas-9 enzyme melts the target DNA sequence is not yet fully understood. The Cas-9 protein is then activated for DNA cleavage, with the HNH domain cleaving the complementary strand and the RuvC domain cleaving the non-complementary strand of the target DNA to produce predominantly blunt-ended DSBs. The DSB is repaired by the host cellular machinery through two main mechanisms: non-homologous end joining (NHEJ) and homology-directed repair (HDR). NHEJ joins DNA fragments through an enzymatic process in the absence of exogenous homologous DNA and is active in all phases of the cell cycle. It is the predominant and efficient cellular repair mechanism, but it is also an error-prone mechanism that may result in small random insertion or deletion (indels) at the cleavage site, leading to the generation of frame shift mutation or premature stop codon. On the other hand, HDR is highly precise and requires the use of a homologous DNA template. It is most active in the late S and G2 phases of the cell cycle. In CRISPR-gene editing, HDR requires a large amount of donor (exogenous) DNA templates containing a sequence of interest. HDR executes the precise gene insertion or replacement by adding a donor DNA template with sequence homology at the predicted DSB site.

BASE EDITING & PRIME EDITING

Some of the most recently developed CRISPR methods are base editing and prime editing. These technologies work on the same principle, however at a more precise scale, inducing single nucleotide substitutions. Importantly, base editing and prime editing do not induce DSBs in the target DNA. Base editing uses either a catalytically dead Cas9 (dCas9) or a nickase Cas9 (nCas9). dCas9 is incapable of cutting DNA, while nCas9 produces 'nicks', or single-stranded breaks (SSBs) in the DNA. By fusing either dCas9 or nCas9 to a DNA modifying enzyme, researchers can alter specific nucleotides. One of the limitations of base editing is that they cannot be used to alter every possible nucleotide, and this is one of the factors that led to the development of prime editing.

Prime editing involves fusing nCas9 to an engineered reverse transcriptase and a prime editing guide RNA (peg-RNA). The peg-RNA contains two sections: one that guides to the region of interest, and another that contains the desired substitution/s for repair after the single-stranded cut has been generated. After one strand has been altered by the prime editor, the complementary strand can also be corrected an additional gRNA and nCas9 will create a nick in the strand and it will be repaired using the previously edited strand as a template. Prime editing is predicted to be capable of treating 89% of genetic mutations in humans.

(A) METHODS FOR CREATING GENE-EDITED ANIMALS

For gene editing methods to have a significant impact on genetic changes in animals, they must be integrated seamlessly with traditional animal breeding programs, which require precise and reliable germ line-editing.

1. Somatic Cell Nuclear Transfer

SCNT has been a major technique for delivering nuclease-mediated genetic modifications in livestock. The advantage of SCNT is that the gene-edited cell line can be genotyped and screened before transfer into the enucleated oocyte (Figure 6) to ensure that only the desired edits, and no off-target edits, have occurred. Several gene-edited animals have been produced using the SCNT cloning technique. The first successful attempt in cattle was made by Tan *et al.* in 2013 who edited the polled gene using TALEN. This breakthrough opened up new possibilities for cattle genome editing. Subsequently, a gene responsible for double muscling was mutated, resulting in the birth of double-muscled cattle. Another success story is the production of *Staphylococcus aureus*-resistant cattle through SCNT by knocking in the human lysozyme gene in bovine fetal fibroblasts. Other examples include editing of bovine lactoglobulin (BLG), human lactoferrin, and MSTN gene in goats. Pig genomes were also edited and propagated through SCNT cloning techniques with respect to MSTN, RELA (v-rel avian reticulo-endotheliosis), and Von Willebrand factor (vWF) gene. Despite the progress made through the SCNT-editing method, certain drawbacks associated with cloning, such as early embryonic losses, postnatal death, and birth defects, cannot be ignored (Ball & Peters, 2004; Campbell, McWhir, Ritchie & Wilmut, 1996; Wilmut & Whitelaw, 1994; Camara *et al.*, 2008).

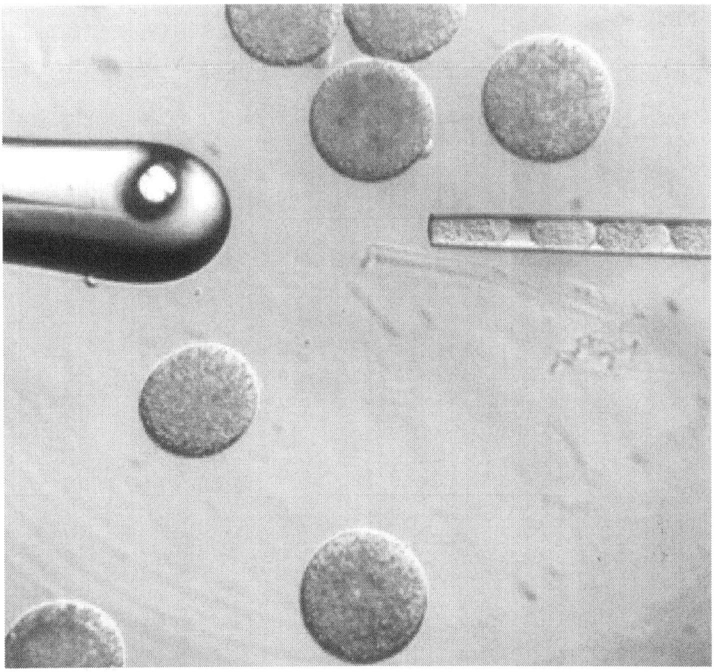

Figure 6: Enucleation in progress

2. Direct Editing of Zygotes

Editing animal genomes through direct editing of zygotes is advantageous as it allows for direct application in the next generation, although not all embryos are edited. It involves two techniques

(i) Electroporation: A method of introducing gene editing machinery into cells by using electric pulses to create pores in cell membrane. It simplifies the generation of gene-edited livestock as it doesn't require micromanipulation skills. With advancements in nanotechnology and micro-technologies, there's a higher demand for this physical transfection method. Nanostructure-mediated electroporation allows for miniaturization and enhances precision and efficiency while causing minimal damage to cells (Lino *et al.*, 2018).

(ii) DNA Microinjection (Figure 7) : Various animal genomes, including those of cattle, sheep, and pigs, have been edited through this method. A study demonstrated that injecting TALEN mRNA into the zygote can produce MSTN gene-edited cattle and sheep. This innovation is critical to the cattle industry, as specific gene-edited offspring can be produced through ovum pickup, in vitro fertilization, and zygote microinjection (OPU IVF-ZM). Similarly, TALEN reagents were directly injected into the zygote to successfully edit PRNP (prion protein) and BLG genes in cattle. Two studies focused on the RELA proto-oncogene gene in pigs, which has been proposed to play a role in resistance against African swine fever. Moreover, more recently, the BMPR/FecB gene was disrupted in sheep embryos by injecting CRISPR/Cas9 reagents into the zygote (Salamone *et al.*, 2012).

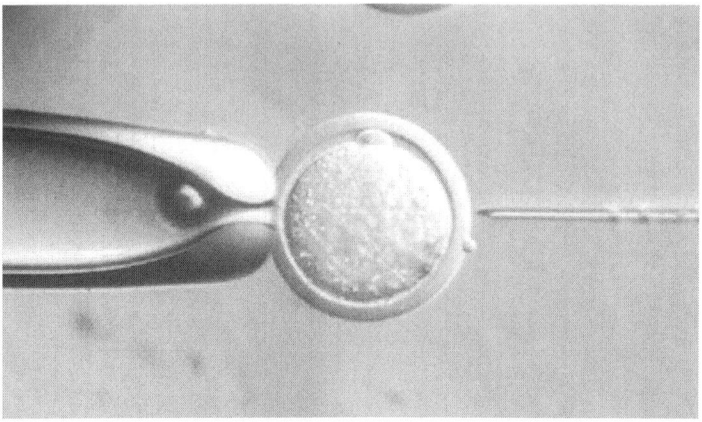

Figure 7: DNA microinjection in progress

(B) GENOME EDITING IN LIVESTOCK

Over the past ten years, genome editing using engineered designer nucleases has emerged as a promising approach. Among these, CRISPR/Cas9 is the simplest and most predictable designer nuclease, with the ability to target multiple genomic sites simultaneously. It's worth noting that CRISPR/Cas9 is being disproportionately used for livestock editing. The CRISPR/Cas9-mediated genome engineering technologies allow performing precise genetic modifications, which dramatically enhance the ease and speed for producing genetically modified livestock (Zhao et al., 2019; Van Eenennaam, 2019; Menchaca et al., 2020; Lee et al., 2020; Navarro-Serna et al., 2020; Bishop and Van Eenennaam, 2020; Dua et al., 2021). In 2020, genome-edited pigs were produced using the CRISPR/Cas9 system in which the von Willebrand factor (vWF) gene was targeted in order to generate a medical model with reduced activity of coagulation factor VIII leading to severe bleeding closely mimicking the human disease (Hai *et al.*, 2014). Thereafter, genome engineering technologies have been applied in many livestock such as cattle, sheep, goat and pig for improvement of growth performance, development of disease-resistant lines, enhancement of animal welfare, and for generation of models for human diseases.

For improvement in the performance of livestock, knockout of the myostatin (MSTN) gene is the most prominent example due to its association with growth and skeletal muscle development. CRISPR/Cas9 technology has been successfully applied to knockout the MSTN from the genomes of sheep (Zhang *et al.*, 2018), goat (He *et al.*, 2018) and pig (Tanihara *et al.*, 2016). Another significant accomplishment has been the production of tuberculosis-resistant cattle and porcine reproductive and respiratory syndrome (PRRS) virus-re-sistant pigs, both of which are economically important in the livestock industry. Tuberculosis-resistant cattle were produced by insertion of natural resistance to infection with intracellular pathogens 1 (NRAMP1) gene into bovine fetal fibroblasts followed by SCNT (Tuggle and Waters, 2015). The genome-edited animal showed higher expression of the NRAMP1 gene and exhibited higher degree of resistance to Mycobacterium bovis infection (Tuggle and Waters, 2015).

Livestock is also assessed as a bioreactor to produce human biological products such as albumin. The blood-derived human serum albumin (HSA) is recommended for a number of severe diseases, such as liver failure and traumatic shock, and is in high demand. Due to the shortage of human blood supplies and the infection risks associated with human blood, alternative ways to produce HSA have long been sought. Success was obtained when CRISPR/Cas9 was used to knock in human albumin cDNA to the pig endogenous albumin locus, leading to transgenic pig-lets with human albumin in their blood (Peng *et al.*, 2015). Due to the similarity in anatomy, size, and physiology of porcine organs with their human counterparts, the pig is considered the most suitable model for human diseases such as atherosclerosis, Parkinson's disease, Huntington's disease, cardiovascular diseases, diabetes, ophthalmological diseases, and neuronal disorders (Garrels et al., 2016; Gün and Kues, 2014; Holm et al., 2016; Schook *et al.*, 2016). To understand the molecular mechanism of human atherosclerosis, LDLR, and apo-lipoprotein E (ApoE) double knockout pigs were produced using CRISPR/Cas9, which exhibited elevated levels of low-density lipoprotein cholesterol (LDL-C), apolipoprotein B, and total cholesterol (TC) in serum (Huang *et al.*, 2017). Researchers created CRISPR/Cas9- mediated double DJ1, PARK2/PINK1, or Parkin/DJ-1 PINK1 triple knockout pigs mimicking Parkinson's dis-ease (Zhou *et al.*, 2015; Yao *et al.*, 2015; Wang *et al.*, 2016)and Huntingtin knock-in pig model for Huntington s disease (Yan *et al.*, 2018), which could help in evaluating the pathology of the disease and for development of the therapeutic intervention. Li *et al.* created mutant pigs for the study of behavioral and neuropsychiatric disorders of humans by deleting tryptophan hydroxylase-2 (TPH2) using CRISPR/Cas9 (Li *et al.*, 2017). The generated pigs were able to produce reduced levels of serotonin which impaired pup survival and growth rates. In another study, tyrosinase (TYR) was bi-allelically mutated with CRISPR/Cas9, resulting in complete loss of pigmentation in the skin, hair, and eyes of the produced pigs that could be useful to elucidate the genetics of human skin pigmentation (Zhou et al., 2015). Recently, Han and coworkers produced a model pig by deletion of Hoxc13 gene for ectodermal dysplasia-9 (ED-9), a human disease characterized by reduced hair follicles, external hair loss, and abnormal hair follicle structure, but normal skin structure, skeleton phenotype, and growth pattern (Han et al., 2017). Recently, Menchaca et al. produced otoferlin gene-edited sheep as a model which may allow a better understanding and development of new therapies for human deafness related to genetic disorders (Menchaca *et al.*, 2020).

(C) CURRENT SCENARIO & FUTURE PERSPECTIVES FOR MORE PRODUCTION IN INDIA

There are at least 16 institutions in India that are actively involved in gene editing research. Most of them work on genome editing in crops. Only a few institutions work in animal genome editing namely ICAR-NDRI, NIAB, ICAR-CIRG and SKUAST-Kashmir. As of now no edited farm animal has been produced in india. ICAR funded consortium project is running for generation of Myostatin edited buffalo, goat and sheep.

Genome engineering in ruminants is majorly focused on subjects such as disease resistance (e.g., tuberculosis), eradicating allergens (e.g., beta-lactoglobulin knock-out), product generation (e.g., meat from male and milk from female), male or female birth specifically (animal sexing), the introduction of desirable phenotypes (e.g., stress tolerance, disease resistance) and their long-term survival (e.g., polled or hornlessness).

Till 2015, a dependable tool for genome altering was inefficiently and not routinely utilised. Since the CRISPR/Cas9 set foot in the gene engineering field, it brings various desires and hopes for the scientific community to reproduce and modify the defects within the gene of interest for the enhancement, even in large animals including livestock.

Genetic improvement of livestock around the globe has been, and will continue to be, an important driver of the sustainability of animal agriculture.

1. Doubling Muscle Mass: Increasing the body weight and accelerating the growth rates of farm animals are very important aims in livestock development (Kalds *et al.*, 2019). Genes that affect these traits are attractive targets for emerging disruptive gene-editing techniques. Myostatin (MSTN) inhibition, which results in the double muscling phenotype due to hyperplasia and hypertrophy of muscle fibers, resulting in advantage in terms of meat production. The myostatin gene has been analyzed in many different species and has been found to be extraordinarily well conserved (Perisse *et al.*, 2021). This mutation is naturally present in Belgian Blue cattle and Texel sheep (Alberio and Wolf, 2021). These genetically modified animals had superior muscles mass compared to their non-modified counter parts (Luo *et al.*, 2014 and Qian *et al.*, 2015). MSTN gene has been subjected to CRISPR/Cas9 targeting by applying gene-editing tools in sheep and goats. No off-target have been detected and enhanced body weight in edited animals as compared to wild-type individuals has been reported (Wang *et al.*, 2016a). A recent report described the application of CRISPR/Cas9-based base editors for the introduction of a point mutation within the suppressor of cytokine signaling 2 (SOCS2) gene in sheep (Zhou *et al.*, 2019). CRISPR/Cas9 has significantly highlighted the functional role of genes related to muscle growth and body weight both in sheep and goats, further emphasizing the potential role of gene editing to provide the farm animal sector with novel breeds that carry desirable and valuable traits. Another potential candidate gene for improving meat production in livestock and for developing therapeutic interventions for muscle diseases is FBXO40 protein coding gene, a member of the F-box protein family and its expression of FBXO40 is restricted to muscles. FBXO40 KO pigs have been reported to exhibited only marginal increase in muscle mass (4%) compared to Wild Type controls (Zou *et al.*, 2018).

2. Promotion of Fiber Length and Growth: Genes associated with fiber quality and quantity are a source of attraction, and many researchers hope to alter these genes in attempts to obtain desired and new fiber properties. The FGF5 gene, which is a dominant inhibitor of fiber length and growth, is an attractive target. It has been reported that the disruption of FGF5 in sheep can lead to an increased wool length and average wool growth rate (Zhang *et al.*, 2019b). Also in goats simultaneous FGF5 disruption at both morphological and genetic levels has been confirmed and an enhancement in fiber length, as well as an increase in the number of secondary hair follicles obtained (Wang *et al.*, 2016b).

3. Disease Resistance: Gene editing has been suggested as a robust tool that can be used to generate disease resistant animals. Consequently, genetically modified resistant farm animals have been produced. These offer good models to investigate and understand disease pathogenesis and offer a potential source for the spread of disease resistance traits in commercial flocks. The PrPc gene associated with the pathogenesis of the transmissible spongiform encephalopathies, PrP-resistant animals can be produced by suppressing the expression of PrP (Golding *et al.*, 2006). CRISPR/ Cas9 has been applied to target PrP in goat fibroblasts with the aim to generate PrP-knockout donor cells that can be used in SCNT for the production of PrPresistant goats (Ni *et al.*, 2014 & Fan *et al.*, 2019). Menchaca *et al.* (2018) indicated the application of the CRISPR/ Cas9 system to induce the loss of function of hyaluronidase 2 (HYAL2), which can be used by Jaagsiekte sheep retrovirus as a cell entry receptor, resulting in ovine pulmonary adenocarcinoma syndrome.CRISPR/ Cas9 system for producing virus-resistant farm animals and will help to investigate the functional roles of HYAL2. The Porcine Reproductive and Respiratory Syndrome (PRRS) virus causes huge economic losses. Knocking out cysteine-rich receptor CD163 in pigs via genome editing makes them completely resistant to PRRS virus (Whitworth *et al.*, 2016), such pigs can be used to reduce the significant economic costs of PRRS and improve the profitability of pig production. In cattle, studies have demonstrated that cattle resistant to *Mycobacterium bovis* infection could be produced via genome editing (Alberio and Wolf, 2021 and Wu *et al.*, 2015). *Mycobacterium bovis* can cause significant economic losses to the livestock industry, and also poses zoonotic risks since humans mostly acquire M. bovis infection through contaminated food or drinks, unpasteurized dairy products, or by direct exposure to infected animals. Studies have demonstrated that Cas9 nickase can be used to overexpress NRAMP1 (natural resistance to infection with intracellular pathogens 1) in cattle, in order to produce *M. bovis* resistant cattle (Gao *et al.*, 2017). The research of genetic engineering via CRISPR systems for the generation of disease-resistant sheep and goats is ongoing, and maybe varieties of genetically modified resistant sheep and goats will be reported soon, thus enriching the field with novel and valuable models. Similar application are likely possible in a variety of other livestock species and even wildlife, in order to improve profitability or reduce biosecurity risks (Kalds *et al.*, 2019 & Perisse *et al.*, 2021).

4. Improved Reproductive Performance: Improving the reproductive performance is an important direction of livestock breeding. Ciccarelli *et al* (2020) introduced the concept of "surrogate sires", validating for pigs, goats, and cattle. It was demonstrated that $NANOS_2$ gene Knock Out males generated by CRISPR/ Cas9 editing have testes that are germline ablated but otherwise structurally normal. Subsequent, spermatogonial stem cell transplantation (SSCT) with allogeneic donor stem cells led to sustained donor derived spermatogenesis. This made a great basis for dissemination of elite livestock genetics. Mutations in the sheep BMPR-IB (FecB) gene has shown to be responsible on an increased ovulation rate and consequently larger litter size (Fabre *et al.*, 2006). In goats, another defined point mutation has also been introduced by in the growth differentiation factor 9 (GDF9) gene, which exerts a large effect on both ovulation rate and litter size (Niu *et al.*, 2018).

(D) THE LEGAL FRAMEWORK OF GENOME-EDITED ANIMALS IN INDIA

In India, the legal framework for genome-edited animals is primarily being regulated using 'Rules for the Manufacture, Use, Import, Export, and Storage of Hazardous Microorganisms, Genetically Engineered Organisms or Cells", 1989 (Rules 1989), under the guidance of the Environment (Protection) Act, 1986. In addition, Prevention of Cruelty to Animals Act, 1960 (PCA Act), the Wildlife Protection Act, 1972, and the Biotechnology Regulatory Authority of India (BRAI) Bill, 2013 are also considered for regulations and ethics approval. The PCA Act provides for the prevention of cruelty to animals and regulates the use of animals in research. The Wildlife Protection Act, 1972, prohibits the hunting of animals, and the possession or trade of any wildlife products, without proper authorization from the government.

The BRAI Bill, 2013, aims to establish a regulatory framework for the development and application of biotechnology products in India. The bill proposes the formation of a regulatory authority to oversee the research and development of biotechnology products, including genome-edited animals. In addition to these laws, India has also ratified the Convention on Biological Diversity (CBD) and the Cartagena Protocol on Biosafety. The CBD aims to promote the conservation and sustainable use of biological diversity, while the Cartagena Protocol seeks to regulate the transboundary movement of genetically modified organisms, including genome-edited animals.

The Department of Biotechnology recently published a draught guideline for gene editing regulation, pro-posing strict regulation of gene-edited organisms. In India, the Genetic Engineering Appraisal Committee (GEAC) is responsible for the approval of genetically engineered organisms for research, development, and cultivation. In Rules 1989, genetic engineering defined as modification, deletion or removal of parts of heritable material which infers that all new gene editing technologies will be subject to regulation under the provision of the Rules, 1989 (Raman, 2017). In view of the present definition, it is expected that regulatory considerations for new and emerging technologies will be on a case by case basis based on the existing regulatory framework. Overall, the legal framework for genome-edited animals in India is still in its nascent stages, with regulations being developed and implemented on a case-by-case basis. However, the existing laws and regulations provide a framework for ensuring the ethical treatment of animals and the safe development and deployment of biotechnology products.

The Indian Ministry of Environment, Forest and Climate Change has decided to exempt products derived through two gene editing techniques, site directed nuclease (SDN)-1 and SDN-2, from the purview of the country's regulations governing genetically modified organisms, national media report. The move allows such products to circumvent biosafety assessments undertaken by the country's apex biotechnology regulatory body, the Genetic Engineering Appraisal Committee (GEAC), besides reassigning the jurisdiction of these products to India's Seeds Act, in lieu of the Environment Protection Act.

SDN creates site-specific double-stranded breaks at defined sequences, typically by recognizing a specific DNA sequence and cleaving DNA within such a sequence or nearby. SDN-1 produces a double-stranded break in the genome of a plant without the addition of foreign DNA. SDN-2 produces a double-stranded break, and while the break is repaired by the cell, a small nucleotide template is supplied that is complementary to the area of the break, which in turn, is used by the cell to repair the break. SDN-3 also induces a double-stranded break in the DNA but is accompanied by a template containing a gene or other sequence of genetic material. While SDN-1 and SDN-2 result either in a random (SDN-1) or intended (SDN-2) modification of a targeted genomic locus without the insertion of foreign DNA, the aim of the SDN-3 approach is to modify the targeted locus by inserting an exogenous DNA template of various lengths.

Following the new rule development in India, requests for approval of SDN1 and SDN2 gene-edited products are to be treated differently from their transgenic counterparts, as both techniques involve "knocking off" or "overexpressing" certain traits within a gene without introducing new genetic material. However, products derived through SDN-3 will still be considered as GMOs as the process involves the introduction of foreign genes.

REFERENCES

Alberio R., Wolf, E., 2021. 25th Anniversary of cloning by somatic-cell nuclear assisted reproductive technologies, and gene editing to drive genetic improvement of cattle. CABI Agriculture and Bioscience (2022) 3:13. https://doi.org/10.1186/s43170-022-00080-z

Chandrasegaran, S., Carroll, D., (2016). Origins of Programmable Nucleases for Genome Engineering. J. Mol. Biol. 428 (5 Pt B), 963–989.

Ciccarelli, M., Giassetti, M. I., Miao, D., Oatley, M. J., Robbins, C., Lopez- Biladeau, B., *et al.* (2020). Donor-derived spermatogenesis following stem cell transplantation in sterile NANOS2 knockout males. Proc. Natl. Acad. Sci. 117, 24195–24204. doi: 10.1073/pnas.2010102117

Cunningham, C.M., Tector, M., Joseph Tector, A., 2016. Silencing porcine genes direct complement regulation. Transgenic Research. 25 (5), 751–759.

Doudna, J. A., and Charpentier, E. (2014). Genome Editing. The New Frontier of Genome Engineering with CRISPR-Cas9. Science 346, 1258096. doi:10.1126/science.1258096

Environmental Sustainability and Poverty Reduction. Front. Genome Ed. 4:863193. doi: 10.3389/fgeed.2022.863193.

Fabre, S., Pierre, A., Mulsant, P., Bodin, L., Di Pasquale, E., Persani, L., *et al.* (2006). Regulation of ovulation rate in mammals: contribution of sheep genetic models. Reprod. Biol. Endocrinol. 4, 20–25. doi: 10.1186/1477-7827-4-20

Fan, Z., Regouski, M., Yang, M., Gash, K., Meng, Q., Davies, C. J., *et al.* (2017). Generation of interferon / receptor knockout sheep using CRISPR/Cas9 and SCNT techniques [Abstract]. In: program and abstracts of the 14th transgenic Golding,

M. C., Long, C. R., Carmell, M. A., Hannon, G. J., and Westhusin, M. E. (2006). Suppression of prion protein in livestock by RNA interference. Proc. Natl. Acad. Sci. 103, 5285–5290. doi: 10.1073/pnas.0600813103

Gaj T, Gersbach CA, Barbas CF. ZFN, TALEN and CRISPR/Cas-based methods for genome engineering. Trends Biotechnol. 2013;31(7):397–405.https:// doi. org/ 10. 1016/j. tibte ch. 2013. 04. 004.

Gao, Y., Wu, H., Wang, Y., Liu, X., Chen, L., Li, Q., Cui, C., Liu, X., Zhang, J., Zhang, Y., 2017. Single Cas9 nickase induced generation of NRAMP1 knockin cattle with reduced off-target effects. Genome Biology.

Gonen, S., Jenko, J., Gorjanc, G., Mileham, A.J., Whitelaw, C.B.A. and Hickey, J.M. (2017) Potential of gene drives with genome editing to increase genetic gain in livestock breeding programs. Genet Selection Evol., 49: 12.

Hensel, G., and Kumlehn, J. (2019). Genome Engineering Using TALENs. Methods Mol. Biol. 1900, 195–215.

Ishii, T., 2015. Germline genome-editing research and its socioethical implications. Trends Mol. Med. 21 (8), 473–481. Lino, C.A.; Harper, J.C.; Carney, J.P.; Timlin, J.A. Delivering CRISPR: A review of the challenges and approaches. Drug Deliv.2018, 25, 1234–1257.

Lino, C.A.; Harper, J.C.; Carney, J.P.; Timlin, J.A. Delivering CRISPR: A review of the challenges and approaches. Drug Deliv.2018, 25, 1234–1257.

Luo, J., Zhang, Y., Guo, Y., Tang, H., Wei, H., Liu, S., *et al.* (2017). TRIM28 regulates Igf2- H19 and Dlk1-Gtl2 imprinting by distinct mechanisms during sheep fibroblast proliferation. Gene 637, 152–160. doi: 10.1016/j.gene.2017.09.048

Maci L. Mueller and Alison L. Van Eenennaam. Synergistic power of genomic selection,

McMurrough, T.A., Brown, C.M., Zhang, K., Hausner, G., Junop, M.S., Gloor, G.B., and Edgell, D.R. (2018). Active site residue identity regulates cleavage preference of LAGLIDADG homing endonucleases. Nucleic Acids Res. 46, 11990–12007

Menchaca, A., Mulet, A. P., dos Santos Neto, P. C., Cuadro, F., Souza, M., Anegon, I., *et al.* (2018). CRISPR in sheep: a southern perspective [Abstract]. In: abstracts from the uc davis transgenic animal research conference xi. Transgenic Res. 27, 467–487. doi: 10.1007/s11248- 018-0086-x

Ni, W., Qiao, J., Hu, S., Zhao, X., Regouski, M., Yang, M., *et al.* (2014). Efficient gene knockout in goats using CRISPR/Cas9 system. PLoS One 9, e106718. doi: 10.1371/journal.pone.0106718

Niu, Y., Zhao, X., Zhou, J., Li, Y., Huang, Y., Cai, B., *et al.* (2018). Efficient generation of goats with defined point mutation (I397V) in GDF9 through CRISPR/Cas9. Reprod. Fertil. Dev. 30, 307–312. doi: 10.1071/RD17068

Perisse IV, Fan Z, Singina GN, White KL and Polejaeva IA (2021) Improvements in Gene Editing Technology Boost Its Applications in Livestock. Front. Genet. 11:614688. doi: 10.3389/fgene.2020.614688 Zhang, R., Wu, H., and Lian, Z. (2019b). Bioinformatics analysis of evolutionary characteristics and biochemical structure of FGF5 Gene in sheep. Gene 702, 123–132. doi: 10.1016/j.gene.2019.03.040

Peter Kalds, Yawei Gao, Shiwei Zhou, Bei Cai, Xingxu Huang, Xiaolong Wang, Yulin Chen, Redesigning small ruminant genomes with CRISPR toolkit: Overview and perspectives, Theriogenology (2020), https://doi.org/10.1016/j.theriogenology.2020.02.015

Polejaeva, I., and Campbell, K. (2000). New advances in somatic cell nuclear transfer: application in transgenesis. Theriogenology 53, 117–126. doi: 10.1016/s0093-691x(99)00245-9

Qian, L., Tang, M., Yang, J., Wang, Q., Cai, C., Jiang, S., Li, H., Jiang, K., Gao, P., Ma, D., Chen, Y., An, X., Li, K., Cui, W., 2015. Targeted mutations in myostatin by zincfinger nucleases result in double-muscled phenotype in Meishan pigs. Sci. Rep. 5, 14435.

Salamone, John D, Bevacqua R, Hiriart MI and Buemo C, *et al.* "Transgenesis in Farm Animals." Anim Reprod 9 (2012): 772-6.

Sayed Haidar Abbas Raza, Abdallah A. Hassanin, Sameer D. Pant d, Sun Bing a, Mahmoud Z. Sitohy e,Sameh A. Abdelnour f, Mashael Alhumaidi Alotaibi g, Tahani Mohamed Al-Hazani h, Ayman H. Abd El-Aziz i,Gong Cheng a, Linsen Zan a Potentials, prospects and applications of genome editing technologies in livestock production Saudi Journal of Biological Sciences 29 (2022) 1928 - 1935

Tian, X.C., Kubota, C., Enright, B. and Xiangzhong Yang Cloning animals by somatic cell nuclear transfer – biological factors. Reprod Biol Endocrinol 1, 98 (2003). https://doi.org/10.1186/1477- 7827-1-98

Wang, X., Cai, B., Zhou, J., Zhu, H., Niu, Y., Ma, B., *et al.* (2016b). Disruption of FGF5 in cashmere goats using CRISPR/Cas9 results in more secondary hair follicles and longer fibers. PLoS One 11, e0164640. doi: 10.1371/journal. pone.0164640

Wang, X., Niu, Y., Zhou, J., Yu, H., Kou, Q., Lei, A., *et al.* (2016a). Multiplex gene editing via CRISPR/Cas9 exhibits desirable muscle hypertrophy without detectable off-target effects in sheep. Sci. Rep. 6, 32271. doi: 10.1038/srep32271

Whitworth, K.M., Rowland, R.R., Ewen, C.L., Trible, B.R., Kerrigan, M.A., Cino-Ozuna, A.G., Samuel, M.S., Lightner, J.E., McLaren, D.G., Mileham, A.J., Wells, K.D., Prather, R.S., 2016. Gene-edited pigs are protected from porcine reproductive and respiratory syndrome virus. 34, 20-22.

Wiedenheft, B., Sternberg, S.H., Doudna, J.A., 2012. RNA-guided genetic silencing

Wu, H., Wang, Y., Zhang, Y., Yang, M., Lv, J., Liu, J., Zhang, Y., 2015. TALE nickasemediated SP110 knockin endows cattle with increased resistance to tuberculosis. Proc. Natl. Acad. Sci. USA 112, E1530–E1539.

Zhang, F., Wen, Y., and Guo, X. (2014). CRISPR/Cas9 for genome editing: progress, implications and challenges. Hum. Mol. Genet. 23 (R1), R40–R46.

Zhang, J.H., Adikaram, P., Pandey, M., Genis, A., and Simonds, W.F. (2016). Optimization of genome editing through CRISPR-Cas9 engineering. Bioengineered 7, 166–174.

Zhou, S., Cai, B., He, C., Wang, Y., Ding, Q., Liu, J., et al. (2019). Programmable base editing of the sheep genome revealed no genome-wide off-target mutations. Front. Genet. 10, 215. doi: 10.3389/fgene.2019.00215

Zou, Y., Li, Z., Zou, Y., Hao, H., Li, N., and Li, Q. (2018). An FBXO40 knockout generated by CRISPR/Cas9 causes muscle hypertrophy in pigs without detectable pathological effects. Biochem. Biophys. Res. Commun. 498, 940–945. doi: 10.1016/j.bbrc.2018.03.085

Chapter 3

Climate Change and Livestock Production: Emerging Concepts and Technologies for Sustenance

V. Sejian[1,*], C. Devaraj[1], M.V.Silpa[2], C.G. Shashank[1] and R. Bhatta[1]

[1]*Centre for Climate resilient Animal Adaptation Studies, ICAR-National Institute of Animal Nutrition and Physiology, Adugodi, Hosur Road, Bangalore-560030*

[2]*Institute of Animal Breeding and Genetics, Justus-Liebig-Universität Gießen, Gießen, Germany*

**E-mail: drsejian@gmail.com*

INTRODUCTION

While climate change is a global phenomenon, its negative impacts are felt more severely by poor people in developing countries, who rely heavily on the natural resource for their livelihoods. In arid and semi-arid areas, livestock are often considered to be one of the most important means of food and economic security for poor and marginal farmers. Elevated ambient temperature and inadequate and low quality feed are the major factors which contribute towards under-production of farm animals in tropical regions. Fig. 1 describes the various impacts of climate change on livestock production.

Given the significance of livestock to the economy of India in particular, efforts are needed to develop new concepts in animal science which could help understand the hidden intricacies of their responses to various environmental stressors which could aid in developing appropriate ameliorative strategies to improve production. This effort is therefore an attempt to project to the farming and scientific communities the various advances associated with climate change and livestock production and to highlight the various technologies available to sustain farm animal production in the changing climate scenario in the country in near future.

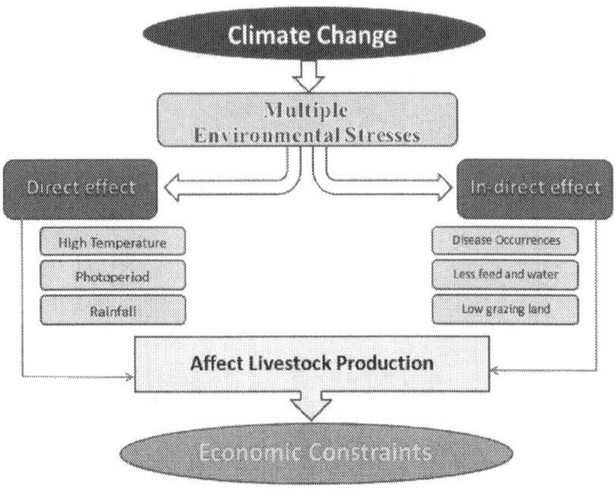

Figure 1: Various impacts of climate change livestock production

EMERGING CONCEPTS IN CLIMATE CHANGE ASSOCIATED LIVESTOCK PRODUCTION

Goat as Ideal Climate Resilient Animal Model

The projected increased temperature and reduction in fodder production can cause detrimental impact on farm animal production. In this context, goat offers greater scope for sustaining livestock production due to its advantages such as higher thermo-tolerance, drought tolerance, ability to survive on limited pastures and high disease resistance over other species. Further, goats possess the ability to walk for long distances in search of limited pastures. All these advantages imparts goat the potential to survive in varied geographical locations and are tipped to be climate resilient animal model in the changing climate scenario. In a recent review Reshma Nair et al. (2021) clearly projected goat to be the species to experience very minimal heat stress level as compared to other farm animals both by 2050 and 2100. Fig.2 projects the advantage of rearing goats over other species in the changing climate scenario.

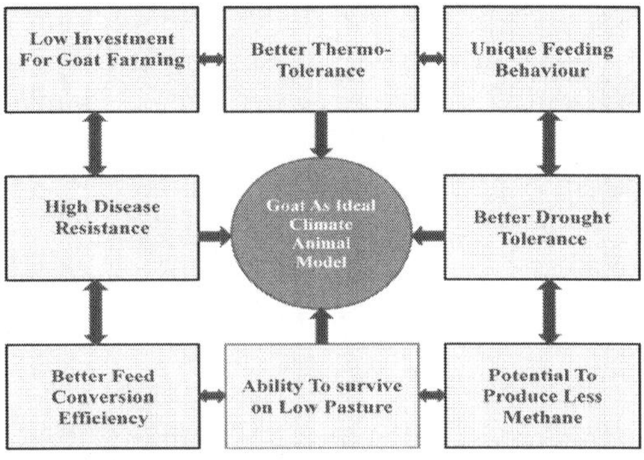

Figure 2: Scientific evidences for considering goat as ideal climate animal model (Information synthesised from International Journal of Biometeorology by Reshma Nair et al., 2021)

CONCEPT OF MULTIPLE STRESSES IMPACTING FARM ANIMALS

When exposed to one stress at a time, animals can effectively counter it based on their stored body reserves and without altering the productive functions. However, if they are exposed to more than one stress at a time, the summated effects of the different stressors might prove detrimental to these animals. Such a response is attributed to animal's inability to cope with the combined effects of different stressors simultaneously. In such a case, the animal's body reserves are not sufficient to effectively counter multiple environmental stressors. Fig. 3 describes the concept of multiple stressors impacting livestock production.

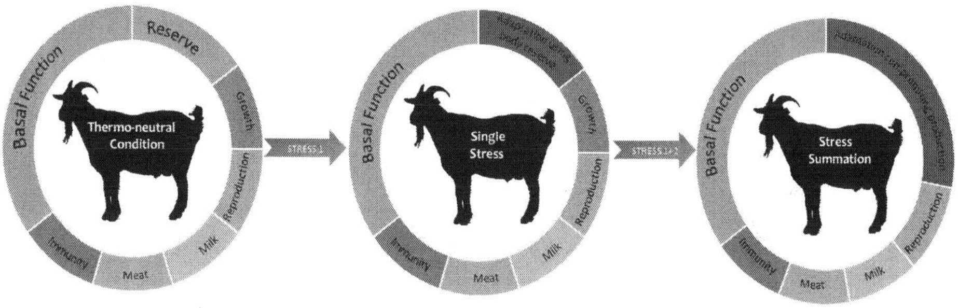

Figure 3: Pictorial representation of concept of multiple stressors on livestock production

Advanced Thermal Indices to Quantify Heat Stress Response

The temperature humidity index (THI) which is being widely used for quantifying heat stress response in farm animals has two drawbacks as it does not take into account solar radiation and wind speed. This has brought the drive in the scientific community to develop advanced thermal indices to address these drawbacks of THI indices. Heat load index is developed as an improvement which overcomes the perceived deficiencies in the THI index. The HLI uses two equations based on the threshold value of black globe thermometer:

- HLI BG 25 = 8:62 + (0.38 X RH) + (1.55 X BG) – (0.5 X WS) + $e^{(2.4 - WS)}$
- HLI BG< 25= 10.66 + (0.28 X RH) + (1.3 X BG) – WS
- Where, BG is the black globe temperature in C, RH the relative humidity in %, WS the wind speed in m/s and e the exponential.

Infrared Thermal Image Applications in Farm Animals

Traditional body temperature measurement requires handling and restraining procedures may increase the average body temperature of the animals. Therefore, there is a need for identifying non-invasive methodology to quantify heat stress response in livestock. Infrared thermography (IRT) is one such non-invasive method which has the potential to record animal body temperature without the need to restrain or relocate animals. Thus, this technology offers scope for understanding in depth the thermo-regulatory mechanisms in heat stressed animals. Fig. 4 describes the different body parts surface temperature using infrared thermography in goat.

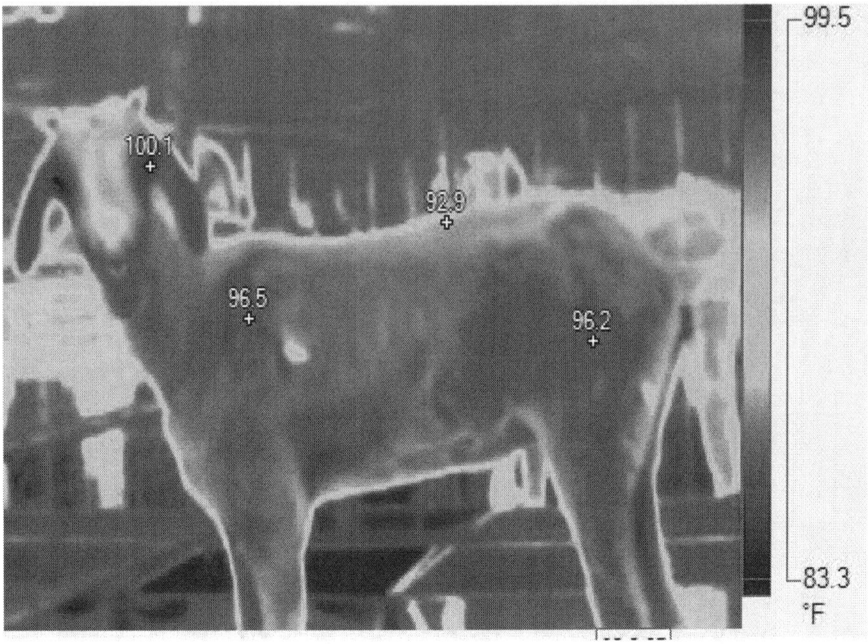

Figure 4: Surface temperature measurement in goat using infrared thermography

Agro-Ecological Zone Specific Breed Identification

Sustaining livestock production in the changing climate scenario requires efforts to identify best indigenous breeds to survive in different agro-ecological zones. Such an effort could ensure that the most suited breeds to specific zones are recommended by the policy makers for dissemination to the local farmers. Therefore, promoting such recommended breeds among the local farmers may prove beneficial in improving their livelihood security. A classic example was provided by our own research which recommends Salem Black breed to be the ideal breed to survive in Southern India. This warrants more research efforts particularly in tropical regions to screen indigenous breeds for their climate resilience and to test their ability to survive in multiple locations.

Rumen Microbes Associate Adaptive Potential

The ruminant animals and gut microbiota has evolved simultaneously while adapting to climatic and pastoral environments. Over the past few years, metagenomics has emerged as a powerful tool to study the rumen microbiome. Recent studies identifying rumen microbial community for novel enzymes, uncultured methanogens, and other metabolic pathways have opened new insights in this area. However, there are very few metagenomics studies conducted on heat stressed animals. This also is a potential area of research which could open up new pathways towards amelioration and mitigation of heat stress in farm animals.

Biomarkers for Heat Stress in Goats

The following genes were found to be associated with thermo-tolerance in indigenous goat breeds. These genes could serve as biological markers for quantifying heat stress response in indigenous goat breeds. These markers are distributed across vital animal functions such as adaptation, growth, reproduction, metabolism and immunity. The identified traits are as follows: (1) Adaptation Traits: Heat shock protein 70 (HSP70), HSP90, HSP27, HSP110 & heat shock factor 1 (HSF1); (2) Growth Traits: Growth Hormone Receptor (GHR), insulin like growth factor 1 (IGF-1), Thyroid Hormone Receptor (THR), leptin receptor (LEPR); (3) Reproduction Traits: Prolactin Receptor (PLR), follicle stimulating hormone receptor (FSHR), leutinizing hormone receptor (LHR), estradiol receptor (ESTR); (4) Immune related traits: toll-like receptor 3 (TLR3), TLR6, TLR8, interleukin 10 (IL10), IL18, tumour necrosis factor α (TNF-α), interferon β (IFN-β), and IFN-γ. Fig. 5 describes the various biomarkers for quantifying heat stress response in goats.

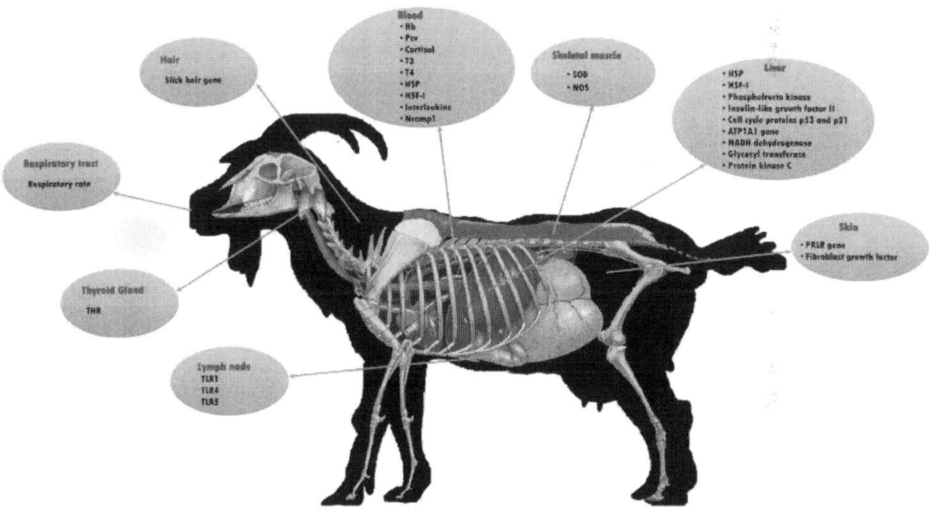

Figure 5: Different biomarkers for heat stress in goats (Source: Sejian et al., 2018)

TECHNOLOGIES TO AMELIORATE HEAT STRESS IN FARM ANIMALS

There are several ameliorative technologies that should be given consideration to prevent economic losses due to environmental stresses. Reducing the impact of climatic stresses on livestock production requires multidisciplinary approaches which emphasize Animal genetics, nutrition, housing, and health. Better management of livestock, may reduce the initiation of thermoregulatory mechanisms which allows for better energy utilisation for growth and/or production. In the face of climate change the continued development of heat stress management tools are needed to ensure the sustainability of animal based agricultural enterprises. Fig. 6 describes the various strategies to sustain livestock production in the changing climate scenario.

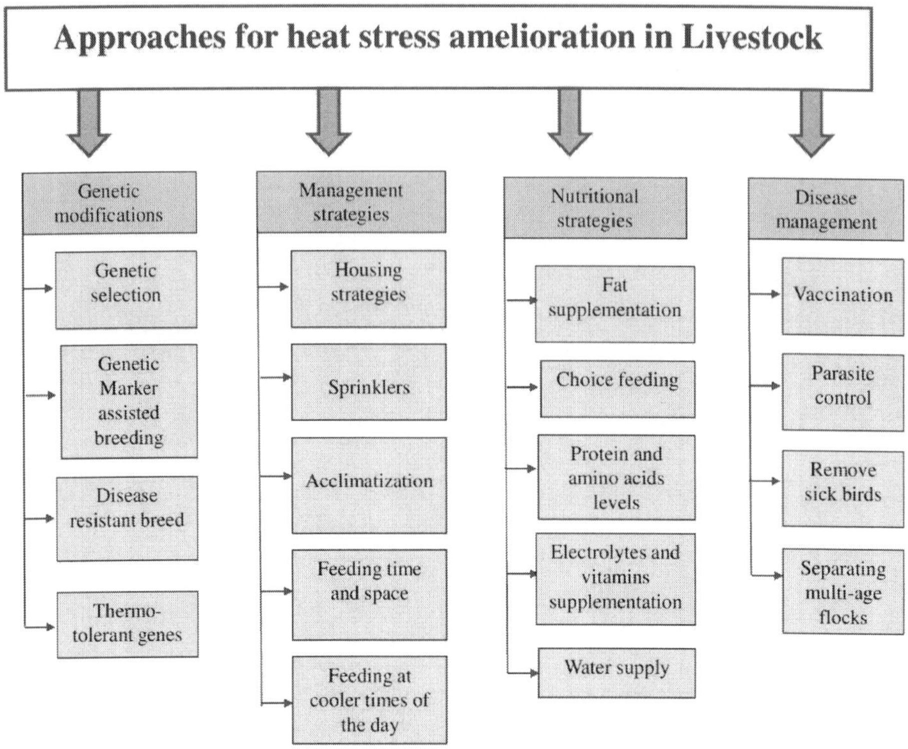

Figure 6: Various technologies to sustain livestock production in the changing climate scenario (Source: Sejian et al., 2018)

CONCLUSION

Responding to the challenges of global warming necessitate a paradigm shift in the practice of agriculture and in the role of livestock within the farming system. Scientific research can help the livestock sector in the battle against climate change. Therefore, the future research efforts involving various stakeholders including the policy makers must ensure the following aspects to sustain livestock production in the country:

- New indices that are more complete than THI to evaluate the climatic effects on each animal species must be developed and weather forecast reports must also be developed with these indices, to inform the farmers in advance.
- Advanced molecular biological tools should be employed to quantify the heat stress response in farm animals.
- The existing breeding programs have concentrated only on production traits. However in an effort to sustain livestock production in the changing climate scenario, the existing breeding programs must be redefined with the amalgamation of production, adaptation and low methane emission traits.

- Research must continue developing new techniques of cooling systems such as thermo-isolation.
- Above all appropriate agro-ecological zone specific breeds needs to be identified to disseminate it to farmers for ensuring optimum economic return which could improve the livelihoods of the poor and marginal farmers across tropical regions.
- Livestock farmers should have key roles in determining what adaptation and mitigation strategies they support if these have to sustain livestock production in changing climate.
- The integration of new technologies into the research and technology transfer systems potentially offers many opportunities to further the development of climate change adaptation strategies.

REFERENCES

Aleena, J., Sejian, V., Bagath, M., Krishnan, G., Beena, V and Bhatta, R (2018). Resilience of three indigenous goat breeds to heat stress based on phenotypic traits and PBMC HSP70 expression. International Journal of Biometerology, 62(11): 1995-2005.

Gaughan, J.B., Sejian, V., Mader, T and Dunshea, F.R (2018). Adaptation strategies: ruminants. Animal Frontiers, vfy029, https://doi.org/10.1093/af/vfy029

Reshma Nair, M.R., Sejian, V., Silpa, M. V., Fonsêca, V. F. C., de Melo Costa, C. C., Devaraj, C., Krishnan, G., Bagath, M., Nameer, P. O & Bhatta, R. (2021). Goat as the ideal climate resilient animal model in tropical environment: Revisiting advantages over other livestock species. International Journal of Biometeorology, DOI: 10.1007/s00484-021-02179-w

Sejian, V., Silpa, M.V., Reshma Nair, M.R., Devaraj, C., Krishnan, G., Bagath, M., Chauhan, S.S., Suganthi, R.U., Fonseca, V.F., König, S., Gaughan, J.B. Dunshea, F.R and Bhatta R (2021). Heat Stress and Goat Welfare: Adaptation and Production Considerations. Animals 11(4), p.1021. https://doi.org/10.3390/ani11041021

Sejian, V., Bagath, M., Krishnan, G., Rashamol, V.P., Pragna, P., Devaraj, C., Bhatta, R (2019). Genes for resilience to heat stress in small ruminants: A review. Small Ruminant Research 173: 42–53.

Sejian, V., Bhatta, R., Gaughan, J.B., Dunshea, F.R and Lacetera, N (2018). Review: Adaptation of animals to heat stress. Animal 12(s2):s431-s444.

Sejian, V., Kumar, D., Gaughan, J.B and Naqvi, S.M.K (2017). Effect of multiple environmental stressors on the adaptive capability of Malpura rams based on physiological responses in a semi-arid tropical environment. Journal of Veterinary Behavior Clinical Applications and Research, 17: 6-13.

Silpa, M.V., König, S., Sejian, V., Malik, P.K., Reshma Nair, M.R., Fonseca, V.F.C., Maia, A.S.C., and Bhatta, R (2021). Climate resilient dairy cattle production: Applications of genomic tools and statistical models. Frontiers in Veterinary Science doi: 10.3389/fvets.2021.625189.

Chapter 4

KP-KiSS1/R System and Livestock Reproduction: Present and Future

Mohan Mondal
Reproductive Physiology Laboratory, ICAR-National Dairy Research Institute, Eastern Regional Station, Kalyani, Nadia, West Bengal-741235, INDIA
Email: drmmondal@gmail.com
Ph: +91 33 25828264

SUMMARY

Kisspeptin (a product of KISS1 gene and potent GnRH secretagogue) is a RF-amide neuropeptide with high affinity to KISS1R (receptor of KISS1 gene), previously called as orphan G protein-coupled receptor (GPR54). Kisspeptin was initially reported to be expressed in non-metastatic melanoma cells with a subsequently powerful suppressor role of the metastatic melanoma. Since its discovery in 1996, kisspeptin is regarded as a potential regulator of hypothalamic-pituitary-gonadal (HPG) axis with expression in many organs and tissues. Therefore, KISS1-KISSR system is reported as one of the important gatekeepers for numerous physiological processes like puberty, various reproductive and metabolic functions, and also some pathophysiology conditions. This chapter provides an overview of our current knowledge on kisspeptin-kisspeptin receptor system with especial focus on the role of kisspeptin-KiSS1/R system in bovine reproduction.

Keywords: Kisspeptin, bovine, hypothalamus, reproduction regulation, puberty

INTRODUCTION

It is well understood since long time that onset of puberty and subsequent reproductive processes are the consequences of interactions of the hypothalamus-pituitary-gonadal (HPG) axis mainly through the stimulation of gonadotrophin-releasing hormone (GnRH). The GnRH is synthesized in the preoptic area of the hypothalamus and then released in to the median eminence from axon terminals in a pulsatile manner to stimulate the secretion of follicle stimulating hormone (FSH) and luteinizing hormone (LH) from the adenohypophysis, which ultimately act on the gonads to boost gametogenesis and synthesis of sex steroids. The GnRH stimulation is provoked by a number of important activating factors that could interact together or partially like phoenixin (Yuan *et al.* 2017), kisspeptin (Hendricks *et al.* 2017), neurokinin B (Navarro *et al.* 2015), leptin (Ohga *et al.* 2017) etc. Out of these GnRH stimulators, kisspeptin is considered to be a most potent GnRH-secretagogue in mammalian species. The regulation of HPG axis by kisspeptin was known later in 2003 than its first known function discovered by Lee et al. (1996) who found that transfecting a full-length KiSS-1 cDNA into metastatic cells could clearly suppress metastasis. Since then, researchers are exploring the influence of kisspeptin in various physiological and pathological events emphasizing its role on reproduction. Therefore, some of these highlight the most recent updates addressing to the metastatic role of KISS1 that was expressed in non-metastatic melanoma cells and was subsequently demonstrated to act as a powerful suppressor of the metastatic potential of malignant melanoma cells in different types of cancer, including breast, pancreatic, ovarian, gastric, prostate and bladder cancer, and esophageal carcinoma (Bhattacharya and Babwah 2015, Wahab *et al.* 2016). Others emphasized the current advancement on molecular diversity and phylogenetic evolution of vertebrate traits of kisspeptin, KiSS1 and KiSS2 and their respective receptor genes i.e. GPR54-1 and GPR54-2 (Kanda and Oka 2013, Yun *et al.* 2014). Furthermore, another group of scientists had focused on the electrical properties of kisspeptin neurons and neurohormonal regulation of kisspeptin activity by its topographic distribution, network connectivity, neurochemistry and burst firing of kisspeptin and kisspeptin-R system (Shannon and Alexander, 2017). Meanwhile, the oscillation of kisspeptin neurons on a circadian basis and its expression clock genes that are thought to regulate its rhythmic activities were also aimed by many researchers (Beymer *et al.* 2016).

Recently, most of the researches on kisspeptin have been associated to delineate its roles in reproduction, where kisspeptin-receptor signaling has been described in various physiological and pathophysiological conditions like during the onset of puberty and in the genital tract, and more for its possible therapeutic application in the treatment of fertility disorders (Okamura *et al.* 2013, Clarke *et al.* 2015, Clarke and Dhillo, 2016, Nejad *et al.* 2017). Other attributed functions to kisspeptin, no less important, were metabolism and stress regulation of kisspeptin in the modulation of reproductive function and sexual, social and emotional brain processing integrated by kisspeptin (Alexander *et al.* 2017, Comninos et al., 2017).

Among all multi-faceted roles of kisspeptin as mentioned above, the present chapter will emphasize specifically the role of kisspeptin in reproduction of livestock species in general and bovines in particular. Finally, we will throw some lights on how kisspeptin, a potent secretagogue of GnRH can be used to address fertility issues of livestock species in future ahead.

DISCOVERY AND STRUCTURE OF KISSPEPTIN

Initially, kisspeptin was been considered as a biomolecule (known then as Metastin) responsible for the suppression of metastasis. This important invention was made in 1996 (Lee et al.) using a "modified subtractive hybridization" method for the purpose of comparing the mRNA expressions through analyzing the cDNAs in metastatic (C8161/MelJuSo) as well as non-metastatic cells/hybrid clones (neo6/

C8161 or neo6/MelJuSo) in chromosome 6/melanoma cell hybrids. The study revealed a suppression of metastasis in an expression-dependent manner when the full-length KiSS-1 cDNA was transfected into C8161 melanoma cells. One year later, the authors confirmed that the KiSS-1, when injected (as transfectant of KiSS-1 clones) into the mammary fat pads of athymic nude mice, acts as a metastasis suppressor gene in some of the human breast cancers tested (Lee and Welch, 1997). The KiSS-1 cDNA was reported to encode a 164 amino acid hydrophilic peptide enriched with a polyproline domain containing a SH3 ligand and a putative protein kinase C-alpha phosphorylation site (Lee *et al.* 1996). Later, a corrected genomic sequence and structure, and refined chromosomal location for KiSS-1 were proposed (West *et al.*; 1998). They reported four exons for this KiSS-1 gene. Of which, the first two are not found to be translated; the third one was reported to have 38 5′ non-coding bases that follow the translational start site with another 100 translated bases. The last exon i.e., terminal one contains 332 translated bases, the translational stop codon, and the polyadenylation signal. Afterwards, other studies were performed showing KiSS-1 with a high affinity natural agonist of GPR54 (Kotani *et al.* 2001) and encoding a carboxy-terminally amidated peptide with 54 amino-acid, primarily isolated from human placenta as the endogenous ligand of GPR54 named as 'metastin' (Ohtaki *et al.* 2001). The GPR54 was identified in the rat brain as an orphan receptor exhibiting high sequence similarity of 45%, 45% and 44%, respectively with the transmembrane regions of galanin receptors GalR1, GalR3 and GalR2 (Lee *et al.* 1999).

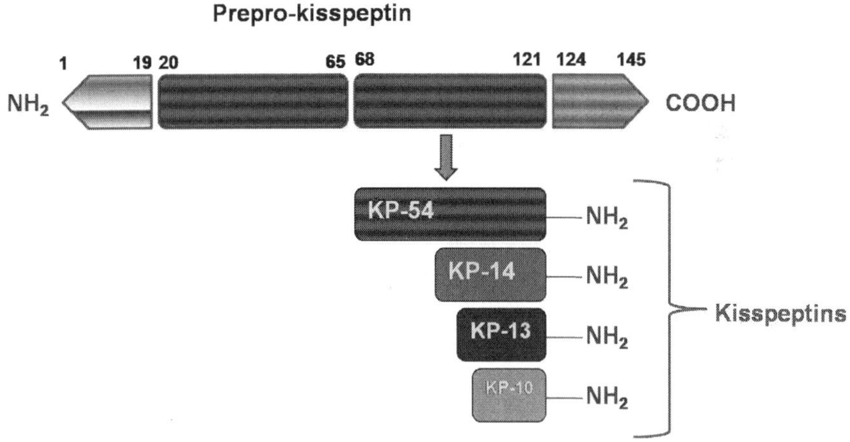

Figure 1: Formation of different types of kisspeptin from its common precursor. Structurally different types of kisspeptin are produced by the cleavage from its common precursor i.e., the prepro-kisspeptin. The prepro-kisspeptin, a peptide of 145 amino acid long, consists of a signal peptide (19-amino acid peptide) and a central 54-amino acid region i.e., kisspeptin-54 (previously known as metastin). Further cleavage of kisspeptin-54 produces kisspeptins of lower molecular weight: Kp-14, Kp-13, and Kp-10. All kisspeptins contain the RF-amide motif that is required to bind and activate KiSS1R. *[Adopted and modified from Hu et al., 2018].*

Furthermore, other kisspeptin fragments that were identified from its precursor were named based on the number of amino acids they contain like kisspeptin-10, kisspeptin-13, and kisspeptin-14 (Bilban *et al.* 2004; Figure 1). And, it was found that all the fragments of kisspeptin staring from kisspeptin-54 to kisspeptin-10 (the shortest kisspeptin fragment) has similar affinity and efficacy on its receptor indicating that the C-terminal part of the peptides is responsible both for the high affinity binding and the activation of GPR54 (Kotani *et al.* 2001). Unlike humans and animals, the identification and characterization of the fish gonadal kisspeptin system revealed four kisspeptin system mRNAs i.e., kiss1, kiss2, and gpr54-1 and gpr54-2 (Fairgrive *et al.* 2016).

LOCALIZATION OF KISS1/KISS1R

Kisspeptin neurons are generally located in the hypothalamus, but kisspeptin receptors are localized in different parts of the brain, pituitary, genital tract and placenta of the vertebrate animals and this localization depends on the species and physiological stage of the animals.

Hypothalamus

Kisspeptin was found in the arcuate nucleus (ARC) and medial preoptic area (mPOA) in sheep where the bed nucleus of the stria terminalis (BNST) was responsible for sexual behavioral onset, whereas; the ARC, ventromedial nucleus (VMN), mPOA and kisspeptin cells located in the ARC and mPOA were found to regulate the positive feedback of estradiol only during the LH surge (Franceschini *et al.*, 2013). Similar distribution map of kissppetin10-immunoreactive (Kp10-ir) cells in the ovine hypothalamus were reported (Franceschini *et al.*, 2006**).** Indeed, high numbers of KP10-ir cells were present in the caudal ARC, mPOA and dorsomedial nucleus, and numerous varicose KP10-ir bers were found in the preoptic area where GnRH neurons reside and in the median eminence, seemingly projecting around small capillaries in its external zone. Expression of KiSS1 in the ARC across the ovine estrous cycle was found to increase in the caudal ARC during the preovulatory period (Estrada *et al.;* 2006). The chronic levels of estrogen and progesterone were found to negatively regulate the expression of the KiSS1 gene in the ARC of the ewe, suggesting that both these steroids may influence GnRH secretion by exerting negative feedback control via altered kisspeptin signaling (Smith *et al.;* 2007). Polkowska *et al.* (2015) reported a decrease of kisspeptin axons extending from preoptic area to medial basal hypothalamus and also in the median eminence in the lambs that were fasted for short-term compared to control animals. Recently, it was demonstrated that the density and proportion of these kisspeptin neurons in ARC and POA were increased with the ram effect in sexually quiescent ewes (Fabre-Nys *et al.* 2017).

Pituitary

Kisspeptin gene is expressed in different cells of the pituitary. KiSS1 and KiSS1R are expressed throughout the gonadal development (Shahi *et al.* 2016). The most recent advances of the role of the Kiss1/Kiss1R system regulating pituitary functions emphasizing the direct role of kisspeptin on pituitary cells and its interactions with other relevant regulators has been reviewed recently (Gahete et al., 2016).

GENITAL TRACT

Kisspeptin/KISS1R is largely expressed in genital tract of male and female (Fairgrieve et al. 2016, Shahi et al. 2016, Rather et al. 2017).

The very first study on KP-KiSS1-KiSS1R system revealed that KiSS-1 and KiSS-1R mRNA expressed more abundantly in the placenta (Lee *et al.* 1996, Muir *et al.* 2001, Bilban *et al.* 2004). Kisspeptin-ir was also found in the cyclic ovaries, where prominent signals were recorded in the theca layer of growing follicles, corpora lutea, interstitial gland, and ovarian surface epithelium (Gaytan *et al.* 2009). KISS1 and KISS1R were also expressed in the uterus, ovary, and oviduct with marked expression in endometrial and oviductal epithelial cells throughout the reproductive cycle (Roman *et al.* 2012). In rodent female, it was found that the WT mouse uterus expresses kisspeptin and KISS1 receptor on day 4 of implantation (Babwah 2015). There are also evidences, which clearly showed that kisspeptin signaling is essential for folliculogenesis, oocyte maturation and ovulation (Gaytan *et al.* 2014; Hsu *et al.* 2014).

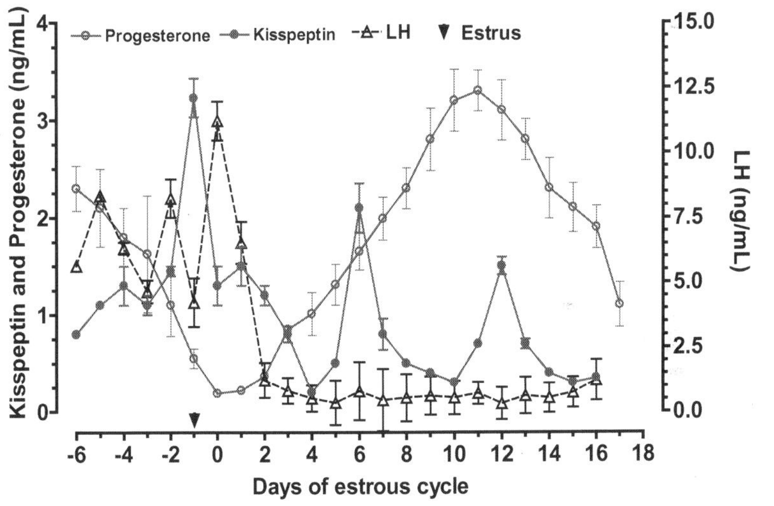

Figure 2: Blood kisspeptin, LH and progesterone profiles (mean±SEM) in cyclic crossbred cows.

On an average, a total of three peaks of kisspeptin were recorded during an entire estrus cycle; the first peak was found to occur on a day before appearance of preovulatory LH surge, the 2nd and 3rd peaks were found on day 6 and 18 of the estrus cycle. Kisspeptin peaks in an estrus cycle vary from 2 to 4. [***Adopted from Mondal et al., 2015]***

Studies conducted in crossbred cows showed for the first time a large and interesting data not only on development of a simple and sensitive assay for kisspeptin determination in plasma but also on kisspeptin concentrations during follicular development and pregnancy (Mondal et al., 2016a). Indeed, these authors recorded three peaks of kisspeptin during an entire estrous cycle; the first peak was found to occur on a day before appearance of preovulatory LH surge, the

2nd and 3rd peaks were found on day 6 and 18 of the estrous cycle (**Figure 2**). This kisspeptin level increased with the follicular development and with the stages of pregnancy. In another study conducted in mithun (*Bos frontalis*) showed that kisspeptin concentrations in follicular fluid increased as the follicles grow and the highest concentrations were found in preovulatory follicles (Mondal et al., 2016b).

In mammalian male, KISS1/KISS1R system plays an important role in the physiology of the genital organ/tract development. KiSS1 and its receptor are expressed mainly in Leydig cells and seminiferous tubules, respectively (Hsu *et al.* 2014). Moreover, the expression of KISS1R was later observed in the gamete, specifically in the acrosome of spermatids and mature sperm. Reduction of serum kisspeptin levels were reported after gonadectomy in males (Salehi *et al.* 2015). Also, Kisspeptin and its receptor were detected in the interstitial compartment and Sertoli cells in the periphery of the seminiferous tubules in adult testes (Irfan *et al.* 2016).

Kisspeptin receptor besides its high presence in placenta and pituitary, was also expressed in pancreas and spinal cord, which clearly indicates its role in the control of the endocrine function (Kotani *et al.* 2001). For the non-vertebrate species, existence and distribution of kisspeptin-like peptides (Kiss-l) and their receptors were discovered in suboesophageal, thoracic ganglia, dorsolateral cluster and ventromedial cluster in the central nervous system (Thongbuakaew *et al.* 2016).

REGULATION OF KISSPEPTIN BY SEX STEROIDS

Research findings showed that kisspeptin neurons are regulated by sex steroids (**Figure 3**). Experiments conducted in ovine species clearly showed that low and high levels of estrogen regulate the kisspeptin neurons in an inhibitory and stimulatory manner, respectively. Progesterone and testosterone were also found to inhibit the kisspeptin neurons as that of low level of estrogen. The concentration of estrogen required to exert a negative feedback on GnRH secretion is also capable to inhibit kisspeptin neurons in the ARC (Lopez et al., 2016). Abundance of transcripts encoding KISS1 gene was found to increase in the ARC during the late follicular phase of the estrous cycle than other phases (Estrada et al., 2006; Li et al. 2015). Treatment of OVX ewes with exogenous estrogens to induce a surge of LH resulted an increase in Foss expression in arcuate kisspeptin neurons thereby neuronal activation (Smith et al. 2009). The activation of kisspeptin neurons was reported to be much higher in estrous animals than the ewes in the luteal phase (Merkley et al., 2015). Hence, unlike female rodents, where the arcuate kisspeptin population being negatively regulated by estrogen (Smith et al., 2005), both a positive and negative regulation of the arcuate population does exist in the ruminants like ewes depending on the circumstances.

Unlike estrogen, less report is available on the regulation of kisspeptin by progesterone. Ovariectomized ewes administered with progesterone showed moderately low level of KISS1 mRNA than to non-OVX animals, which had very insignificant effect than those treated with estrogen (Smith et al., 2007). Very limited studies have been conducted in large ruminants like cattle to compare the population of kisspeptin neuron during follicular and luteal phases of the estrous cycle. Studies revealed that population of kisspeptin cell in the preoptic (Hassaneen et al., 2016) and arcuate area (Tanco et al., 2016) were higher during the follicular than luteal phase of the bovine estrous cycle. These studies suggested that progesterone generally inhibits kisspeptin expression in the arcuate nucleus.

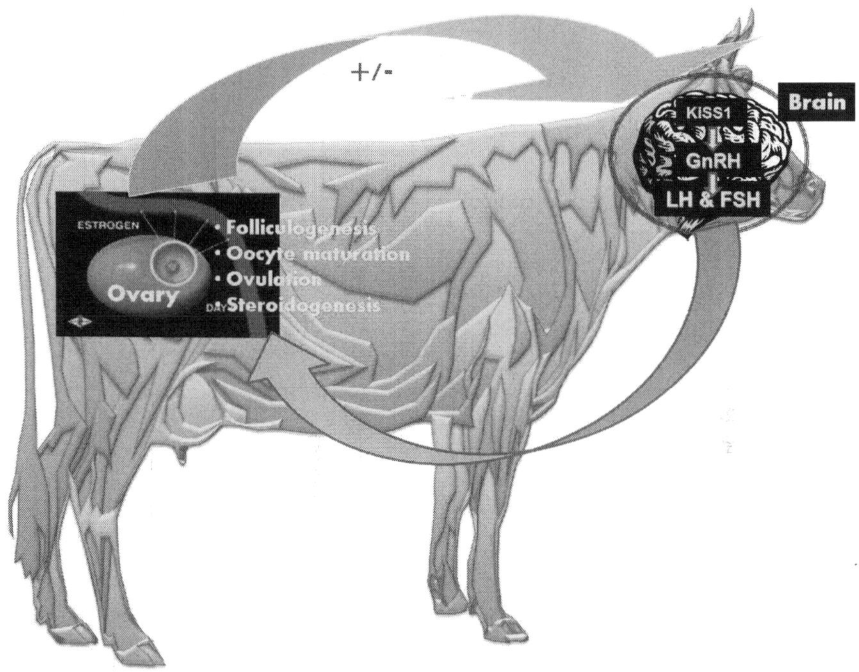

Figure 3: Influence of kisspeptin on ovarian functions and its control through steroid feedback mechanism in bovine species. The main functions of kisspeptin in domestic animals on ovary are folliculogenesis, oocytes maturation, ovulation and steroidogenesis. Kisspeptin neurons are found to be controlled by the levels of estrogen. Low level acts as inhibitory and high-level acts as stimulatory of the kisspeptin neurons. Progesterone always exerts inhibitory action like that of low level of estrogen.

KISSPEPTIN AND REPRODUCTION

Puberty

"Puberty is major developmental event in the lifespan of any individual, which culminates with the attainment of sexual (somatic, psychological) maturity and reproductive capacity. This intricate maturational phenomenon is grounded on early differentiation events (starting *in utero*), and involves a complex series of morphological, functional, endocrine, behavioral and psychological changes, which ultimately lead to the acquisition of a complete adult phenotype" (Parent et al., 2003). Physiologically, puberty in animals could be considered as "the developmental processes, which begins with the first sign of ovarian activity that terminates with the onset of the first reproductive cycle" (Blaustein *et al.* 2016). This growth phase in the vertebrates begin with the increased pulsatile secretion of GnRH that ultimately results in gonadal function activation required for the onset of puberty (Teles *et al.*

2011). While the multifactorial control of GnRH neurons is well established, and GnRH secretion have been reported to be regulated by several neuropeptides and transmitters, kisspeptin has recently been considered as a potential regulatory signal to control the onset of puberty in mammalian species (Pinilla et al., 2012). It has been seen that for final activation of GnRH neurons during pubertal process, higher expression of hypothalamic KiSS1 mRNA and kisspeptin peptide are utmost essential. Enhanced kisspeptin pulsatility with higher frequency and amplitude has been recorded during pubertal onset in crossbred cows (Mondal et al., 2021- *unpublished data*). Repeated administration of kisspeptin-10 in prepubertal crossbred heifers hastens puberty at least two months earlier than control animals (Mondal et al., 2021- *unpublished data*). Similarly, early activation of the gonadotrophic axis and induction of precocious vaginal opening was possible in immature female rats treated with repeated doses of exogenous kisspeptin-10 (Navarro *et al.* 2004b) and showed an increased Kiss-1 mRNA coinciding with the pubertal onset (Navarro *et al.* 2004a). The expression of hypothalamic Kiss-1 mRNA reached the highest level on the day when the animal attained puberty. On the other hand, the population of kisspeptin-ir cell in both ARC and PeN was found to decrease, but the population of the cell was increased in POA during the post-pubertal period (Sun *et al.*, 2007). And also, it was seen increasing the number of kisspeptin cells in ARC nucleus, periventricular nucleus and POA and Kiss1 mRNA in the hypothalamus as soon as puberty is attained (Takase *et al.* 2009, Cui *et al.* 2015). This action of kisspeptin on puberty is possible by modulating the activity of estrogen circuits at the onset of puberty (Cui *et al.* 2015). Expression of KiSS1 and KiSS1R has been increased during the transition period from prepubertal to pubertal stage in crossbred cows and sheep (Redmond et al. 2011; Mondal et al., 2021- *unpublished data*). KiSS1 mRNA levels were also found to increase across the early stages of puberty in the preoptic area in OVX ewe lambs treated with estrogen and a high positive correlation that was found to exist between the number of KISS1-expressing cells and the frequency of LH clearly indicates their active involvement with the process of onset of puberty (Redmond et al. 2011).

Regulation of Gonadotropins, LH Surge and Ovulation by Kisspeptin

Most of the research in the field of kisspeptin biology of domestic animals has been concentrated on the effects of exogenous kisspeptin administration on its efficacy to release plasma LH. Single intravenous kisspeptin administration has been found to increase blood LH in females from all livestock species studied so far like cattle (Kadokawa et al. 2008), goats (Hashizume et al. 2010), sheep (Caraty et al. 2007), horses (Magee et al. 2009) and pigs (Lents et al. 2008). Kisspeptin probably acts three places to stimulate plasma LH: a) stimulating GnRH secretion through acting on the GnRH neurons present in the POA or ARC nucleus, b) stimulating on GnRH terminals present in the median eminence and c) stimulating LH secretion by directly acting on adenohypophysis (anterior pituitary). And, all these can act as GnRH/LH pulse generator and also have influence on the preovulatory GnRH/LH surge.

A number studies revealed that exogenous administration of kisspeptin always resulted in increased release of follicle stimulating hormone (FSH) and luteinizing hormone (LH) in the blood. In goats, it was seen that the average concentrations of plasma LH and FSH in the treatment group were significantly higher 6 h after kisspeptin analog treatment than those in the control group. And also, for the second ovulation, ovulatory follicles in the treatment group were significantly smaller in maximal diameter than in the control group (3.8 ± 0.5 vs 5.4 ± 0.2 mm, $p < 0.05$) (Goto *et al.*, 2014). The timing of surge-like release of these hormones after kisspeptin injection is associated with the estrous cycle (Endo *et al.* 2015, Rahayu *et al.* 2017). Because during the luteal phase, a surge-like release of LH with a peak was observed at 12.5±1.0h after administration of exogenous kisspeptin but in the follicular phase, a surge-like release of LH occurred immediately after kisspeptin administration with a peak at 6.0±3.5h (Endo *et al.* 2015). Furthermore, significant increases in plasma LH concentration were detected during the periods of 3 to 5 h and 2 to 5 h after 50 µg kisspeptin analogue injection in female goats with early luteal phase and mid luteal phase, respectively (Rahayu *et al.* 2017). But, these increased peripheral concentrations of both LH and FSH in mares were always rapid, transient and failed to induce ovulation, even when kisspeptin was perfused for prolonged periods (Decourt *et al.* 2014). Similar observations were made by McGrath and his team 2016, when they found that, a 30 hours infusion of kisspeptin at a low and high rate ([88 µg] and [130 µg] per hour, respectively) in mares increased LH secretion but was not able to stimulate an LH surge for follicle ovulation. Also, administration of 500 µg and 1.0 mg rodent kisspeptin (rKP-10) exhibited LH and FSH peak, although a single injection of 1.0 mg rKP-10, IV was not enough to induce ovulation in the estrous mare (Magee *et al.* 2009).

A significant stimulation of LH and FSH release was observed in kisspeptin treated young calves with peaks of their plasma concentrations reached at 20 – 40 min after kisspeptin injections (Ahmed *et al.* 2009). The area under the LH and FSH curve for a 120-min period post-Kp10 administration was significantly higher in the males than females ($P<0.05$). And this LH and FSH release is greater after an IV than an IM injection of Kp10 in calves (Ahmed et *al.*, 2009).

Kisspeptin Regulation of Estrous Cycle

Literature on the influence of kisspeptin in estrous cycle of domestic animals is limited. A few studies have been conducted on kisspeptin during rat estrous cycle. Experiments in cattle revealed that kisspeptin concentrations varied significantly ($P<0.05$) during different days of bovine estrous cycle. A mean of three kisspeptin peaks of varying amplitudes were recorded during the entire bovine estrous cycle. The highest peak of kisspeptin was obtained on two days before the onset of estrus (day -2). On an average, the 2nd and 3rd peak of kisspeptin were found to occur on day 6 and 12, respectively. The number of peaks for blood KP was recorded to vary between two to four in individual cows (Mondal et al., 2015; **Figure 2**).

Abundance of transcripts encoding KiSS1 gene was found to be significantly different ($P<0.01$) during different stages of bovine estrous cycle. The highest expression of KiSS1 gene was found during proestrus stage of the estrous cycle.

Abundance of transcript encoding KiSS1R gene was similar (P>0.05) during different stages of estrous cycle (Mondal et al., 2021- *unpublished data*).

One study conducted in Japanese Black beef cows showed that exogenous kisspeptin-54 accelerated the follicular development of the first DF and this effect was mediated by kisspeptin-induced LH release (Naniwa et al., 2013). Full-length kisspeptin was also capable of inducing ovulation (Naniwa et al., 2013). Thus, keeping in view the great potential of kisspeptin as a 'biomolecule of promise' for reproduction augmentation, it can be considered as a novel drug of choice to stimulate the follicular growth and development, and ovulation in livestock species in general and bovine in particular.

Kisspeptin and Assisted Reproduction

Kisspeptin controls secretion of GnRH and gonadotropins thereby control the functions of gonads, and this is the basis for using kisspeptin in assisted reproduction in almost all mammalian species including livestock (Macedo et al., 2014, 2015, 2019; Mondal et al., 2015, 2016; Decourt et al., 2016; Northup et al., 2020). Exogenous kisspeptin administration was reported to increase endogenous LH secretion and resulted with better ovulation synchronization than GnRH in crossbred dairy heifers (Mondal et. al., 2015) and crossbred beef heifers and cows (Leonardi, 2018). Bovine full length kisspeptin induced LH release and growth of the dominant follicle during first follicular wave in Japanese Black beef cows (Naniwa et al., 2013). Similarly, continuous 48h administration of kisspeptin through osmotic minipump during proestrus increased growth of the follicles and rate of ovulation in anestrous Nelore cows (Macedo et al., 2015).

Recently, kisspeptin analogue, called C6, has pharmacological advantages over endogenous kisspeptin in terms of having a long-lasting effect and increased activity following intramuscular injection (Decourt et al., 2019). The C6 influenced plasma LH and FSH in the Alpine goat during the breeding, non-breeding season and at the onset of the breeding season and trigger successful ovulation. The C6 has also been reported to advance puberty in female mice when administered for five consecutive days (Decourt et al., 2016). Hence, C6 or any other kisspeptin analogues can potentially be used for early attainment of puberty and fertility management in livestock species. All the evidences as cited herein clearly revealed that the kisspeptin either natural or its analogue can stimulate inactive or partially active GnRH neurons thereby initiation of reproductive processes.

KISS1/KISS1R was found to be localized in the follicular cells (granulosa and theca cells), and oocytes, and kisspeptin was also reported to present in the follicular fluid (Mondal et al., 2015; **Figure 4**). We can, therefore, suggest from these findings that kisspeptin and KiSS1/KiSS1R system may have autocrine/paracrine actions within the follicles. Kispeptin-ir has also been detected in bovine corpus luteum (CL). Young CL was found to contain higher kisspeptin than the mid- or late-cycle CL (Mondal et al., 2015; **Figure 5**). Supplementation of kisspeptin in the culture media was reported to enhance in vitro maturation of oocytes (Byri et al., 2017) and increased blastocysts formation (Soares et al., 2018) in sheep, cattle and buffaloes (Rajesh et al., 2018).

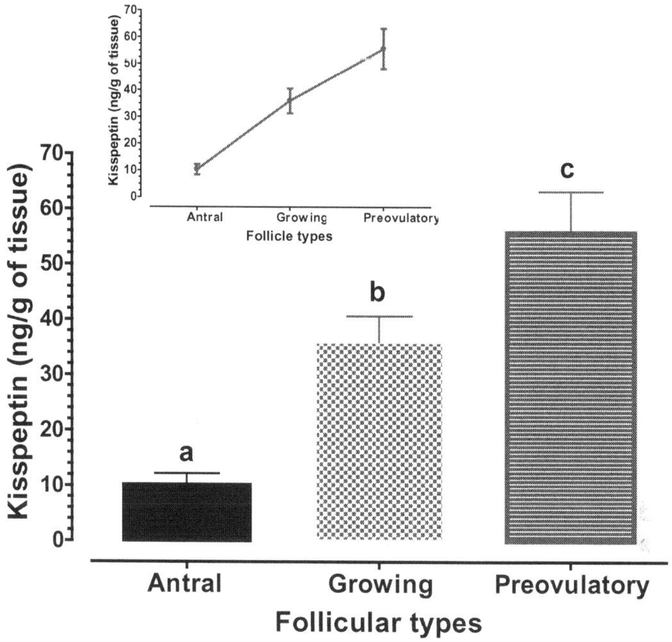

Figure 4: Mean (±SEM) content of kisspeptin in the follicles of different stages of development. A total of 10 grams of antral (5-6 mm), growing (8-10 mm) and preovulatory (15-16 mm) follicles were extracted (n=4). Bars indicated with different letters (a,b,c) differ (P<0.001). ***[Adopted from Mondal et al., 2015]***

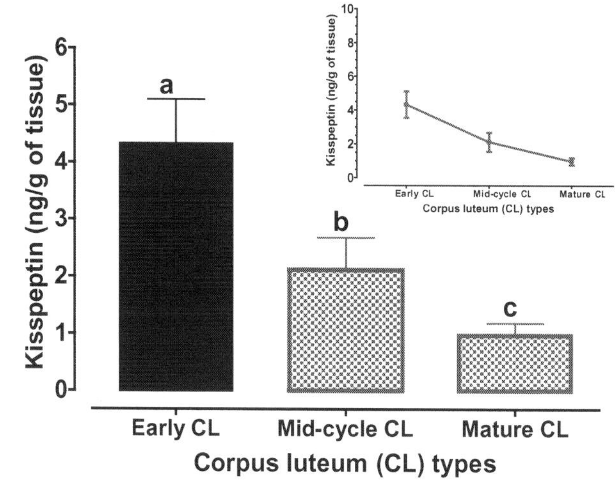

Figure 5: Mean (±SEM) content of kisspeptin in the bovine corpus luteum (CL) during different stages of development. A total of 10 grams of early, mid-cycle and mature CL tissues were extracted (n=4). Bars indicated with different letters (a,b,c) differ (P<0.001).

Kisspeptin and Pregnancy

In female genital tract, KISS1/KISS1R system plays an important role in regulating implantation of the mammalian embryo, placentation and maintenance of pregnancy (Lee *et al.* 1996, Bilban *et al.* 2004). Moreover, it has been demonstrated that the WT mouse uterus expresses kisspeptin and KISS1 receptor on day 4 of implantation (Babwah et al. 2015). Furthermore, in human, KISS1 and KISS1R are expressed in the placenta in the syncytiotrophoblast during the first trimester of pregnancy (Bilban *et al.* 2004). And, it was seen that the decreased kisspeptin and PIBF (progesterone-induced blocking factor) expressions in trophoblasts and deciduas were associated with recurrent spontaneous abortion (RSA) because expressions of these molecules in syncytiotrophoblasts and cytotrophoblasts were decreased in RSA women than controls (Wu *et al.* 2014). Moreover, reduced trophoblast invasiveness was associated with the development of preeclampsia as there were lower circulating serum kisspeptin concentrations in women pregnancies complicated by preeclampsia than in healthy pregnancies (Matjila *et al.* 2016).

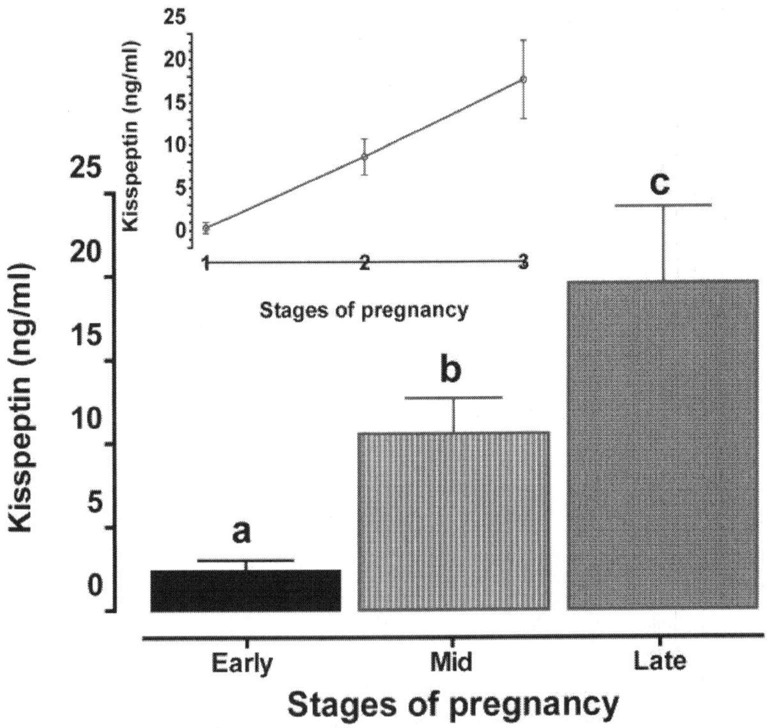

Figure 6: Mean (±SEM) profiles of blood kisspeptin in pregnant cows during different stages of pregnancy viz., early (<10 weeks; n=6), mid (>10 to <20 weeks; n=6) and late (>20 to 36 weeks; n=6) stages of pregnancy. Bars indicated with different letters (a,b,c) differ (P<0.001). ***[Adopted from Mondal et al., 2015]***

In bovines, it was seen that kisspeptin-1r/kisspeptin system plays a crucial role during pregnancy by regulating the proliferation of cells of bovine placental cotyledon cell lines isolated during the first trimester of pregnancy, but it was not involved in modulating placental progesterone secretion during this stage of pregnancy (Martino *et al.* 2015). Mondal *et al.* (2016b) reported higher plasma kisspeptin levels in early pregnant than non-pregnant mithun (*Bos frontalis*) cows. Plasma kisspeptin concentrations were found to increase as the pregnancy advances in crossbred cows (Mondal et al., 2015; **Figure 6**) and placental kisspeptin levels were also found to increase with the advancement of bovine pregnancy (Mondal et al., 2015; **Figure 7**). And in small ruminants, KiSS-1 gene affected litter size in goats because it was seen that the single nucleotide polymorphism in goat KiSS-1 gene had significant effects on litter size (Hou *et al.* 2011).

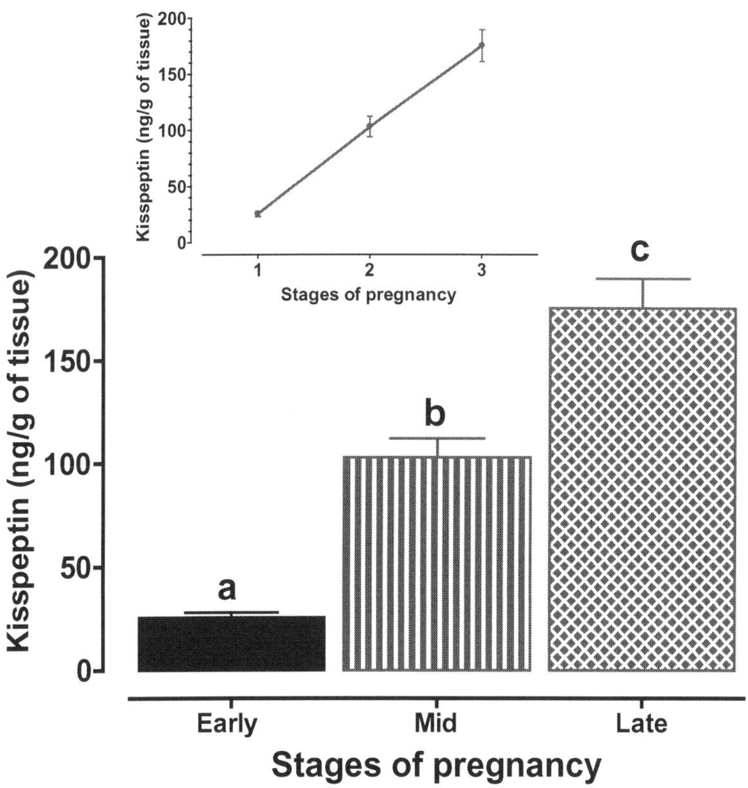

Figure 7: Mean (±SEM) content of kisspeptin in bovine placental tissues collected from animals of different stages of pregnancy. A total of 10 grams of placental tissues were extracted (n=6). Bars indicated with different letters (a,b,c) differ (P<0.001). ***[Adopted from Mondal et al., 2015]***

CONCLUSIONS

During the first decade of kisspeptin discovery, it is interesting to underline its revolutionary characteristics that have registered the kisspeptin-KiSS1/KiSS1R system in the top priority of research in a variety of mammalian species including livestock. From its classical function as a melanoma suppressor agent to a potential gatekeeper of the hypothalamic-pituitary-gonadal axis proved its multi-faceted functions. Kisspeptin controls pubertal onset, follicular development, emergence of follicular waves and ovulation. There are also evidences that support its active participation in the autocrine/paracrine regulation of ovarian function, early embryonic development, implantation, placentation and maintenance of pregnancy. Though most of the research has been conducted in rat and human model, a good quantum of work has already been initiated in livestock species, which clearly showed that kisspeptin is a potent secretagogue of GnRH and can potentially be used in assisted reproduction. It can be used to induce puberty in prepubertal animals. Similarly, kisspeptin can be used as a wonder molecule for estrus synchronization protocol for timed AI. It can also be used as an ovulation inducer in anovulatory cases and for enhancing follicular growth. Additionally, kisspeptin holds promise in the field of *in vitro* maturation (IVM) of oocytes, *in vitro* fertilization (IVF) and *in vitro* culture (IVC) of embryos. Furthermore, use of recently available kisspeptin analogue like C6 that have an extended half-life and high biological potency can be used for fertility management in livestock species in general and bovine in particular. A lot of research is needed to be undertaken in the field of kisspeptin biology in livestock species particularly the kisspeptin analogues and its role in embryo implantation, placentation, IVM, IVF, IVC etc. It is interesting to note that the research in the field of kisspeptin biology, which was started with its metastasis suppressor function has now been reached to reproduction as a stimulator of GnRH, and still, we have to travel a lot to unravel its role in the assisted reproduction particularly embryo survival and IVF.

REFERENCES

Ahmed, E, A, Saito H, Sawada T, Yaegashi T, Yamashita T, Hirata T, Sawai K, Hashizume T. Characteristics of the stimulatory effect of kisspeptin-10 on the secretion of luteinizing hormone, follicle-stimulating hormone and growth hormone in prepubertal male and female cattle. J Reprod Dev. 2009 Dec;55(6):650-4. Epub 2009 Sep 29.

Alexander N. Comninos and Waljit S. Dhillo. Emerging Roles of Kisspeptin in Sexual and Emotional Brain Processing. Neuroendocrinology 2017. DOI: 10.1159/000481137.

Alreja M. Electrophysiology of kisspeptin neurons. Adv Exp Med Biol. 2013;784:349-62. doi: 10.1007/978-1-4614-6199-9_16

Babwah AV. Uterine and placental KISS1 regulate pregnancy: what we know and the challenges that lie ahead. Reproduction 2015 ; Oct;150(4):R121-8. doi: 10.1530/REP-15-0252. Epub 2015 Jul 16.

Beymer M, Henningsen J, Bahougne T, Simonneaux V. The role of kisspeptin and RFRP in the circadian control of female reproduction. Mol Cell Endocrinol. 2016 Dec 15;438:89-99. doi: 10.1016/j.mce.2016.06.026. Epub 2016 Jun 27.

Bhattacharya M, Babwah AV. Kisspeptin: beyond the brain. Endocrinology. 2015 Apr;156(4):1218-27. doi: 10.1210/en.2014-1915. Epub 2015 Jan 15.

Bilban M, Ghaffari-Tabrizi N, Hintermann E, Bauer S, Molzer S, Zoratti C, Malli R, Sharabi A, Hiden U, Graier W, Knöfler M, Andreae F, Wagner O, Quaranta V, Desoye G. Kisspeptin-10, a KiSS-1/metastin-derived decapeptide, is a physiological invasion inhibitor of primary human trophoblasts. J Cell Sci. 2004; 117(Pt 8):1319-28.

Blaustein JD, Ismail N, Holder MK. Review: Puberty as a time of remodeling the adult response to ovarian hormones. J Steroid Biochem Mol Biol. 2016 Jun;160:2-8. doi: 10.1016/j.jsbmb.2015.05.007. Epub 2015 May 21.

Byri P, Gangineni A, Reddy KR, Raghavender KBP. Effect of kisspeptin on in vitro maturation of sheep oocytes. Vet World 2017;10:276–280.

Caraty A, Smith JT, Lomet D, Ben Saïd S, Morrissey A, Cognie J, Doughton B, Baril G, Briant C & Clarke IJ 2007 Kisspeptin synchronizes preovulatory surges in cyclical ewes and causes ovulation in seasonally acyclic ewes. Endocrinology 148 5258–5267. (https://doi.org/10.1210/en.2007-0554)

Clarke H, Dhillo WS, Jayasena CN. Comprehensive Review on Kisspeptin and Its Role in Reproductive Disorders. Endocrinol Metab (Seoul). 2015 Jun;30(2):124-41. doi: 10.3803/EnM.2015.30.2.124.

Clarke SA, Dhillo WS. Kisspeptin across the human lifespan:evidence from animal studies and beyond. J Endocrinol. 2016 Jun;229(3):R83-98. doi: 10.1530/JOE-15-0538.

Comninos AN, Wall MB, Demetriou L, Shah AJ, Clarke SA, Narayanaswamy S, Nesbitt A, Izzi-Engbeaya C, Prague JK, Abbara A, Ratnasabapathy R, Salem V, Nijher GM, Jayasena CN, Tanner M, Bassett P, Mehta A, Rabiner EA, Hönigsperger C, Silva MR, Brandtzaeg OK, Lundanes E, Wilson SR, Brown RC, Thomas SA, Bloom SR, Dhillo WS. Kisspeptin modulates sexual and emotional brain processing in humans. J Clin Invest. 2017 Feb 1;127(2):709-719.

Cui P, Yang C, Zhang K, Gao X, Luo L, Tian Y, Song M, Liu Y, Zhang Y, Li Y, Zhang X, Su S, Fang F, Ding J. Effect of estrogen on the expression of GnRH and kisspeptin in the hypothalamus of rats during puberty, *Theriogenology* (2015), doi: 10.1016/j.theriogenology.2015.08.004.

Decourt C, Robert V, Anger K, Galibert M, Madinier JB, Liu X, Dardente H, Lomet D, Delmas AF, Caraty A, Herbison AE, Anderson GM et al. A synthetic kisspeptin analog that triggers ovulation and advances puberty. Nat Sci Rep 2016;6:26908.

Decourt C, Caraty A, Briant C, Guillaume D, Lomet D, Chesneau D, Lardic L, Duchamp G, Reigner F, Monget P, Dufourny L, Beltramo M, Dardente H. Acute injection and chronic perfusion of kisspeptin elicit gonadotropins release but fail to trigger ovulation in the mare. Biol Reprod. 2014 Feb 20;90(2):36. doi: 10.1095/biolreprod.113.114157. Print 2014 Feb.

Endo N, Tamesaki C, Ohkura S, Wakabayashi Y, Matsui H, Tanaka A, Watanabe T, Okamura H, Tanaka T. Differential changes in luteinizing hormone secretion after administration of the investigational metastin/kisspeptin analog TAK-683 in goats. Anim Reprod Sci. 2015 Aug;159:87-93. doi: 10.1016/j.anireprosci.2015.05.016. Epub 2015 May 29.

Estrada KM, Clay CM, Pompolo S, Smith JT & Clarke IJ 2006 Elevated KiSS-1 expression in the arcuate nucleus prior to the cyclic preovulatory gonadotrophin-releasing hormone/lutenising hormone surge in the ewe suggests a stimulatory role for kisspeptin in oestrogen-positive feedback. Journal of Neuroendocrinology 18 806–809. (https://doi.org/10.1111/j.1365-2826.2006.01485.x)

Fabre-Nys C, Cognié J, Dufourny L, Ghenim MS, Martinet S, Lasserre O, Lomet D, Millar RP, Ohkura S, Suetomi Y. The two populations of kisspeptin neurons are involved in the ram induced LH pulsatile secretion and LH surge in anestrous ewes. Endocrinology. 2017 Sep 1. doi: 10.1210/en.2017-00429.

Fairgrieve MR, Shibata Y, Smith EK, Hayman ES, Luckenbach JA. Molecular characterization of the gonadal kisspeptin system: Cloning, tissue distribution, gene expression analysis and localization in sablefish (Anoplopoma fimbria). Gen Comp Endocrinol. 2016 Jan 1;225:212-223. doi: 10.1016/j.ygcen.2015.07.015. Epub 2015 Sep 16.

Franceschini I, Lomet D, Cateau M. Kisspeptin immunoreactive cells of the ovine preoptic area and arcuate nucleus co-express estrogen receptor alpha. Neuroscience. Letters 2006; 401 (3), 225–230.

Franceschini I, Desroziers E. Development and Aging of the Kisspeptin-GPR54 System in the Mammalian Brain: What are the Impacts on Female Reproductive Function? Front Endocrinol (Lausanne). 2013 Mar 28;4:22. doi: 10.3389/fendo.2013.00022. eCollection 2013.

Gahete MD, Vázquez-Borrego MC, Martínez-Fuentes AJ, Tena-Sempere M, Castaño JP, Luque -RM. Role of the Kiss1/Kiss1r system in the regulation of pituitary cell function. Mol Cell Endocrinol. 2016 Dec 15;438:100-106. doi: 10.1016/j.mce.2016.07.039. Epub 2016 Jul 29.

Gaytan F, Garcia-Galiano D, Dorfman MD, Manfredi-Lozano M, Castellano JM,Dissen GA,Ojeda SR & Tena-Sempere M. Kisspeptin receptor haplo-insuficiency causes premature ovarian failure despite preserved gonadotropin secretion. Endocrinology 2014; 155: 3088–3097.

Gaytán F, Gaytán M, Castellano JM, Romero M, Roa J, Aparicio B, Garrido N, Sánchez-Criado JE, Millar RP, Pellicer A, Fraser HM, Tena-Sempere M. KiSS-1 in the mammalian ovary: distribution of kisspeptin in human and marmoset and alterations in KiSS-1 mRNA levels in a rat model of ovulatory dysfunction. Am J Physiol Endocrinol Metab. 2009 Mar;296(3):E520-31. doi: 10.1152/ajpendo.90895.2008. Epub 2009 Jan 13

Goto Y, Endo N, Nagai K, Ohkura S, Wakabayashi Y, Tanaka A, Matsui H, Kusaka M, Okamura H, Tanaka T. Ovarian and hormonal responses to follicular phase administration of investigational metastin/kisspeptin analog, TAK-683, in goats. Reprod Domest Anim. 2014 Apr;49(2):338-42. doi: 10.1111/rda.12283. Epub 2014 Feb 1.

Hashizume T, Saito H, Sawada T, Yaegashi T, Ezzat AA, Sawai K & Yamashita T 2010 Characteristics of stimulation of gonadotropin secretion by kisspeptin-10 in female goats. Animal Reproduction Science 118 37–41. (https://doi.org/10.1016/j.anireprosci.2009.05.017)

Hassaneen A, Naniwa Y, Suetomi Y, Matsuyama S, Kimura K, Ieda N, Inoue N, Uenoyama Y, Tsukamura H, Maeda KI, et al. 2016 Immunohistochemical characterization of the arcuate kisspeptin/neurokinin B/dynorphin (KNDy) and preoptic kisspeptin neuronal populations in the hypothalamus during the estrous cycle in heifers. Journal of Reproduction and Development 62 471–477. (https://doi.org/10.1262/jrd.2016-075)

Hendriks E, Prentice P, Williams R. Disorders of puberty. Medicine (2017), http://dx.doi.org/10.1016/j.mpmed.2017.06.011.

Hou JX, An XP, Wang JG, Song YX, Cui YH, Wang YF, Chen QJ, Cao YB. New genetic polymorphisms of KiSS-1 gene and their association with litter size in goats. Small Ruminant Research *96 (2011) 106–110.*

Hsu MC, Wang JY, Lee YJ, Jong DS, Tsui KH, Chiu CH. Kisspeptin modulates fertilization capacity of mouse spermatozoa. Reproduction 2014;147(6):835-45.

Hu KL, Zhao H, Chang HM, Yu Y, Qiao J. Kisspeptin/kisspeptin receptor system in the ovary. Front Endocrinol 2018;8:365.

Irfan S, Ehmcke J, Shahab M, Wistuba J, Schlatt S. 2016. Immunocytochemical localization of kisspeptin and kisspeptin receptor in the primate testis. J Med Primatol.;45(3):105-11.

Kadokawa H, Matsui M, Hayashi K, Matsunaga N, Kawashima C, Shimizu T, Kida K & Miyamoto A 2008 Peripheral administration of kisspeptin-10 increases plasma concentrations of GH as well as LH in prepubertal Holstein heifers. Journal of Endocrinology 196 331–334. (https://doi.org/10.1677/JOE-07-0504)

Kanda S, Oka Y. Structure, synthesis, and phylogeny of kisspeptin and its receptor. Adv Exp Med Biol. 2013;784:9-26. doi: 10.1007/978-1-4614-6199-9_2.

Kotani M, Detheux M, Vandenbogaerde A, Communi D, Vanderwinden JM, Le Poul E, Brezillon S, Tyldesley R, Suarez-Huerta N, Vandeput F, Blanpain C, Schiffmann NS, Vassart G, and Parmentier M. The Metastasis Suppressor Gene KiSS-1 Encodes Kisspeptins, the Natural Ligands of the Orphan G Protein-coupled Receptor GPR54. J. Biol. Chem. 2001, 276:34631-34636. doi: 10.1074/jbc.M104847200 originally published online July 16, 2001.

Lee JH, Miele ME, Hicks DJ, Phillips KK, Trent JM, Weissman BE, Welch DR. KiSS-1, a novel human malignant melanoma metastasis-suppressor gene. J Natl Cancer Inst. 1996 Dec 4;88(23):1731-7.

Lee JH, Welch DR. Suppression of metastasis in human breast carcinoma MDA-MB-435 cells after transfection with the metastasis suppressor gene, KiSS-1. Cancer Res. 1997 Jun 15;57(12):2384-7.

Lee DK, Nguyen T, O'Neill GP, Cheng R, Liu Y, Howard AD, Coulombe N, Tan CP, Tang-Nguyen AT, George SR, O'Dowd BF. Discovery of a receptor related to the galanin receptors. FEBS Lett. 1999 Mar 5;446(1):103-7.

Lents CA, Heidorn NL, Barb CR & Ford JJ 2008 Central and peripheral administration of kisspeptin activates gonadotropin but not somatotropin secretion in prepubertal gilts. Reproduction 135 879–887. (https://doi.org/10.1530/REP-07-0502)

Leonardi CEP. Kisspeptin function in female bovine reproduction. 2018. PhD Thesis. University of Saskatchewan, Saskatoon, Canada; https://harvest.usask.ca/handle/10388/9597

Li Q, Millar RP, Clarke IJ & Smith JT 2015 Evidence that neurokinin B controls basal gonadotropin-releasing hormone secretion but is not critical for estrogen-positive feedback in sheep. Neuroendocrinology 101 161–174. (https://doi.org/10.1159/000377702)

Lopez JA, Bedenbaugh MN, McCosh RB, Weems PW, Meadows LJ, Wisman B, Coolen LM, Goodman RL & Hileman SM 2016 Does dynorphin play a role in the onset of puberty in female sheep? Journal of Neuroendocrinology 28. (https://doi.org/10.1016/j. psyneuen.2016.07.080)

Macedo GG, Carvalho NAT, Soares JG, Santos RM, Jacomini JO, Baruselli PS. Kisspeptin stimulates LH release in buffalo cows in the breeding and nonbreeding season. Anim Reprod 2014;11:460–460. https://www.animal-reproduction.org/article/5b5a6041f7783717068b4663/pdf/animreprod-11-3-447.pdf

Macedo GG, Mingoti RD, Batista EOS, Monteiro BM, Vieira LM, Barletta RV, Wiltbank MC, Nogueira GP, Renno FP, Maio JR, Baruselli PS. Profile of LH release in response to intramuscular treatment with kisspeptin in Bos indicus and Bos taurus prepubertal heifers. Theriogenology 2019;125:64–70.

Macedo GG, Sala RV, Martins LF, Baruselli PS. Kisspeptin slowly administered during proestrus improves follicle growth and ovulation in anestrous cows. Reprod Fert Develop 2015;28:133–133.

Magee C, Foradori CD, Bruemmer JE, Arreguin-Arevalo JA, McCue PM, Handa RJ, Squires EL & Clay CM 2009 Biological and anatomical evidence for kisspeptin regulation of the hypothalamic-pituitarygonadal axis of estrous horse mares. Endocrinology 150 2813–2821. (https://doi.org/10.1210/en.2008-1698)

Martino N, Rizzo A, Pizzi F, Dell'Aquila M, Sciorsci R. Effects of Kisspeptin-10 on in vitro proliferation and Kisspeptin receptor (Kiss-1R) expression in primary epithelial cell cultures isolated from bovine placental cotyledons of embryos/fetuses at the first trimester of pregnancy. *Theriogenology* (2015), doi: 10.1016/j.theriogenology.2014.11.033.

Matjila M, Millar R, Spuy Z, Katz A. Elevated placental expression at the maternal–fetal interface but diminished maternal circulatory kisspeptin in preeclamptic pregnancies. Pregnancy Hypertension: An International Journal of Women's Cardiovascular Health 6 (2016) 79–87.

McGrath BM, Scott CJ, Wynn PC, Loy J, Norman ST. Kisspeptin stimulates LH secretion but not ovulation in mares during vernal transition. Theriogenology. 2016 Oct 1;86(6):1566-1572. doi: 10.1016/j.theriogenology.2016.05.016. Epub 2016 May 25.

Merkley CM, Coolen LM, Goodman RL & Lehman MN 2015 Evidence for changes in numbers of synaptic inputs onto KNDy and GnRH neurones during the preovulatory LH surge in the ewe. Journal of Neuroendocrinology 27 624–635. (https://doi.org/10.1111/jne.12293)

Mondal M, Baruah KK, Ghosh MK, Karunakaran M, Dutta TK. Kisspeptin modulates reproduction in ruminants. J Vet Sci Tech 2016;5:7–12.

Mondal M, Baruah KK, Karunakaran M, Ghosh MK, Dutta TK. Development of a new kisspeptin based method of ovulation synchronization for crossbred dairy heifers. Research and reviews. J Dairy Sci Tech 2015;4:12–16.

Mondal M, Baruah KK, Prakash BS. Determination of plasma kisspeptin concentrations during reproductive cycle and different phases of pregnancy in crossbred cows using bovine specific enzyme immunoassay. Gen Comp Endocrinol. 2016a; 1(224):168-75.

Mondal M, Karunakaran M, Baruah KK. Development and Validation of a Sensitive Enzymeimmunoassay for Determination of Plasma Metastin in Mithun (Bos frontalis). J Immunoassay Immunochem. 2016b; 37(2):201-16.

Muir AI., Chamberlain L, Elshourbagy NA, Michalovich D, Moore DJ, Calamari A, Szekeres PG, Sarau HM, Chambers JK, Murdock P, Steplewski K, Shabon U, Miller JE, Middleton SE, Darker JG, Larminie CGC, Wilson S, Bergsma DJ, Emson P, Faull R, Philpott KL, Harrison DC. *J. Biol. Chem. 2001;* 276, 28969–28975.

Naniwa Y, Nakatsukasa K, Setsuda S, Oishi S, Fujii N, Matsuda F, Uenoyama Y, Tsukamura H, Maeda K, Ohkura S. Effects of full-length kisspeptin administration on follicular development in Japanese Black beef cows. J Reprod Develop 2013;59:588–594.

Navarro VM, Bosch MA, León S, et al. The integrated hypothalamic tachykinin-kisspeptin system as a central coordinator for reproduction. Endocrinology. 2015; 156:627–37.

Navarro VM, Castellano JM, Fernandez-Fernandez R, Barreiro ML, Roa J, Sanchez-Criado JE, Aguilar E, Dieguez C, Pinilla L, TenaSempere M. Developmental and hormonally regulated messenger ribonucleic acid expression of KiSS-1 and its putative receptor, GPR54, in rat hypothalamus and potent luteinizing hormone-releasing activity of KiSS-1 Peptide. Endocrinology 145 (2004a) 4565–4574.

Navarro VM, Fernandez-Fernandez R, Castellano JM, Roa J, Mayen A, Barreiro ML, Gaytan F, Aguilar E, Pinilla L, Dieguez C,Tena-empere M. Advanced vaginal opening and precocious activation of the reproductive axis by KiSS-1 peptide, the endogenous ligand of GPR54. J. Physiol. 561 (2004b) 379–386.

Nejad ZS, Tehrani RF, and Zadeh-Vakili A. The Role of Kisspeptin in Female Reproduction. Int J Endocrinol Metab. 2017; 15(3):e44337.

Northup SL, Coffman EA, Strickland LG, Pohler KG, Daniel JA, Whitlock BK. Intravenous infusion of kisspeptin increased serum luteinizing hormone acutely and decreased serum follicle stimulating hormone chronically in prepubertal bull calves. Theriogenology 2020; 144:1–7.

Ohga H, Adachi H, Matsumori K, Kodama R, Nyuji M, Kato K, Yamamoto S, Yamaguchi A, Matsuyama M, Selvaraj S. mRNA levels of kisspeptins, kisspeptin receptors, and GnRH1 in the brain of chub mackerel during puberty. Comparative Biochemistry and Physiology, Part A 179 (2015) 104–112.

Ohtaki T, Shintani Y, Honda S, Matsumoto H, Hori A, Kanehashi K, Terao Y, Kumano S, Takatsu Y, Masuda Y, Ishibashi Y, Watanabe T, Asada M, Yamada T, Suenaga M, Kitada C, Usuki S, Kurokawa T, Onda H, Nishimura O, Fujino M. Metastasis suppressor gene KiSS-1 encodes peptide ligand of a G-protein-coupled receptor. Nature 2001;411, 613–617.

Okamura H, Tsukamura H, Ohkura S, Uenoyama Y, Wakabayashi Y, Maeda K. Kisspeptin and GnRH pulse generation. Adv Exp Med Biol. 2013;784:297-323. doi: 10.1007/978-1-4614-6199-9_14.

Parent, A.S., Teilmann, G., Juul, A., Skakkebaek, N.E., Toppari, J. & Bourguignon, J.P. (2003) The timing of normal puberty and the age limits of sexual precocity: variations around the world, secular trends, and changes after migration. Endocr Rev 24, 668-693.

Pinilla, L., Aguilar, E., Dieguez, C., Millar, R.P. & Tena-Sempere, M. (2012) Kisspeptins and reproduction: physiological roles and regulatory mechanisms. Physiol Rev 92, 1235-1316.

Polkowska J, Cie lak M, Wa kowska M, Wójcik-Gładysz A. The effect of short fasting on the hypothalamic neuronal system of kisspeptin in peripubertal female lambs. Anim Reprod Sci. 2015 Aug;159:184-90. doi: 10.1016/j.anireprosci.2015.06.016. Epub 2015 Jun 24.

Rahayu LP, Behiry ME, Endo N, Tanaka T. Effect of investigational kisspeptin/metastin analog, TAK-683, on luteinizing hormone secretion at different stages of the luteal phase in goats. J Reprod Dev. 2017 Jun 21;63(3):221-226. doi: 10.1262/jrd.2016-183.

Rajesh K, Swathi B, Kumari GA, Shanmugam M. Effect of different concentrations of kisspeptin on in vitro maturation rate of buffalo oocytes. Pharm Innov J 2018;7:375–378.

Redmond JS, Baez-Sandoval GM, Spell KM, Spencer TE, Lents CA, Williams GL & Amstalden M 2011 Developmental changes in hypothalamic Kiss1 expression during activation of the pulsatile release of luteinising hormone in maturing ewe lambs. Journal of Neuroendocrinology 23 815–822. (https://doi.org/10.1111/j.1365-2826.2011.02177.x)

Roman CA, Pinto FM, Dorta I, Almeida TA, Hernandez M, Illanes M, Tena-Sempere M & Candenas L. Analysis of the expression of neurokinin B, kisspeptin, and their cognate receptors NK3R and KISS1R in the human female genital tract. Fertility and Sterility 2012; 97:1213–1219.

Salehi S, Adeshina I, Chen H, Zirkin BR, Hussain MA, Wondisford F, Wolfe A, Radovick S. Developmental and endocrine regulation of kisspeptin expression in mouse Leydig cells. Endocrinology. 2015 Apr;156(4):1514-22. doi: 10.1210/en.2014-1606. Epub 2015 Jan 30.

Shahi N, Singh AK, Sahoo M, Mallik S K, Thakuria D. Molecular cloning, characterization and expression pro le of kisspeptin1 and kisspeptin1 receptor at brain-pituitary-gonad (BPG) axis of golden mahseer, Tor putitora (Hamilton, 1822) during gonadal development. Comparative Biochemistry and Physiology, Part B (2016), doi:10.1016/j.cbpb.2016.11.010.

Shannon B. Z. S and Alexander S. K. Regulation and possible functions of kisspeptin in the medial amygdale. Front. Endocrinol. 2017; 8:191.doi: 10.3389/fendo.2017.00191

Smith JT, Clay CM, Caraty A & Clarke IJ 2007 KiSS-1 messenger ribonucleic acid expression in the hypothalamus of the ewe is regulated by sex steroids and season. Endocrinology 148 1150–1157. (https://doi.org/10.1210/en.2006-1435)

Smith JT, Cunningham MJ, Rissman EF, Clifton DK & Steiner RA 2005 Regulation of Kiss1 gene expression in the brain of the female mouse. Endocrinology 146 3686–3692. (https://doi.org/10.1210/en.2005-0488)

Smith JT, Li Q, Pereira A & Clarke IJ 2009. Kisspeptin neurons in the ovine arcuate nucleus and preoptic area are involved in the preovulatory luteinizing hormone surge. Endocrinology 150 5530–5538. (https://doi.org/10.1210/en.2009-0712)

Soares MM, Antonino DC, Oliveira M, Junior JM, Peixoto LR, Maia TS, Alves KA, Jacomini JO, dos Santos RM, Macedo GG. The role of kisspeptin in bovine in vitro embryo production. Semin Cienc Agrar 2018;49:621–630.

Sun Y, Tian Z, Zhao H, Wong TCS, Chen B. Characteristic of hypothalamic kisspeptin expression in the pubertal development of precocious female rats. Neuroscience Letters 420 (2007) 12–17.

Takase K, Uenoyama Y, Inoue N, Matsui H, Yamada S, Shimizu M, Homma T, Tomikawa J, Kanda S, Matsumoto H, Oka Y, Tsukamura H, Maeda KI. Possible role of oestrogen in pubertal increase of Kiss1/kisspeptin expression in discrete hypothalamic areas of female rats. J Neuroendocrinol. 2009 Jun;21(6):527-37. doi: 10.1111/j.1365-2826.2009.01868.x.

Tanco VM, Whitlock BK, Jones MA, Wilborn RR, Brandebourg TD & Foradori CD 2016 Distribution and regulation of gonadotropinreleasing hormone, kisspeptin, RF-amide related peptide-3, and dynorphin in the bovine hypothalamus. PeerJ 4 e1833. (https://doi.org/10.7717/peerj.1833)

Teles MG, Silveira LF, Tusset C, Latronico AC. New genetic factors implicated in human GnRH-dependent precocious puberty: the role of kisspeptin system. Mol Cell Endocrinol. 2011 Oct 22;346(1-2):84-90. doi: 10.1016/j.mce.2011.05.019. Epub 2011.

Thongbuakaew T, Saetan J, Suwansa-ard S, Kankoun W, Sumpownon C, Parhar I, Meeratana P, Sobhon P, Sretarugsa P. The existence of kisspeptin-like peptides and effects on ovarian development and maturation in the giant freshwater prawn Macrobrachium rosenbergii. Aquaculture 455 (2016) 50–62.

Wahab F, Atika B, Shahab M, Behr R. Kisspeptin signalling in the physiology and pathophysiology of the urogenital system. Nat Rev Urol. 2016 Jan;13(1):21-32. doi: 10.1038/nrurol.2015.277. Epub 2015 Dec 1.

West A, Vojta PJ, Welch DR, Weissman BE. Chromosome localization and genomic structure of the KiSS-1 metastasis suppressor gene (KISS1). Genomics. 1998 Nov 15;54(1):145-8.

Wu S, Zhang H, Tian J, Liu L, Dong Y, Mao T. Expression of kisspeptin/GPR54 and PIBF/PR in the first trimester trophoblast and decidua of women with recurrent spontaneous abortion. Pathol Res Pract. 2014 Jan;210(1):47-54. doi: 10.1016/j.prp.2013.09.017. Epub 2013 Oct.

Yuan T, Sun Z, Zhao W, Wang T, Zhang J, Niu D. Phoenixin: A Newly Discovered Peptide with Multi-Functions. Protein Pept Lett. 2017;24(6):472-475. doi: 10. 2174/0929866524666170207154417.

Yun S, Kim DK, Furlong M, Hwang JI, Vaudry H, Seong JY. Does Kisspeptin Belong to the Proposed RF-Amide Peptide Family? Front Endocrinol (Lausanne). 2014 Aug 13;5:134. doi: 10.3389/fendo.2014.00134. eCollection 2014.

Chapter 5

Recent Advancements in Animal Cloning Vis-à-Vis Buffalo

P S Yadav*, Swati Thakur and Dharmendra Kumar
Animal Physiology and Reproduction Division, ICAR-Central Institute for Research on Buffaloes, Hisar-125001, Haryana, India
**psycirb@gmail.com*

Buffalo, an important dairy animal contributes significantly to milk, meat and draught power. India is home to almost 56% of world's buffalo population (109.85 million) and contribute about 20.45% of total livestock population of India (20th Livestock census, DAHD, 2019). There is as increase of 1.1% in total buffalo population and female buffalo population increased by 8.61%, whereas, male buffalo population has declined by 42.35% over previous Livestock Census (2012). Buffaloes contribute about 49% in country's milk production, however, the number of high milk producing buffaloes is still limited and one of the major obstacles is shortage of proven bulls for genetic upliftment of this valuable animal. Presently, the country has about 1200 breeding buffalo bulls and about 40 million semen doses for artificial insemination are produced annually. It is estimated that by 2024-2025, India shall require 5600 bulls to produce 140 million semen doses annually for inseminating 70 million breedable buffaloes. For compensating the shortage of superior male germplasm in short time interval as compared to conventional breeding system, the assisted reproductive techniques (ART) especially animal cloning can be foreseen for faster propagation of elite and superior germplasm.

Animal cloning is a technique of producing genetically indistinguishable copies of desired animals. Animal cloning, also known as somatic cell nuclear transfer (SCNT) is a technique in which nucleus of a somatic cell (donor) is transferred into an enucleated metaphase-II oocyte (recipient) for the generation of a new individual which is genetically identical to donor by the process called nuclear reprogramming (Campwell, 1996; Wilmut, 1997). Nuclear reprogramming is a process in which terminally differentiated cell is reverted back to totipotent stage (potential of an embryonic cell to develop into all cell types of an organism) i.e. the genes inactivated during tissue differentiation can be reactivated. SCNT is one of the most advanced ART that can be used for production of multiple copies of elite and desired germplasm, to produce transgenic animals for pharmaceuticals or xenotransplantation, conservation of endangered animal species, biomedical research, therapeutic and reproductive purposes (Keefer, 2015; Selokar et al., 2018, Selokar et al., 2019). SCNT is of two types: micromanipulator based and hand made cloning (HMC). Micromanipulator based cloning involves removal of nucleus of oocyte (M-II) and introduction of donor cell or nucleus in ooplasm with fusion or direct injection with the help of microinjection. Micromanupulator based SCNT requires skilled expertise and expensive micromanipulators. HMC, also known as zona free cloning or hand guided cloning is an advanced procedure of enucleation of zona free mammalian oocyte by hand bisection using a metal blade or by density gradient centrifugation or by chemicals. Micromanipulator based SCNT is also known as traditional cloning in which zona pellucida will be intact unlike HMC which is zona free. Birth of first cloned mammal, Dolly sheep is major breakthrough in animal cloning (Wilmut et al., 1996) and since then more than 20 animal species have been cloned including buffaloes. Since then, there are many advancement occurs in the refinement of the protocols, uses of the donor cell, understanding of reprogramming process, etc which have improved the success rate of the cloning then also live calf birth rate is low efficiency (0-10%) and incidences of developmental anomalies which are due to incomplete reprogramming of epigenetic markers.

Animal cloning mainly involves the following steps:

- **Selection of donor cell**: Somatic cells from desired animal to be cloned are isolated and cell lines are maintained. Most commonly used donor cell is fibroblasts. The cells are to be in G_0/G_1 stage of cell cycle.
- **Enucleation**: The nucleus of recipient oocyte is removed so that its genetic information (DNA) is lost and now is termed as ooplasm.
- **Nuclear transfer**: Somatic cell is introduced into enucleated oocyte to produce reconstruct/zygote.
- **Stimulation**: The reconstruct/zygote is stimulated through electric current.
- ***In-vitro* culture**: The reconstruct/zygote are cultured for 7-8 days for blastocyst formation
- **Embryo transfer**: The blastocysts formed on 7-8 days of in-vitro culture are transferred in to synchronised surrogate female for calf production.

STATUS OF ANIMAL CLONING WORLD WIDE

Dolly sheep was the first mammal cloned in 1996 at The Roslin Institute by using adult mammary gland cell, after that a no. of other species including eight mammals has been cloned. These include pigs in 2000 by PPL pharmaceuticals (five female piglets from adult pig cell), Rhesus monkey in 2000, Noah gaur in 2001, CC cat in 2001 and white-tailed deer from skin cells of deceased white deer in 2003 at Texas A and M University, female horse in 2003 in Italy, Snupy dog in 2005 at Seoul National University and endangered grey wolf from ear cells in 2005 in South Korea, Gene cow calf produced at American Breeders Service facilities in Deforest in 2007, Wisconsin, United States, mice in 2008, Pyrenean ibex (wild goat) in 2009. World's first swamp buffalo clone was produced in Chine in 2007 using SCNT method whereas, Murrah cloned buffalo born in India on 6th Feb 2009 by "Hand guided cloning" at NDRI, Karnal, however, it died within seven days of birth. Subsequently, second buffalo cloned which survived was born on 6th June 2009 at NDRI, Karnal. World's first pashmina goat, Noori was born at SKUAST, Kashmir.

Table 1: Different animal species cloned worldwide and the organizations involved

S. No.	Company Name	Country	Animals being cloned
1	Sinogene	USA	Dog, Cat, Horse
2.	Viagen	USA	Dog, Cat, Equine
3.	Trans Ova Genetics	USA	Bovine, Ovine, Caprine, Porcine
4.	Sinogene	China	Dog
5	Sooam Biotech	South Korea	Dog
6	Tianjin Animal cloning Centre	China	Cattle, Dog, Horses, Endangered & extinct species
7	Camel Reproductive Centre	Dubai	Camel
8	Advanced cell technology	USA	Cattle and Pig
9	Bio Sidus	Argentina	Cattle
10	BresaGen	Australia	Cattle, Pig and dog

STATUS OF BUFFALO CLONING IN INDIA

World's as well as India's first Murrah buffalo clone (Samrupa) was born on 2009 at NDRI, Karnal, and thereafter several cloned buffaloes have been produced by using different types of somatic cells. ICAR-CIRB, Hisar became the second centre for producing buffalo clone named Hisar-Gaurav on 11th December 2015. In 2017, Assamese cloned bull was produced in field conditions by ICAR-CIRB. Thereafter, seven clones from a single superior bull named M-29 and a re-clone of Hisar Gaurav were born between October 2019 to January 2020. All the produced clones have normal physiological and reproductive health. In addition to that, recently, NDRI, Karnal produced two clones: female (Karnika) and male (Gantantra) in December 2021 and January 2022, respectively from somatic cells of elite male and female buffaloes. Female calf has been produced from cell of the buffalo, which has given 6,089-kg milk in fifth lactation.

Table 2: Different donor cells and efficiency rate of different animal species

S. No.	Species	Donor cell type	Birth rate of transferred embryo (%)
1	Buffalo	Fetal fibroblast and granulosa cells	11.9
2	Cow	Fetal fibroblast (transgenic)	14.29
		Oviductal cells	75
		Adult cumulus cells	83.33
3	Sheep	Adult mammary epithelium	3.45
4	Goat	Fetal fibroblast (transgenic)	2.08
5	Camel	Adult cumulus cells	3.85
6	Pig	Granulosa cells	6.94
7	Horse	Adult skin fibroblast	4.55
8	Mule	Fetal fibroblast	0.88
9	Dog	Adult skin fibroblast	0.18
10	Cat	Adult cumulus cells	33.3
11	Rabbit	Adult cumulus cells (transgenic)	1.62
12	Mouse	Adult cumulus cells	15.56
13	Ferret	Adult cumulus cells	0.53

Salient Achievement of Buffalo Cloning in India

In last 14 years, 21 cloned buffaloes have been produced in India using donor cell derived from their milk, ears, urine, blood and semen.

- NDRI, Karnal has cloned over 25 animals of which 11 are alive and are in good health and productive.
- ICAR-CIRB, Hisar produced 10 cloned buffalo bulls and they are good in health and productive.
- Sach-Gaurav, second cloned bull and first Assamese buffalo clone in surrogate Murrah under field conditions 100 km from cloning lab at High Tech Sach Dairy Farm by ICAR-CIRB, Hisar.
- All cloned males at ICAR-CIRB producing semen which is comparable in terms of motility, viability, fertility and freezability with breeding bulls. From cloned bulls 11000 frozen semen doses cryopreserved and some of them utilize for AI purpose and 25 progenies of Hisar-Gaurav born with normal health and 1200 semen doses of Sach-Gaurav are also in stock.
- Cloned animals have fertility similar with donor as well as non-cloned breeding bulls
- For future prospective of buffalo cloning, we have a somatic cell banks of various buffalo breeds at ICAR-CIRB which could be used for propagation of these elite animals.

Chapter 6

Strategies for Enhancing Transfection Efficiency Through Electroporation in Difficult to Transfect Animal Cells – A Physiological Perspective

Iqbal Hyder[1], Wilfried Kues[2]

[1]*Department of Physiology & Biochemistry, College of Veterinary Science, Garividi, Andhra Pradesh – 535 101.*

[2]*Department of Biotechnology, FLI-Institute of Farm Animal Genetics, Neustadt, Germany – 31535.*

Transfection studies are useful and often considered as powerful analytical tools to ascertain the gene functions and their products in various cell types. Some of the applications of transfection include gene therapy, generation of induced pluripotent stem cells (iPSCs), knocking out certain selective genes in a cell to decipher its function, production of certain desired products and generation of cell culture models for any desired studies of physiological phenomena.

Of late, the transfection studies have gained lot of importance in livestock biotechnology and editing endogenous genes or knocking-in genes-of-interest into primary cells, is one of the techniques that precedes further advanced procedures like animal cloning via SCNT. The few best examples of application of transfection technologies include establishment of genetically modified livestock with economically significant traits like transgenic 'Enviropig' that could produce recombinant phytase in the saliva to enable more effective digestion of phytate, the form of phosphorus found feed ingredients, like corn and soybeans, transgenic pig with salivary specific expression of β-glucanase to reduce the negative effects of β-glucan on nutrient absorption and growth, and a triple transgenic pig that can express three microbial enzymes, β-glucanase, xylanase, and phytase in the salivary glands for digestion of non-starch polysaccharides (NSPs) and phytate have created transgenic pigs that expresses. Apart from economical significant traits in pigs, some studies in cattle include production of triple transgenic cattle using the Sleeping Beauty system that allowed multiplex transgenesis into the bovine genome. Our research group recently also produced a rat salivary cell model that can produce bacterial ligninase protein specifically driven by salivary promoter, an application that can be used to produce transgenic ruminants that can breakdown lignin in plants.

As on date there are wide varieties of techniques available for stable transfection in cells that include physical methods like microinjection, electroporation, laserfection; biological methods like adeno or retroviral mediated transfection; chemical transfection using cationic lipids and calcium phosphates etc. However, the commonly used, economical and widely preferred method still is the use of high-voltage electric shocks different molecules can be introduced into cells, a procedure called as electroporation. In electroporation, an electric field that can disrupt cell membrane capacitance is used to create temporary but reversible disruption in cell membrane permeability that can allow translocation of different molecules into the cell.

Though transfection studies have been extensively applied to various cell and tissue types, in livestock science, the primary cells especially easily obtainable fibroblasts are the most preferred cells given the routine nature of applications as described above. However, primary cells pose a particular challenge for electroporation-mediated gene transfer, since they are more vulnerable than immortalized cells, and have a limited proliferative capacity. Moreover, it is also necessary to ensure that treatment of electroporation results in lower levels of cellular toxicity, minimal effects on normal physiology if the cells are to be used for further downstream processes. It was also observed from various studies that even a common cell type from different species respond differently to similar treatments thereby increasing the complexity in understanding the cell behaviour to apply the knowledge in transfection studies.

Therefore, the success of transfection by electroporation depends upon optimization of various factors, such as the electroporation medium, cuvette type (path width, and length), as well as the pulsing method which includes the amount, number, duration, and interval of pulses. In principle, two distinct wave forms of a pulse can be generated in a bulk electroporation setting, that are "exponential decay pulse" and "square wave pulse". Whereas both wave forms can be used for electroporation, the latter was proven to be optimal for mammalian cells since it allows the experimenter to control both voltage and pulse duration, and can produce rapidly repeating pulses.

In our experiments with bovine and murine fibroblasts, induced Pluripotent stem cells (iPSCs) we observed that the most important factor that determines ionic strength on the cells and thereby the viability of cells post electroporation is the electroporation buffer. Whereas, some studies recommend to maintain hypo-osmolar conditions owing to easier and controlled electroporation, other studies are recommending iso-osmolar conditions to promote efficient DNA uptake and cell viability.

Our research group did considerable studies on optimizing the electroporation technique in difficult to transfect cells like fibroblasts, iPSCs and testing of most commonly used and widely available buffers proved that buffers that contain reduced serum with other ingredients like glutamine and its derived products like L-alanine-L-glutamine, and polymers like poly-L-glutamate can increase efficacy and reduce toxicity of electroporation

Whereas high transfection rate is no doubt a desired outcome in electroporation especially when dealing with primary and difficult to transfect cells, the other desirable outcome is to have post-handling viability that largely depends upon the number of pores formed during the electroporation since large number of pores or large size of pores can coalesce leading to cell death. The number and size of pores formed largely depends upon strength, duration and interval between pulses (if multiple pulsations are used). Though both microsecond and milli-second pulses can be used for electroporation, the desirable results have been observed by researchers with the use of millisecond pulses in primary cells the most ideal being 10 millisecond pulse. This apart, the voltage of pulse also seems to be a critical factor since high voltage can easily disrupt cells. However, the significance of voltage of the pulse cannot be seen in isolation since it has to be always considered along with the size of the cuvette used for electroporation. The size of the cuvette is best indicated by the distance between two electrodes and the commonly available sizes include 1mm, 2mm and 4mm cuvettes. Though all these cuvettes produce considerable field strength at experimental voltages, all of them do not produce identical field strength at similar voltage. For example, a 500 V with 4 mm cuvettes produce same field strength (1.25 kV/cm) as 250 V with 2 mm cuvettes. Interestingly, irrespective of same field strength, the efficiency of transfection is better in 4 mm cuvettes owing to the greater distance of cells from electrodes since the proximity of cells to electrodes is lethal for the cells. Therefore, the benefit of using large diameter cuvettes is that they produce high electric strength that will ensure that cell membranes become less resistive to pulsation and simultaneously less lethal to cells.

Apart from the above parameters, the one parameter which is speculated to play a role in transfection efficiency is "temperature". Since the electroporation increases the temperature of the reaction mixture which can harm the cells, attempts were also made to assess if pre-cooling of cuvettes can enhance the transfection efficiency. However, pre-cooling can drastically decrease transfection efficiency and viability as it will affect membrane fluidity apart from the other reason that it is found to effect resealing of membrane after pore formation during the voltage pulse.

From the studies performed so far, though it is true that primary cells are difficult to transfect, but necessary interventions at critical steps can enhance the transfection outcomes that will ensure ideal results in further downstream processes.

REFERENCES

Golovan, S.P., Meidinger, R.G., Ajakaiye, A., Cottrill, M., et al. 2001b. Pigs expressing salivary phytase produce low-phosphorus manure. Nature Biotechnology,19(8), 741-745.

Hyder, I., Eghbalsaied, S. and Kues, W.A. 2020. Systematic optimization of square-wave electroporation conditions for bovine primary fibroblasts. BMC Mol and Cell Biol21, 9.

Zhang, X., Li, Z., Yang, H., Liu, D., at al. 2018. Novel transgenic pigs with enhanced growth and reduced environmental impact.Elife7, e34286.

Guan, L. Z., Cai, J. S., Zhao, S., Sun, Y. P., et al. 2017. Improvement of anti-nutritional effect resulting from β-glucanase specific expression in the parotid gland of transgenic pigs.Transgenic Research 26(1), 1-11.

Gehl J. Electroporation: theory and methods, perspectives for drug delivery, gene therapy and research. Acta Physiol Scand. 2003;177(4):437–47

Garrels, W., Talluri, T.R,. Apfelbaum, R., Carratala, et al. 2016. One-step multiplex transgenesis via sleeping beauty transposition in cattle. Sci Rep. 6, 21953.

Kotnik T, Rems J, Tarek M, Miklavici D. 2019. Membrane electroporation and electropermeabilization: mechanisms and models. Annu Rev Biophys. 48:63–91

Eghbalsaied, S., Hyder, I. and Kues, W.A. 2020. A versatile bulk electrotransfection protocol for murine embryonic fibroblasts and iPS cells. Sci Rep10, 13332

Hyder I, Kues W. 2023. Transgenic mammalian salivary cells expressing ligninase as a proof-of-concept model for enhanced lignocellulose degradation to generate future resilient livestock. Journal of Cleaner Production 393, 136226

Kim, T.K., Eberwine, J.H. 2010. Mammalian cell transfection: the present and the future. Anal Bioanal Chem. 397(8):3173-8.

Chapter 7

Advances in Genomics for Improved Production and Reproduction Performance in Indian Bovines

Sheikh Firdous Ahmad*, Celus C.S., Sakshi Vaishnav, Subodh Kumar, Amit Kumar, Gyanendra Kumar Gaur and Triveni Dutt

ICAR-Indian Veterinary Research Institute, Izatnagar, Bareilly 243122, Uttar Pradesh, India

Correspondence: firdousa61@gmail.com

INTRODUCTION

Agriculture and Livestock sectors are challenged by increased food demands projected by ever-increasing human population along with the competition for similar resources with animals. The *'livestock revolution'* is currently impacting agriculture in all its major dimensions. The increasing demand for animal protein and nutritional requirements must be fulfilled by cutting-edge technologies and innovations. Genomics is one of the sustainable and fast-growing technologies that can ensure food safety and security by stabilizing the livestock sector. Lately, *'precision livestock farming'* has gained more attention with continuous monitoring of animals using cameras, microphones, and sensors to understand and predict animal health, production, reproduction, behaviour, environmental impact, and welfare. Livestock genomics has made significant strides in recent years towards accelerating the selection response and improving the selection accuracy. The development of genotyping arrays has enabled researchers to identify and select novel traits, with particular emphasis on functional and adaptive traits. As *'phenomics'* and *'genomics'* go together, a vast amount of data ("big data") is routinely generated in the field of livestock genomics. With the advent of new sequencing tools, it is estimated that the amount of data generated will only continue to grow, potentially reaching beyond the scale of zettabytes in the future.

Genomics is one of the emerging sustainable technologies that promise to ensure food safety and security by stabilizing the output from livestock sector. India is home to a diverse inventory of animal germplasm with more than 202 registered breeds of farm animals and gods. India is capable to use advanced genomic techniques to improve and conserve the unique gene pool of farm animals. Single nucleotide polymorphisms (SNPs) are commonly used to characterize livestock breeds, study genetic diversity in animal populations and make genomic predictions on them. The latest techniques have enabled the evaluation of population structure, admixture levels, haplotype structure, selection signatures, copy number variations, GWAS and other genetic parameters. The progress has been contributed by progress in accessibility and use of improved statistical and Bioinformatics tools. Genomic selection (GS) implies the usage of genomic estimated breeding value (GEBV) to make precise breeding decisions, while genome-wide association studies are used to find marker-trait associations in different economically relevant traits. To upgrade genomics research in India, high-throughput omics technologies should be integrated for comprehensive data analysis, and hurdles for implementing the GS should be removed. In near future, genome editing technologies may complement these tools to create transgenic facilities for production of disease-resistant animals, improve production and reproduction performance, and enhance meat and milk composition, thereby increasing the production capacity of various livestock species.

IMPORTANCE OF IMPROVING PRODUCTION AND REPRODUCTION PERFORMANCE

According to FAO-Domestic Animal Diversity Information System, there are around 8800 breeds of livestock worldwide. India is home to 53 diverse cattle breeds and many other species. Though renowned as 'dairy leader of the world,' a significant number of animals are poor to average milk producers due to varying environmental and physiological factors. It is estimated that the average milk yield per day for an indigenous animal is around 3.4 kg; meanwhile, exotic animals produce 8.5 kg/day in India. Surprisingly, 10% of the total milk production comes from non-descript cattle and almost the same from the indigenous population. Lowered reproductive efficiency and lactation disorders are the other main reasons for increasing the risk of culling. In bulls, nutritional deficiency leads to reduced libido and spermatogenesis whereas, in females, postpartum negative energy balance induces reproductive failure. Improving the production and reproduction status of animals will benefit the farmers through revenue arising from the selection of sires and dams which yield a higher *'lifetime profitability index'*. This may be achieved by synergies of genomic selection; assisted reproductive technologies (ARTs) including artificial insemination, *in-vitro* embryo production, sexing of semen, and MOET; and genome editing. Livestock genomics offers a wide range of applications for genetic improvement in Indian cattle which is illustrated in Fig. 1. In addition, genetic diversity studies and conservation efforts are urgently needed to maintain the variability and genetic wealth for the coming generations.

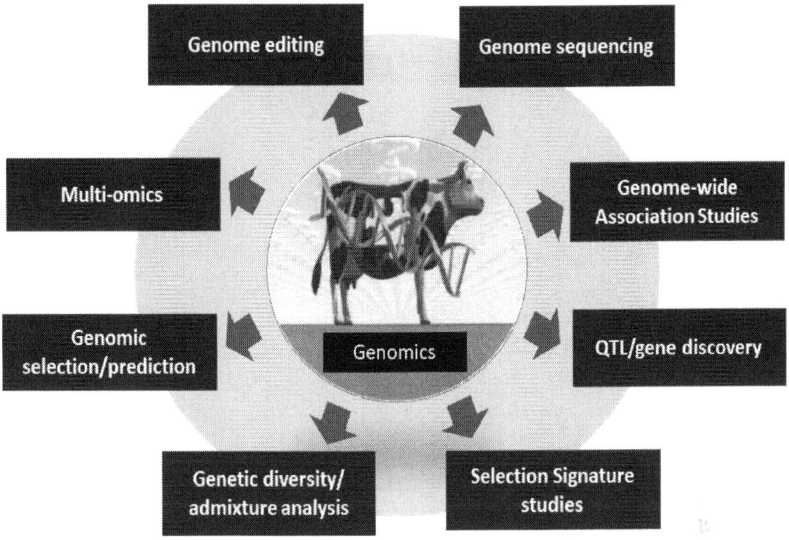

Figure 1: Overview of Applications of Genomics for Genetic improvement in Cattle

GENETIC LANDSCAPE OF INDIAN CATTLE THROUGH GENOMIC STUDIES

Genetic Improvement Through Genomic Selection

Meuwissen *et al.* (2001) introduced the concept of genomic selection (GS), which utilizes genomic estimated breeding value (GEBV) or molecular breeding data to make precise decisions by capturing almost all the variance across the SNP markers. This technique has the potential to double the rate of genetic gain and reduce the genetic interval. However, the accuracy of GS is influenced by several factors such as heritability, marker density, and the size and constitution of the reference population. With changing agro-climatic trends across the globe, recurrent outbreaks in livestock species are propelling the cost of production to a greater extent, coupled with high production losses (5–15%) and lowered conception rates in cattle. GS for heat tolerant or resilient animals is a partial solution along with proper management of nutrition and other pressing factors. Moreover, GS is effective for other traits such as disease resistance, heat tolerance, and for boosting the fertilizing capacity of cattle. In addition, adopting genomic prediction (GP) models and machine learning algorithms have been reported to improve the accuracy of GS in various studied populations.

Recently, NDDB has decided to expand the reference population by performance recording of 1.9 lakh animals and genotyping of 80,000 important cattle breeds (Gir and Kankrej), crossbred cows and buffalo breeds (Mehsana, Jaffarabadi, and Murrah) in India. A non-governmental organization named BAIF Development Research Foundation is involved in implementation of genomic selection to improve milk production in these populations. However, the need for superior quality phenome, a significant reference population, effective collaboration between farmers and laboratory personnel, the absence of appropriate genetic infrastructure, and the challenges associated with generating data and data curation hinder GS in India, which may take a prolonged timeline to achieve successful implementation.

The earlier attempts to create linkage maps have expedited the use of marker-assisted breeding programs in cattle. With time, second-generation and radiation hybrid maps were introduced, which enabled the markers to be spread along the chromosome according to the physical distances between them. The current sequencing technology originated with the attempt to purify the first DNA molecule. Development of livestock genomics has been greatly influenced by the techniques and tools used in human genomics research, most importantly with the discovery of Sanger's sequencing technology. Subsequently, drafts of whole genomes have been released for various animals starting with chicken and bovines. Though the development of dideoxy method of sequencing was a significant achievement and contributed immensely to development of biological sciences, the limitations necessitated further novel sequencing technologies. Commercially available next-generation sequencing platforms and more sensitive third-generation platforms (PacBio, and Oxford nanopore) currently produce great impact on animal genomic research leading to lower cost per base (genotyping or sequencing). Recently, four native cattle breeds were completely sequenced for the first time (Kasargod Dwarf & Kapila, Vechur, and Ongole) by researchers of IISER, Bhopal.

Synergies of GS With Reproductive Technologies

Assisted reproductive technologies (ARTs) possess the potential to help in ensuring significant genetic enhancements in animal populations when combined with genomic selection. Concurrent use of genomic selection with multiple ovulation embryo transfer (MOET) technology potentiates the advantages over using it alone. It allows for the selection of the best heifers for flushing, and early identification of the best males from the flushing. ON application of multi-omics approach for studying the different facets of oocytes and embryo traits related to the *in-vitro* production of embryos, embryo transfer, and pregnancy rates, scientists have identified biomarkers that indicate successful outcomes. Genomic screening of embryos confirms the genetic merit before embryo transfer, and this increases selection intensity as it chooses the best embryos from a larger pool. This synergistic power accelerates the genetic gain and reduces the generation interval substantially.

Breed Characterization, Population Structure and Genetic Diversity

Post the introduction of next generation sequencing (NGS) platforms, whole genome sequencing (WGS) has become accessible to many researchers around the world. For example, Illumina made a major achievement in cattle genetics by developing the 'BovineSNP50K' (around 54,609 SNPs) and 'BovineHD BeadChip' (770K with more than 7 Lac SNPs), which are helpful to analyze both *Bos indicus* and *Bos taurus* populations and their crossbreeds. Availability and easy handling made them increasingly popular for various purposes across different breeds, such as genomic selection, QTL detection, linkage disequilibrium-based analyses, comparative genomics, genetic diversity, and breed characterization. Identification of molecular markers (SNPs) that explain the significant part of genetic variation is instrumental in selecting the best bull for artificial insemination. The same SNPs will be useful for several other purposes.

In the endeavour of initiating genomic selection in Indian livestock populations, National Dairy Development Board (NDDB) developed customized *"INDUSCHIP"* for genotyping the Indian cattle breeds and their crosses in 2015. Another chip *"IndiGau"*, featuring 11,496 SNPs more (in number only, not similar) than the 777K chip (developed originally for *taurine* breeds) was developed by the National Institute of Animal Biotechnology (NAIB), Hyderabad and is in use for many studies. Despite these developments, India still lags in producing the necessary genotypic data. Consequently, the breed composition of cattle populations is not fully and reliably determined. Considering this, the National Bureau of Animal Genetic Resources (NBAGR) at Karnal is undertaking measures for breed identification, evaluation, characterization, and conservation. The institute has successfully characterized 35 breeds genetically and 37 breeds phenotypically, according to their current progress (web source: https://nbagr.icar.gov.in/en/achievements/; accessed on 16th March, 2023). The genetic diversity of different cattle breeds (Tharparkar, Kherigarh, Tho-tho, Gir, and Sahiwal) has been studied using either SNP arrays or genotyping-by-sequencing (GBS) methods by different researchers.

Genomic techniques have enabled the evaluation of population structure and admixture levels in crossbred cattle in India. Studies have been conducted on Vrindavani crossbred cattle developed by Indian Veterinary Research Institute (IVRI), Izatnagar (Uttar Pradesh), utilizing SNP data to determine animal and population-wise admixture levels. Similarly, the admixture level in Frieswal crossbred cattle was evaluated through different software (STRUCTURE, ADMIXTURE, and frappe) pretested on confirmed crossbred populations. In addition, discriminant analysis of principal components (DAPC), a technique integrating the principal component analysis and discriminant analysis, is also utilized for estimating admixture and ancestry inheritance levels in Vrindavani cattle. Similarly, studies have been undertaken in various other crossbred and composite varieties in India.

SELECTION SIGNATURE STUDIES

Domestication and genomic selection have greatly impacted the genetic makeup of livestock, leaving behind evidence of selective pressure in the form of selection signatures. Continuous selection has caused certain mutations that control specific traits to become fixed (or nearly fixed), resulting in a reduction of genetic diversity. Understanding these patterns provide insights into phenotypic adaptation and evolutionary trajectories. Different methods have been utilized for the identification of selection signatures such as inter or intra-population statistics relying on the concepts of linkage disequilibrium (e.g., iHS), site frequency spectrum (e.g., Tajima's D), reduced local variability (e.g., runs of homogeneity, ROH), and haplotype characteristics (e.g., XP-EHH).

The availability of SNP arrays and high throughput sequencing technologies has allowed for genome-wide scans for selection signatures in the major livestock species. As a result, many studies have revealed thousands of genes affecting thermotolerance, adaptation, disease resistance, and production performances in cattle and other species. Interestingly, attempts are not limited to SNP data; but recent studies have utilized copy number variations (CNVs) too for the purpose. A study by Dixit *et al.* (2020) on seven Indian cattle noticed that genes in ROH islands vary between draft and dairy cattle. Illa et al. (2021) genotyped Sahiwal cattle using *'INDUSCHIP2'* and revealed the selection signatures involved in genes related to sperm membrane integrity; milk composition; reproduction; and coat color. Importantly, the genomic regions and the genes under selection identified by genome-wide selection signature studies can be exploited for future breed improvement and conservation programs.

Genome-Wide Association Studies

Genomics provides an opportunity to identify QTLs associated with various performance traits. In Indian cattle, the majority of the GWAS studies have been targeted at milk production traits (peak yield, test day milk yield), milk composition traits (milk fatty acids, proteins, minerals), coat color, and reproduction traits (age at first calving, service period). Unlike the traditionally recorded reproductive traits focusing on conception and calving, male fertility and female maturation have started appearing in recent GWA studies. The external udder characteristics such as teat length, udder depth, teat thickness, etc. in Gir cattle, traits related to mastitis, as well as growth traits in Sahiwal cattle, have also been examined. On the other hand, research in developed countries emphasizes on health traits, disease resistance, susceptibility to mastitis, bovine paratuberculosis, tick resistance, and foot and mouth disease (FMD) in large cattle populations. These studies yield significant SNPs and QTLs, determining the variation of the mentioned traits.

Reference Genome and Pangenomics

Deciphering the genetic architecture of traits to estimate even the smaller effects of mutations requires sequencing of a large resource population. However, the approach is expensive as well as challenging in many aspects. As an alternative approach, 1000 Bull Genomes Project was initiated, which aims to compile the WGS of a large group of ancestors to create a global reference set for genomic research and breeding programs. To date, many reference genome assemblies are publicly available for *taurine* (e.g., UMD3.1.1 and Btau_5.0.1) and *indicine* cattle (Bos_indicus_1.0 and ASM293397v1). Rosen *et al.* (2020) demonstrated a new *de novo* assembly of the reference genome 'ARS-UCD1.2' that showed considerable improvement in sequence continuity and per-base accuracy as compared to known cattle assemblies. Nevertheless, linear reference genomes have a drawback in that downstream analyses can be biased due to the alleles and haplotypes found in the reference sequence.

The *'pangenome'* concept was proposed to overcome the inadequacy of using single reference genomes for genomic research. Pangenomes constitute a *'core genome'* (common in all individuals) and a *'dispensable genome'* (variable among individuals conferring specific adaptations). Unlike the single reference genome, they capture complete genomic diversity within a particular species. Zhou *et al.* (2022) demonstrated a cattle pangenome representing 57 breeds of cattle with

3.1% novel sequence over reference. Another promising development is the 'graph genome' which potentiates genetic variant detection by incorporating data from many animals into a graph genome representing the universal animal diversity (Talenti *et al.*, 2022). These reference sets may enable the imputation of variants for genomic prediction and GWAS as well as for the discovery of causal mutations.

Genomic Databases: Tools for Managing Genomic Data

Databases serve as a reference resource for genomic data enabling data storage, management, systemic retrieval, and quality analysis. There are several databases that are widely used in genomics research, for example, Bovine Genome Database (web source: http://BovineGenome.org) that integrates data mining, curation, and genome annotation tools using graphical browsers constructed upon genome assemblies. Other public databases such as GenBank, ENA (European Nucleotide Archive), DDBJ (DNA Databank of Japan), and UniProt provide extensive resources for accessing nucleotide and protein sequences as well as structural information. Additionally, there are specific databases dedicated to structural, functional, and comparative annotation such as NONCODE and miRbase. The Gene Ontology (GO) resource is one of the popular databases for describing gene function. After gene annotation, the data has successfully been incorporated into many recent genomic prediction (GP) models to improve accuracy.

The identification of QTLs has greatly enhanced the possibility of genetic advancement. AnimalQTLdb offers a means to associate specific genomic segments with different phenotypes. Currently, the database comprises 193,641 QTL/eQTL/associations in cattle for 686 different traits (web source: https://www.animalgenome.org/cgi-bin/QTLdb/BT/summary; accessed on 15th March, 2023) as per the latest release. Majority of them represent milk composition traits, reproduction, and growth; however, QTLs for limb traits, sensory characteristics, feed intake, and semen quality is also growing with the number of publications.

Revisiting Marker-Assisted Selection

Marker-assisted selection (MAS) is an indirect process of selecting breeding individuals using markers linked with traits of interest. This is considered the best choice for sex-limited, low heritable, and slaughter traits, and for those expressed later in life, difficult and expensive to measure traits. However, with increased support for infinitesimal modal of genetic variation, the pace of MAS for genetic improvement has declined. Despite this, some recent articles discuss the need for revisiting the MAS together with GWAS and other genomic methodologies to identify candidate genes, underlying pathways, and significantly associated markers accounting for all relevant effects on traits. Through this, the most accurate and significant markers can be included in MAS, especially for the selection of bull fertility traits.

Multi-Omics and Applications

High-throughput omics technologies allow for a comprehensive analysis of data, leading to genetic improvement in different traits. Omics-scale data helps to identify genes, regulatory genes, networks, and markers responsible for complex traits and explains the effect of variants on performance. Many studies have focused on identifying differentially expressed genes, for instance, during lactation and heat stress in cattle. This may help to understand the pathophysiology in diverse tissues and at various points in physiological development.

The link between bull fertility and methylation signature has been explored in previous research using epigenetic and transcriptomic profiling. By combining the results of methylome analysis with GWAS, it may be possible to identify important genetic regions and potential candidate genes. Several researchers have conducted proteomic profiling to investigate the underlying reasons for variations in bull fertility. This has led to the identification of numerous proteins that play a crucial role in processes such as sperm production, maturation, motility, induction of capacitation, and other markers associated with bull fertility. Milk transcriptome pro le of Sahiwal cows has also been attempted by NBAGR. Similarly, by studying the metabolome of different body fluids, researchers have identified numerous potential biomarkers for milk production and quality. Metagenomics, on the other side, may enable the designing of rumen machinery for limiting methane production, improving feed efficiency, and predicting intake levels in near future. Some studies have used machine learning approaches in conjunction with multi-omics data analysis, thus improving selection efficiency. Though many advancements have been made in this field, the biggest challenge lies in integrating the structural, functional, and other '*-omic*' sciences to detect genotypic-phenotypic associations.

Genome Editing

Genetic engineering is a complementary approach to genomic selection. The field has been significantly impacted by the emergence of genome editing systems especially through clustered regularly interspaced short palindromic repeats (CRISPR) with Cas9 protein (CRISPR/Cas) system. CRISPR/Cas creates cuts at targeted locations of the genome utilizing the guide RNA. Though it is not extensively used for '*genetic designing*' of animals, it may be employed in the future for targeted modification of genes affecting economically relevant traits. Genome editing technologies potentiate the production capacity of various livestock species, by creating disease-resistant animals, improving the (re)production performance, and enriching the meat and milk composition.

FUTURE PERSPECTIVES AND CONCLUSION

Scientific research in livestock, in Indian context, has mainly focused on traditional traits related to production and reproduction. However, a transition to automated systems equipped with electronic devices could allow for the high-frequency recording of novel traits that could be exploited for GWAS. A large amount of genotyping data should be generated alongside precise performance data to enhance genomic selection and genomic prediction efficiency. Using bioinformatic tools, statistical approaches, and machine learning algorithms, it is now possible to make accurate predictions, interpretations, and informed decisions. Further research is necessary to explain the 'missing heritability' that is not accounted-for by other genetic variations. To effectively propagate superior germplasm, cost-effective genome selection can involve reproductive technologies such as artificial insemination and *in-vitro* fertilization. Tools such as genome sequencing, variant mapping, expression arrays, and genomic databases are becoming increasingly vital in the genomic toolbox. These tools enable breed characterization, estimation of genome diversity, and selection signatures. Identifying QTLs and genetic variants for disease resistance in livestock could be the next challenge for domestic animal genomics.

REFERENCES

Bouquet, A. and Juga, J., 2013. Integrating genomic selection into dairy cattle breeding programmes: a review. *Animal,* 7(5), pp.705-713.

Dixit, S.P., Singh, S., Ganguly, I., Bhatia, A.K., Sharma, A., Kumar, N.A., Dang, A.K. and Jayakumar, S., 2020. Genome-wide runs of homozygosity revealed selection signatures in Bos indicus. *Frontiers in Genetics, 11,* p.92.

Illa, S.K., Mukherjee, S., Nath, S. and Mukherjee, A., 2021. Genome-wide scanning for signatures of selection revealed the putative genomic regions and candidate genes controlling milk composition and coat color traits in Sahiwal cattle. *Frontiers in Genetics, 12,* p.699422.

Meuwissen, T.H., Hayes, B.J. and Goddard, M., 2001. Prediction of total genetic value using genome-wide dense marker maps. *genetics,157*(4), pp.1819-1829.

Qanbari, S. and Simianer, H., 2014. Mapping signatures of positive selection in the genome of livestock. *Livestock science,166,* pp.133-143.

Raza, S.H.A., Hassanin, A.A., Pant, S.D., Bing, S., Sitohy, M.Z., Abdelnour, S.A., Alotaibi, M.A., Al-Hazani, T.M., Abd El-Aziz, A.H., Cheng, G. and Zan, L., 2022. Potentials, prospects and applications of genome editing technologies in livestock production. *Saudi Journal of Biological Sciences, 29*(4), pp.1928-1935.

Rosen, B.D., Bickhart, D.M., Schnabel, R.D., Koren, S., Elsik, C.G., Tseng, E., Rowan, T.N., Low, W.Y., Zimin, A., Couldrey, C. and Hall, R., 2020. De novo assembly of the cattle reference genome with single-molecule sequencing. *Gigascience, 9*(3), p.giaa021.

Seetan, R.I., Bible, J., Karavias, M., Seitan, W. and Thangiah, S., 2016, December. Consensus Clustering: A Resampling-Based Method for Building Radiation Hybrid Maps. In *2016 15th IEEE International Conference on Machine Learning and Applications (ICMLA)* (pp. 240-245). IEEE.

Suravajhala, P., Kogelman, L.J. and Kadarmideen, H.N., 2016. Multi-omic data integration and analysis using systems genomics approaches: methods and applications in animal production, health and welfare. *Genetics Selection Evolution, 48*(1), pp.1-14.

Talenti, A., Powell, J., Hemmink, J.D., Cook, E.A., Wragg, D., Jayaraman, S., Paxton, E., Ezeasor, C., Obishakin, E.T., Agusi, E.R. and Tijjani, A., 2022. A cattle graph genome incorporating global breed diversity. *Nature communications, 13*(1), p.910.

Wang, J., Yang, W., Zhang, S., Hu, H., Yuan, Y., Dong, J., Chen, L., Ma, Y., Yang, T., Zhou, L. and Chen, J., 2023. A pangenome analysis pipeline provides insights into functional gene identification in rice. *Genome Biology*, *24*(1), pp.1-22.

Zhou, Y., Yang, L., Han, X., Han, J., Hu, Y., Li, F., Xia, H., Peng, L., Boschiero, C., Rosen, B.D. and Bickhart, D.M., 2022. Assembly of a pangenome for global cattle reveals missing sequences and novel structural variations, providing new insights into their diversity and evolutionary history. *Genome Research*, 32(8), pp.1585-1601.

Chapter 8

Advancing Age, Human Male Fertility, and Functional Proteomics

Mohd A. Beg[1],*, Abrar O. Ismail[1,2], Ishfaq A. Sheikh[1]

[1]*Reproductive Biology Laboratory, King Fahd Medical Research Center, King Abdulaziz University, Jeddah, Saudi Arabia.*

[2]*Biomedical Sciences, Clinical Embryology and Reproductive Biology, College of Medicine, Alfaisal University, Riyadh, Saudi Arabia.*

**Correspondence (mabeg51@gmail.com)*

ABSTRACT

Ageing is a natural phenomenon. Paternal age is a significant factor for a couple's chances of conceiving and the outcome of their pregnancy. Men experience a decrease in fertility associated with advancing age which includes decreased pregnancy rate, increased time to conception, higher risk of miscarriage, and adverse pregnancy outcomes along with increased health risks to their newborn children. The age-associated decreased paternal fertility is attributed to qualitative and quantitative changes in semen parameters such as sperm count and concentration, motility, morphology, DNA fragmentation, etc., and decreased androgen levels. In addition, the decreased fertility could be due to dysregulated molecular and biological pathways associated with functional genomics (proteome, metabolome, transcriptome, epigenome) of spermatozoa and seminal plasma. Studies on advancing age in men and functional genomics of reproductive function have been given very little attention. Age related reproductive research is of critical importance for both the couples who are struggling with fertility issues and for the clinicians/ scientists to develop novel methods and lifestyle strategies to improve sperm health and fertility in older men. In the present manuscript, we present a brief review of the age-associated changes in the reproductive function and fertility in men including testicular histomorphology, semen characteristics, oxidative stress, varicocele, obesity, genetic and epigenetic consequences, paternal effects on pregnancy and miscarriage, and functional proteomics of spermatozoa. In addition, we also briefly summarize the results from our recent studies on age-related proteomic changes in human spermatozoa.

INTRODUCTION

"In youth we run into difficulties. In old age difficulties run into us — Josh Billings."

Advancing age is one of the most important factors affecting fertility in men (Martins da Silva and Anderson, 2022; Setti et al., 2022; Zhang et al., 2022). Men typically never stop producing sperms, but as men get older their spermatozoa undergo changes in form and function which affect a man's ability to procreate (Haidl et al., 1996; Kühnert and Nieschlag, 2004; Verón et al., 2018; Bhasin et al., 2022). Many of the age-associated fertility problems in men are related to testosterone levels (Yang et al., 2011), spermatozoa count and quality (Zhu et al., 2011), DNA fragmentation (Condorelli et al., 2020), and integrity of the spermatozoa cell membrane including alterations in membrane proteins, cholesterol levels, fatty acid composition, etc. (Yang et al., 2011; Yatsenko and Turek, 2018; Pennings et al., 2021). Additionally, as men get older, they are more likely to have health conditions such as diabetes, heart disease, obesity, etc., which can also adversely affect spermatozoa production and quality (Johnson et al., 1987; An et al., 2018). Also, with age there is more likelihood of chromosomal abnormalities which may have important implications for the early embryo, fetal, and neonatal development (Schmid et al., 2013).

With rapid industrialization and adoption of modern lifestyles, globally more people delay having children to gain financial security, to pursue a suitable career or higher education, to cover increased childcare costs, or just to enjoy life (George and Kamath, 2010; Smith, 2015; Pennings et al., 2021). This is a public health issue for potential adverse impact of paternal and maternal age on the health of the next generation, including genetic risks, and effects on reproduction, and fertility among other things (George and Kamath, 2010; Smith, 2015). In this regard, the National Center for Health Statistics in the United States has documented an almost 25% increase in the number of men in the age group of 35–54 years fathering children since 1980 (Sloter et al., 2004). According to a 2017 survey, the average age of first-time fathers in the United States has risen from 27 to 30 years (Khandwala et al., 2017). Further, the average age of spermatozoa donors for assisted reproductive techniques (ART) in the United Kingdom has climbed from 26 to 34 years since 2005(Smith, 2015). The data for other countries including Saudi Arabia also trend in the similar direction because of the industrialization and social changes together with more population from both the genders going into higher education and entering into public and private workforce (Abusaaq, 2015; Karlin et al., 2016; Al-Khraif et al., 2020).

In comparison to advanced maternal age, the impact of advanced paternal age on fertility and the risk of unfavorable reproductive outcomes has been given less attention (along the lines of infertility in men) and, thus, this research area is less understood. Previous studies have reported many advanced age-associated effects in men such as increase in the incidence of infection and inflammation, oxidative stress or higher reactive oxygen species (ROS), higher body mass index (BMI), decline of male libido, increase in sperm DNA fragmentation, sperm DNA mutations, time needed to conceive pregnancy and miscarriage rate, decline of seminal fluid amount and quality (sperm count, motility, and morphology), and decline in assisted reproductive technologies outcomes (De La Rochebrochard et al., 2003; Hassan and Killick, 2003; Colasante et al., 2019; Takeshima et al., 2020). Ageing also has importance for couples with undetected infertility. By the time such couples are ready to have children and employ natural or assisted reproductive strategies they may have already wasted precious time and in all this age effects also start factoring in complicating the condition further. In this regard, a study on 21,960 injected oocytes from an intracytoplasmic sperm injection (ICSI) program (3837 ICSI cycles) revealed that for every 1-year increase in paternal age, the odds ratio of a live-birth decreased by 1% in women aged 37 years, 1.6% in 38 years, 2.4% in 39-years, and 5% in 42-years (Setti et al., 2022). In addition, the slopes of maternal age for blastulation, blastocyst quality and implantation, pregnancy, miscarriage, and live-birth rate significantly worsened for every year of increase in paternal age.

Therefore, ageing is one of the critical factors regulating the fertility in men. It is essential to undertake the age-related studies in human male reproductive research to gain fundamental understanding of the effects and mechanisms by which the age is interacting with the regulation of male reproductive function.Especially, the age-related studies on the molecular aspects of regulatory mechanisms such as effects on the functional genomics including proteomics, transcriptomics, metabolomics, etc., of the semen constituents need to be undertaken. Such studies have been given very little attention.Currently, the research in our laboratory is focused on age-related proteomic changes in human spermatozoa. Very limited studies are available on advancing age and proteomic changes in human semen.The limited literature available on this topic pertains to the functional importance of targeted individual proteins such as PATE1 (role in fertilization in sperm and oolemma fusion, etc.), PLCz (role in Ca2+ oscillations in the oocyte and oocyte activation), HSPA1L (molecular chaperone function), etc.,which showed age related altered expression of these proteins in human spermatozoa (Liu et al., 2015; Yeste et al., 2016; Liu et al., 2022b). Recently, a global proteomic analysis on retrospectively collected patient sperm samples in two age groups (26–30 years and 45–54 years) were reported (Guo et al., 2023). A total of 2369 proteins were identified in both groups of which 80 proteins were significantly altered with 64 upregulated and 16 downregulated proteins in the aged group compared to the young group. The differentially expressed proteins included semenogelin2 and clusterin which were upregulated and testis-specific H1 histone and cilia- and flagella associated protein 44 which were downregulated in the aged group. The enriched dysregulated pathways included Parkinson disease pathway, cholesterol metabolism, inositol phosphate metabolism, ubiquitin mediated pathway, regulation of actin cytoskeleton, and oxidative phosphorylation. However, information about the fertility/infertility status in these men and detailed proteomic characterization were not available in this study. In the present manuscript we present a brief review of the age-associated changes in the reproductive function and fertility in men including testicular histomorphology, semen characteristics, oxidative stress, varicocele, obesity,geneticand epigenetic consequences, paternal effects on pregnancy and miscarriage, and functional genomics of spermatozoa. In addition, results from our recent studies on age-related proteomic changes in human spermatozoa are briefly presented.

AGEING, REPRODUCTIVE FUNCTION AND TESTICULAR MORPHOHISTOPHYSIOLOGY

Advancing age has a profound effect on the gross testicular morphology and testicular histology in men (Yang et al., 2011; Gunes et al., 2016). Ultrasonography and other imaging techniques demonstrated that between the ages of 11 and 30 years mean testicular volume tended to increase, remained constant between the ages of 30 and 60 years, and gradually decreased after the age of 60 years in human male subjects (Yang et al., 2011). The average testicular volume in men over the age of 75 years has been shown to be 31% lower than in men between the ages of 18 and 40 years (Gunes et al., 2016). Histological changes in testis associated with age included reduction in the number of Sertoli cells, Leydig cells and germ cells, thickening of seminiferous tubule basal membrane and reduction in seminiferous epithelium, and vacuolization of Sertoli and Leydig cells (Guttenbach et al., 2000; Sartorius and Nieschlag, 2010). Leydig cell number was shown to significantly decrease after 45 years of age (Colasante et al., 2019). Ageing was associated with multi-nucleation, immature nuclei, and sparse cytoplasmic organelles in Sertoli cells (Gunes et al., 2016). Age-associated decrease in the number of Leydig cells was associated with significantly greater mean serum gonadotropin levels resulting through effects of lower serum testosterone on hypothalamic-hypophyseal-gonadal feedback pathways (Mahmoud et al., 2003; Sartorius and Nieschlag, 2010; Well et al., 2007). Increased follicle-stimulating hormone (FSH) levels were associated with germ cell degeneration during meiosis which had a detrimental impact on daily spermatozoa production due to decreased Sertoli cell function (Johnson et al., 2008). The levels of testosterone and its precursors (pregnenolone, progesterone, 17 alpha-hydroxyprogesterone, 17 alpha-hydroxypregnenolone, androstenedione, androstenediol, de-hydroepiandrosterone, and dehydroepiandrosterone sulfate) were significantly lower in spermatic vein plasma and tissues of older men (Feldman et al., 2002). Due to the reduction of androgen levels, men suffered from erectile dysfunction. Decline in male sexual activity was reported as the frequency of intercourse decreased with age (Liu et al., 2011). Erectile dysfunction on an average affected about 52 percent of men aged 40 to 70, and it got worse with age (O'leary et al., 2003). Many age-related illnesses, including arterial systemic hypertension, diabetes mellitus, heart disease, obesity, and the metabolic syndrome, have been linked to erectile dysfunction (Sampson et al., 2007; Eisenberg and Meldrum, 2017). Age related increase in oxidative stress was also associated with erectile dysfunction (through reduction of vascular nitric oxide) and damage to intracellular proteins, lipids, and cellular structures (Agostini et al., 2011).

AGEING AND SEMEN CHARACTERISTICS

Advancing age in men has been associated with profound adverse changes in semen quality including ejaculate volume, sperm count, and sperm morphology. Advanced age has been associated with a decrease in accessory gland secretion resulting in a decrease in seminal fluid volume (Sharma et al., 2015; Johnson et al., 2015). Seminal volume declines roughly 0.22 ml for every 5 years of age (Beguería et al., 2014). In this regard, at the age of 35 an inverse association between age in men and seminal fluid volume became obvious (Verón et al., 2018). Several studies have found an inverse association between advanced age and spermatozoa count (Johnson et al., 2015; Verón et al., 2018; Pino et al., 2020) and the count of spermatozoa began to decline at the age of 41 (Verón et al., 2018; Pino et al., 2020). In addition to semen volume and sperm concentration, reduction in spermatozoa motility in association with advanced age has been also reported (Beguería et al., 2014; Johnson et al., 2015; Verón et al., 2018). Both the progressive spermatozoa motility and total spermatozoa motility were inversely related with advanced age (Verón et al., 2018). Similar association of older age and a negative relationship in progressively motile spermatozoa was also shown recently (Chen et al., 2022). In the same study, older age was also associated with higher DNA fragmentation index in spermatozoa. Further, advanced age was negatively associated with spermatozoa viability with a decline starting at the age of 41 years (Brahem et al., 2011; Verón et al., 2018). Reduced physical activity in older men raises the risk of obesity and obesity was associated with poor seminal fluid volume, poor spermatozoa quality, including spermatozoa count, concentration, motility, and seminal fluid volume (Duits et al., 2010; Sermondade et al., 2013; Belloc et al., 2014) along with increased aberrant spermatozoa count (Macdonald et al., 2010; Sermondade et al., 2013). The adipose tissue deposition in men was associated with lower total and free testosterone and higher estrogen levels in the blood (Hammoud et al.,2008). This hormonal shift was associated with a decrease in spermatozoa count and progressively motile spermatozoa (Hammoud et al., 2008). Further, age associated comorbidities such as diabetes mellitus, heart disease,etc. are also associated with lower seminal fluid volume, spermatozoa concentration, and total spermatozoa count (An et al., 2018). Taken together, advanced age has been reported to be associated with abnormal spermiogram.

AGEING, OXIDATIVE STRESS, VARICOCELE, AND OBESITY

Ageing has been linked to higher levels of ROS in seminal fluid and DNA damage in spermatozoa (Cocuzza et al., 2008; Nikitaras et al., 2021). Overproduction of ROS, such as superoxide anions, peroxides, and hydroxyl radicals, and an imbalance in the amounts of ROS and the antioxidants necessary to neutralize them causes oxidative stress (Bakos et al., 2011). Higher oxidative stress was reported to promote lipid peroxidation, motility loss, and reduced spermatozoa–oocyte interactions as well as DNA damage resulting in harmful effects for pregnancy and offspring health (Koppers et al., 2010; Nikitaras et al., 2021). During spermiogenesis, spermatozoa lose majority of their antioxidant properties due to cytoplasmic shedding leaving them vulnerable to oxidative attack (Brandt et al., 2019). In addition, oxidative stress in semen has also been shown to increase due to infections and elevation of ROS levels and higher incidence of infections have been reported to cause functional changes of spermatozoa by changing the biochemical composition of the seminal plasma or spermatozoa membrane (Cocuzza et al., 2008). Another reproductive clinical condition, varicocele, is more common as people get older (Avellino et al., 2017). Varicocele is associated with blood reflux and an increase in local temperature in the testis area, all of which lead to an increased ROS and a decreased antioxidant defense (Hassanin et al., 2018). With age, the varicocele grade is also reported to worsen leading to increased ROS levels resulting in increased sperm DNA damage and decreased fertility (Hassanin et al., 2018). Similarly, studies have shown that obesity, like varicocele, increased with age and was connected to recurring inflammatory disorders and ROS production (Paick, 2000). Worldwide obesity rate was shown to be steadily growing; men of reproductive age had three-fold increase in obesity in the last 30 years (Sermondade et al., 2013). Obesity has been reported to effect semen parameters such as spermatozoa count per ml, total count per ejaculate, motility, and morphology of spermatozoa (Sermondade et al., 2013). Alteration in spermatozoa physiology including aberrant mitochondrial function and a decrease in spermatozoa DNA integrity are also associated with obesity (Mitchell et al., 2011).

AGEING AND GENETIC CONSEQUENCES

The American Society for Reproductive Medicine and the British Andrology Society have adopted the upper age limit of a sperm donor as 40 years based on the increased risk of genetic abnormalities in children of older men (Sartorius and Nieschlag, 2010). An increase was shown in aneuploidies and mutations frequency, DNA fragmentation, chromosomal and genetic imprinting abnormalities in spermatozoa with age (Crow, 2000).The accumulation of mutations in spermatozoa from old men may be responsible for inheritance of many genetic abnormalities (Crow, 2000; Hassold and Hunt, 2001). Advancing age is thought to be a primary source of novel mutations in humans (Crow, 2000). It is possible that this is due to changes in age-related processes like DNA replication and repair (Plastira et al., 2007). Whole genome sequencing of 78 parent-offspring pairs for single nucleotide polymorphisms (SNPs) revealed that the mutation transmission to offspring is mostly paternally inherited and linked to paternal age (De Kluiver et al., 2017). Advanced age was linked to an increase in several autosomal dominant diseases, autistic disorders, and schizophrenia (Crow, 2000; De Kluiver et al., 2017). Apert syndrome and achondroplasia are two single base mutations, the risk of which increases with paternal age (Sartorius and Nieschlag, 2010; Goriely and Wilkie, 2012; Nybo Andersen and Urhoj, 2017). Aneuploidy, alteration in number of chromosomes, is considered the most common chromosomal heritable anomaly and the primary reproductive cause of spontaneous abortion (Sartorelli et al., 2001). Analyses of fetal abortion data showed that 60% of all aneuploidies involve 45, XO monosomy and chromosomes 16, 21, and 22 trisomies (Sartorelli et al., 2001). Significant relationship has been shown between maternal age and trisomy incidence; however, paternally derived trisomy cases are low in number and limited studies are available in this area (Sartorelli et al., 2001). A comparative study between advanced age men donors (between 59 and 74 years old) and young men donors (between 23 and 39 years old) reported a significant higher incidence of hyperploid spermatozoa in advanced age donors (Guttenbach et al., 2000). In another study on men aged over 50 years, two to three-fold higher risk of carrying 24,XY spermatozoa than in younger males was reported (Dakouane et al., 2005). Another study found that as paternal age increases, trisomy 21 and other trisomies increased, trisomy 13 decreased, and trisomy 18 remained unchanged (Eisenberg et al., 2012). Population-based research revealed no link between advanced age and structural chromosomal abnormalities, however, case investigations found that structural abnormalities occurred spontaneously in children conceived by elderly men (Sloter et al., 2004). In this regard, with advanced age the frequency of spermatozoa with centromeric deletions in chromosome 1 increased (McInnes et al., 1998), and the frequency of spermatozoa with centromeric and subtelomeric duplications and deletions of chromosome 9 increased (McInnes et al., 1998; Bosch et al., 2003).Another genetic abnormality, spermatozoa DNA fragmentation, could lead to cell impairment and has been reported to be associated with abnormal chromatin packaging, fragmentation and protamine deficiency (Rosiak-Gill et al., 2019). Many studies have found that DNA damage rate in spermatozoa is positively correlated with paternal age (Plastira et al., 2007; Belloc et al., 2009; Rosiak-Gill et al., 2019). Various intrinsic explanations for DNA fragmentation in spermatozoa have been proposed over the years, including faulty chromatin condensation during spermiogenesis, apoptosis-like changes in spermatozoa, and an ROS and antioxidant capability imbalance (García-Peiró et al., 2011; Lettieri et al., 2020). In this regard, oxidative stress caused by external factors such as ageing, radiation illnesses, medicines, stress, pollution, or the presence of varicocele potentially results in genetic damage at various stages of spermatogenesis (Barati et al., 2020). In addition, ROS generation, varicocele, stress, pollution exposure, and other variables all rise with age, and it is probable that these factors are to account for the age-associated increase in spermatozoa DNA damage (Belloc et al., 2009). Moreover, changes in the efficiency of DNA repair mechanisms might be co-factors for age-related DNA damage (Plastira et al., 2007). In 2019, a study on 1124 men revealed a seminal fluid volume decrease and an increase in spermatozoa DNA fragmentation index in older males (≥ 40 years) compared to younger males (Rosiak-Gill et al., 2019). Another age-related genetic defect involves telomeres. Telomere length has been found to increase with age in spermatozoa, affecting the offspring of older males (inheritance of longer telomeres) (Kimura et al., 2008), whereas in somatic cells telomeres undergo gradual shortening with age (Kimura et al., 2008; De Meyer et al., 2007). Longer telomere length was discovered to be a paternally inherited trait passed down through many generations (Kimura et al., 2008; Eisenberg et al., 2012). Although the exact function of telomeres is unknown, It is known that they play a critical role in protection of DNA from degradation, fusion, and recombination (De Meyer et al., 2007; Kimura et al., 2008; Eisenberg et al., 2012).

AGEING AND EPIGENETIC CONSEQUENCES

Despite the compelling data surrounding the adverse effects of advanced paternal age, the cause of age-related effects on fertility and the higher frequency of many illnesses in the offspring of elderly dads is still not clear (Jenkins et al., 2018a). Age-associated epigenetic changes in spermatozoa can accumulate over time and affect fertility, embryogenesis, and even offspring health. The epigenomic factors such as DNA methylation, nuclear protein composition specifically alterations to histone protein tails, and different RNA species can control gene expression and have been reported to affect the embryo after fertilization (Balhorn, 2007; Jenkins et al., 2018b). Genomic imprinting uses methylation pathways to silence allele expression whether it is inherited maternally or paternally (Oakes et al., 2007). Newborns conceived through assisted reproduction were found to have increased imprinting abnormalities in a study on the paternal involvement in transmitting imprinting diseases (Marques et al. 2004). The effect of paternal age on the methylation process was proven in rats and similar etiology was suggested in humans for some disorders such as Alzheimer's disease, schizophrenia, Huntington disease, and autism (Oakes et al., 2003; Sartorius and Nieschlag, 2010). Age-associated methylation defects found in such disorders were reported in regulatory or promoter regions of genes that control psychiatric, neurological, and behavioural disorders, and have been linked to older fathers (Jenkins et al., 2014; D'onofrio et al., 2014). Like methylation, nuclear protein composition can also affect gene expression. During spermatogenesis, most histones in spermatozoa are displaced by transition proteins which after a short time get substituted by protamine proteins 1 and 2 (PRT1 and PRT2) (Balhorn, 2007). These protamine proteins produce a toroidal structure that is 6 to 20 times more densely packed than the nucleosome bound nucleus when they function together in a 1:1 ratio. Both the spermatozoa activity and fertility are influenced by the expression patterns of these proteins. Uneven expression of the PRT1 and 2 has been linked to impaired spermatozoa function, DNA damage, lower fertilization rates, and lower implantation rate all of which are associated with advancing age (Balhorn, 2007; Jenkins et al., 2018b).

AGEING, PREGNANCY, AND MISCARRIAGE

The effect of advanced paternal age on time to conceive pregnancy (TTP) is another area of fertility that is less well studied and still not clear. In addition to advanced mother's age, advanced paternal age has also been reported to significantly reduce the rate of pregnancy (Klonoff-Cohen and Natarajan, 2004). Analysis of a large population data set on TTP found that majority of men who took more than 12 months to impregnate their partners were substantially older than men who took less than 12 months (Ford et al. 2000). In another retrospective analysis of data on 6188 women, after 12 months of conception failure paternal age over 40 years was revealed to be a major risk factor for infertility (De La Rochebrochard et al., 2003). Further, a retrospective analysis of 2,627 cycles of intracytoplasmic sperm injection (ICSI) found that advanced paternal age is negatively correlated with the number of high-quality embryos (Wu et al., 2017). In a retrospective analysis of 2414 pregnancies with a 12.2% rate of spontaneous miscarriage, advanced paternal age (35 years or more) was found to substantially increase the risk of spontaneous miscarriage (Slama et al., 2003). Increased paternal age is linked to chromosomal abnormalities in spermatozoa, which probably was the cause of spontaneous miscarriages (Sartorelli et al., 2001; Luetjens et al., 2002). In another study on 13,865 couples, advanced paternal age (40 years or more) had a 60% higher risk of spontaneous miscarriage than the control group (25–29 years) (Klonoff-Cohen and Natarajan, 2004). Furthermore, older men had a lower live birth rate with IVF (decreased by 26% for every 5-year rise in paternal age) (Robertshaw et al., 2014). In men over the age of 50 years, ART resulted in reduced fertilization and blastocyst formation rates and increased pregnancy loss (Frattarelli et al., 2008; Luna et al., 2009). A recent study on 21,960 injected oocytes from 3837 ICSI cycles revealed that for every 1-year increase in paternal age, the odds ratio of a live-birth decreased by 1% in women aged 37 years, 1.6% in 38 years, 2.4% in 39-years, and 5% in 42-years (Setti et al., 2022). Taken together, majority of the studies showed an adverse effect of age in men on TTP, pregnancy rate, fertilization, blastocyst formation and conception.

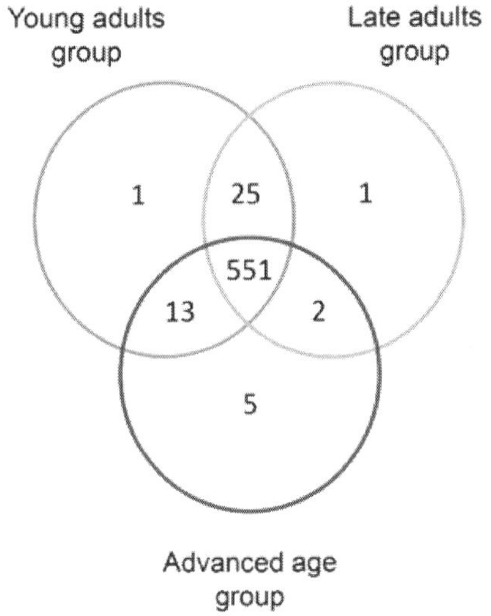

Figure 1: Venn diagram distribution of global proteomic profile the sperms from three age groups of men, i.e., young adult group (21-30 years; n=6), late adult group (31-40 years; n-7), and advanced age group (41-51 years; n=5).

AGEING AND SPERMFUNCTIONAL PROTEOMICS

A complete complement of proteins in a tissue, cell or body fluid is called a proteome. Understanding the spermatozoa fertility also requires an understanding of the proteomic composition of the both the cellular (spermatozoa) and the liquid (seminal plasma) components of semen. The importance of seminal plasma for sperm physiology has been detailed in several studies as it plays a significant role in the survival, maintenance, and functionality of spermatozoa (Pilch and Mann, 2006; Sharma et al., 2013b; Martins et al., 2020). During sperm transport and ejaculation, many seminal plasma proteins interact with spermatozoa membrane, triggering biochemical and structural changes connected to spermatozoa activity and gamete interaction. Proteomics of semen including the spermatozoa and seminal plasma is a novel technique of finding the changes in protein profile of semen that affect male fertility resulting in a more accurate definition of spermatozoa functional pathways as well as how different clinical variables, such as age, infection, obesity, etc., impact male fertility (Fernandez-Encinas et al., 2020). Proteomic studies on human spermatozoa have been done in normal fertile men and in relation to infertility phenotypes and other general disease conditions such as normozoospermia, asthenozoospermia, unexplained fertility, idiopathic oligoasthenozoospermia (Siva et al., 2010; Giacomini et al., 2015; Panner Selvam et al., 2019; Liu et al., 2022a); post-vasectomy, non-obstructive azoospermia (Batruch et al., 2012; Légaré et al., 2013; Korbakis et al., 2017); oxidative stress (Hamada et al., 2013; Sharma et al., 2013a; Sharma et al., 2013c; Intasqui et al., 2015); varicocele (Agarwal et al., 2016);

unexplained infertility (Liu et al., 2019); primary / secondary infertility (Martins et al., 2020); cancer (Panner Selvam et al., 2020), etc. Early spermatozoa proteomic research concentrated on the entire proteome of the spermatozoa, however, subcellular proteomics studies of sperm cell organelle have also recently been reported (Agarwal et al., 2020). Subcellular proteomic analysis is based on separating spermatozoa into fractions (tail, head, membrane, nucleus, etc.) by differential centrifugation, and then subjecting each fragment to proteomic analysis which supplies clear information on spermatozoa proteins as well as their localization (de Mateo et al., 2011; Nixon et al., 2011; Amaral et al., 2013; Agarwal et al., 2020). As mentioned in Introduction section, limited studies related to advanced age and proteomic changes in human sperm and seminal plasma have been reported. Most of the available literature on this topic pertains to the functional importance of individual proteins in relation to seminal plasma and spermatozoa except a recent study (Guo et al., 2023) which details global proteomic analysis of sperm proteins in two age groups of men (26–30 years and 45–54 years). However, as indicated above, information about fertility/ infertility status in these men and detailed characterization of proteomic signatures was lacking in this study.

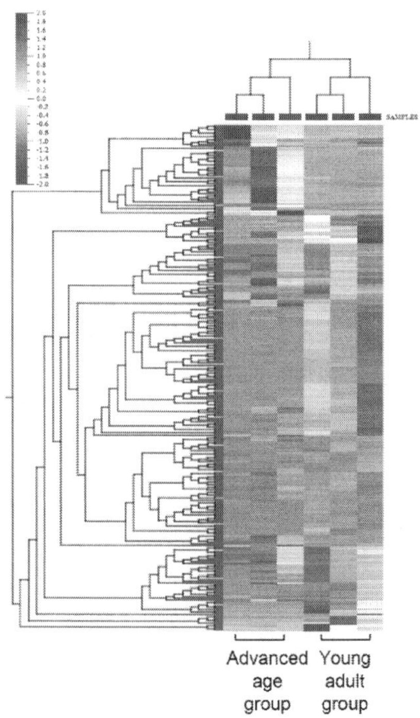

Figure 2. Hierarchical cluster analysis and heat map of 289 differentially expressed proteins of sperms in men for advanced age group (41-51 years; n=5) compared to young adult group (21-30 years: n=6). The 52 upregulated proteins are shown in red color and 237 downregulated proteins are shown in blue color. The criteria for differential expression were probability of P<0.05 and 2-fold change in the protein abundance between two age groups.

In our recent study, healthy fertile Arab men (n=18) were classified into a young adult group (21–30 years, n=6), a late adult group (31–40 years, n=7), and an advanced age group (40–51 years, n=5). The semen samples from men in all three groups were analyzed by routine semen analysis. Semen samples were centrifuged to separate spermatozoa from seminal plasma. The separated spermatozoa were gradient purified. Proteomic analysis of the spermatozoa was performed using quantitative label-free Liquid Chromatography–tandem Mass Spectrometry (LC-MS/MS). Venn diagram was used to illustrate the specific or shared distribution of identified proteins among the three groups. Total detected proteins were filtered and differentially expressed proteins between pairwise groups were analysed using ANOVA at a significance of ($P<0.05$) and a fold change of more than two. The PANTHER Classification System was used for annotation, functional classification, and enrichment analysis of the identified proteins. The mean (±SD) ages of men were different ($P<0.05$) among the three groups (27.8±2.6, 34.3±2.9, and 47.2±4.2 years). A total of 598 proteins were identified in the sperms of the three groups with 551 proteins shared by all three groups, constituting the core-proteins of the human sperm regardless of the age (Fig. 1). Among the remaining identified proteins, one unique protein (MYLK4) was identified in the young adult group and one unique protein (PRSS57) was identified in the late adult group, whereas five unique proteins (KRT4, MGRN1, LPGAT1, HMGB4 and OXCT2) were identified in the advanced age group. Pairwise comparison among groups showed that majority of the proteins dysregulated in advanced age group were common compared to both the young adult and late adult groups. A total of 289 proteins were significantly ($P<0.05$) dysregulated in advanced age group compared to young adult group, and of these dysregulated proteins 52 proteins were upregulated and 237 proteins were downregulated (Fig. 2). PANTHAR analysis revealed that the upregulated proteins were enriched for GO terms associated with cellular component (axonemal central apparatus, axonemal central pair, axonemal outer doublet, axoneme, endomembrane system, envelope, membrane, and microtubule organizing center); GO terms for molecular function (catalytic activity, binding and structural molecule activity); GO terms for biological processes (cellular process and biological regulation, reproduction, reproductive process, and developmental process); and pathways such as inflammation mediated by chemokine and cytokine signaling pathway, angiogenesis, Parkinson disease, Alzheimer disease-presenilin pathway, and ubiquitin proteasome pathway (Fig. 3). Likewise, the downregulated proteins were enriched for GO terms associated with cellular component (actin filament bundle, axonemal central apparatus, axonemal central pair, axonemal outer doublet, axoneme, cell junction, chromatin, distal axon, envelope, membrane, microtubule organizing center, sperm principal piece); GO terms for molecular function (catalytic activity, binding, ATP-dependent activity, transporter activity, molecular adaptor activity, transcription regulator activity, molecular transduce activity, structural molecule activity, molecular function regulator, and translation regulator activity); GO terms for biological processes such as cellular process (actin filament-based process, cell adhesion, cell death, cellular developmental process, cellular homeostasis, cellular process involved in reproduction in multicellular organism, exocytic process, microtubule-based process, movement of cell or subcellular component, transmembrane transport, vesicle-mediated transport), metabolic process (ATP biosynthetic process, ATP generation from ADP, oxidative phosphorylation, and NADP metabolic process), reproduction and reproductive process (developmental process involved in reproduction, fertilization, meiotic cell cycle, sperm motility, sperm-egg recognition), developmental process (anatomical structure development, anatomical structure formation involved in morphogenesis, anatomical structure morphogenesis, cellular developmental process, developmental growth, germ cell development, sex differentiation, spermatid differentiation, spermatogenesis, sperm capacitation, reproductive structure development, developmental process involved in reproduction), and localization (Fig. 4).

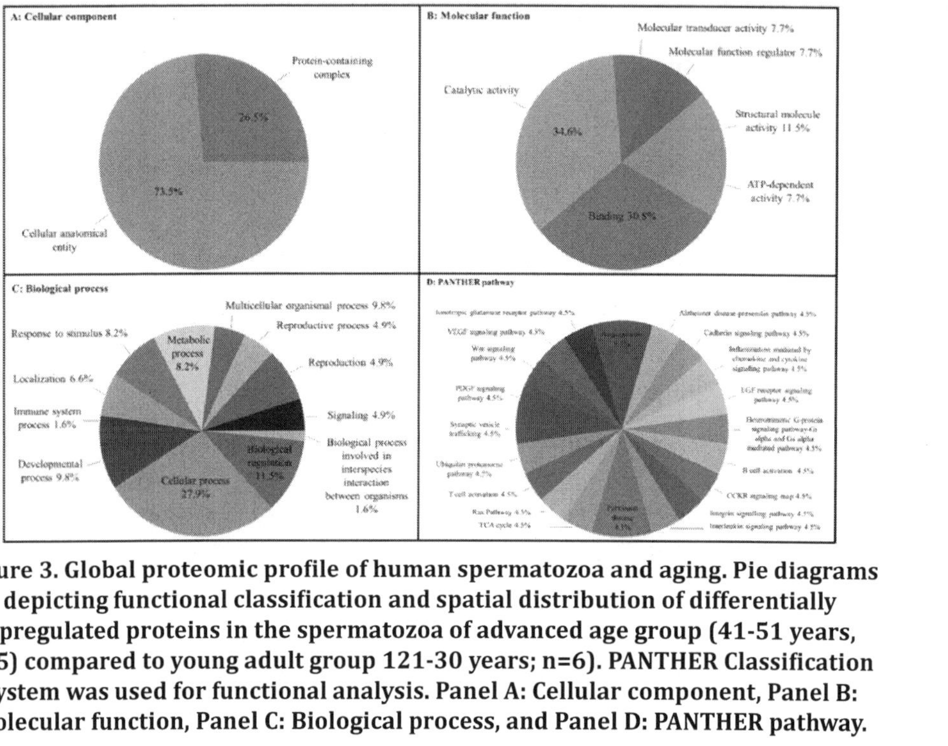

Figure 3. Global proteomic profile of human spermatozoa and aging. Pie diagrams depicting functional classification and spatial distribution of differentially upregulated proteins in the spermatozoa of advanced age group (41-51 years, n=5) compared to young adult group 121-30 years; n=6). PANTHER Classification System was used for functional analysis. Panel A: Cellular component, Panel B: Molecular function, Panel C: Biological process, and Panel D: PANTHER pathway.

Downregulated pathways included glycolysis, pyruvate metabolism, ATP synthesis, cytoskeletal regulation by Rho GTPase, cadherin signaling pathway, inflammation mediated by chemokine and cytokine signaling pathway, neurodegenerative diseases pathways (Parkinson disease, Huntington disease, Alzheimer disease-presenilin pathway), integrin signaling pathway, nicotinic acetylcholine receptor signaling pathway, gonadotropin-releasing hormone receptor pathway, and ubiquitin proteasome pathway. Summarizing the important upregulated proteins of spermatozoa in advanced age group compared to young adult group, this study found upregulated proteins for cytoskeleton (KRT4, HMGB4, AKAP3, PMFBP1, ACTRT3); lysosome trafficking (MGRN1); energy metabolism (LPGAT1); spermatogenesis (FAM170A); antioxidation (HSP90B2P, HSP90AA4P); sperm function (WNT2, SEMG1, TCP11); and proteolysis activity (PSMA7,

PSMB3). The downregulated proteins included those for energy metabolism and mitochondrial structure (MYLK4, MT-CO2, SPATA18); fertilization (CPNE2, TEX101, SPACA1, SPESP1, LYZL4); spermatogenesis (MRTO4, PGK2, SPO11, CETN1, ADAM21); immune response (ANXA1, ANXA13, S100A9); cytoskeleton (TMCO2, CISD1, SQLE, ARHGEF38, SEPTIN4, RPS16, RSPH9, PTK2, ACTB, ACTG1, ACTBL2, ACTA1, SPATA6); nuclear organization (SMYD1, H2AC20); sperm motility (CFAP161, AKAP4, TEKT3, TEKT4, TEKT5, ODF2, ODF3); cellular senescence (CDC73); and protein trafficking and proteolytic activity (PSMA5, PSMA6, HSPA1A, HSPA5, HSPA8).

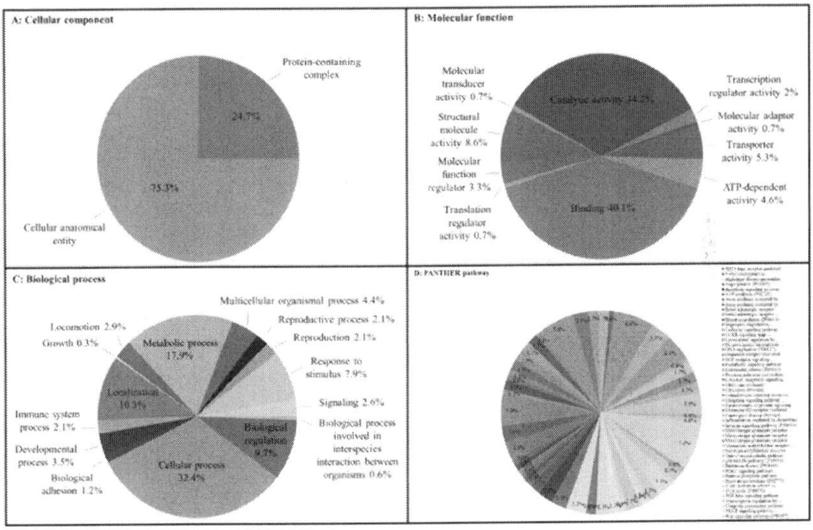

Figure 4. Global proteomic profile of human spermatozoa and aging. Pie diagrams depicting functional classification and spatial distribution of differentially downregulated proteins in the spermatozoa of advanced age group (41-51 years; n=5) compared to young adult group (21-30 years: n=6). PANTHER Classification System was used for functional analysis. Panel A: component, panel : Molecular function, Panel C: iological process, and D: PANTHER pathway.

CONCLUSIONS

In conclusion, ageing is one of the critical factors affecting fertility in men. Advancing age in men is associated with structural and functional alterations of the reproductive axis with profound adverse effects on fertility and fecundity. Paternal ageing adversely impacts the testicular histomorphology,semen characteristics, oxidative stress, genetics, epigenetics, pregnancy, and sperm functional genomics. This research area is still less understood due to less attention given to the effects of aging on male fertility.Age-related studies in human reproductive research are essential to gain a comprehensive understanding of the mechanisms and effects that the aging process has on the regulation of reproductive function. Especially, the studies on the age-related functional genomic signatures (proteome, metabolome, transcriptome) of spermatozoa need to be undertaken. Our proteomic studies indicated a rich repertoire of several hundred proteins in human sperms.Many of these proteins showed dynamic changes with advancing age, potentially impacting sperm physiology, structure, motility, metabolism, and fertilization.

ACKNOWLEDGEMENT

The authors extend their appreciation to the Deputyship for Research & Innovation, Ministry of Education in Saudi Arabia for funding this research work through project number 1132.

REFERENCES

Abusaaq HI. *Saudi Arabian Monetary Agency*, Kingdom of Saudi Arabia, 2015. (https://www.sama.gov.sa/en-US/EconomicResearch/WorkingPapers/population%20aging%20in%20saudi%20arabia.pd)

Agarwal A, et al. *Int J Mol Sci.* 2020;21(5):1621. doi: 10.3390/ijms21051621.

Agarwal A, et al. *Asian J Androl.* 2016;18(2):282–91. doi: 10.4103/1008-682X.170445.

Agostini LC, et al. *Int J Impot Res.* 2011;23(3):115–21. doi: 10.1038/ijir.2011.15.

Al-Khraif R, et al. *SAGE Open.* 2020;10:1–13. https://doi.org/10.1177/2158244020914556.

Amaral A, et al. *Mol Cell Proteomics.* 2013;12(2):330–42. doi: 10.1074/mcp.M112.020552.

An T, et al. *Mol Reprod Dev.* 2018;85(1):7–16. doi: 10.1002/mrd.22930.

Avellino G, et al. *Fertil Steril.* 2017;107(2):305–11. doi: 10.1016/j.fertnstert.2016.12.008.

Bakos HW, et al. *Int J Androl.* 2011;34(5 Pt 1):402–10. doi: 10.1111/j.1365-2605.2010.01092.x.

Balhorn R. *Genome Biol.* 2007;8(9):227. doi: 10.1186/gb-2007-8-9-227.

Barati E, et al. *Cell Mol Life Sci.* 2020;77(1):93–113. doi: 10.1007/s00018-019-03253-8.

Bhasin S, et al. *Endotext [Internet].*2023,South Dartmouth (MA): MDText.com, Inc.; 2000. Bookshelf ID: NBK278998.

Batruch I, et al. *J Proteome Res.* 2012;11(3):1503–11. doi: 10.1021/pr200812p.

Beguería R, et al. *Hum Reprod.* 2014;29(10):2114–22. doi: 10.1093/humrep/deu189.

Belloc S, et al. *Reprod Biomed Online.* 2009;19(2):264–9. doi: 10.1016/s1472-6483(10)60083-1.

Belloc S, et al. *Fertil Steril.* 2014;102(5):1268–73. doi: 10.1016/j.fertnstert.2014.07.1212.

Bosch M, et al. *Eur J Hum Genet.* 2003;11(10):754–9. doi: 10.1038/sj.ejhg.5201049.

Brahem S, et al. *J Assist Reprod Genet.* 2011; 28(5) 425–32.doi: 10.1007/s10815-011-9537-5.

Brandt JS, et al. *Prenat Diagn.* 2019;39(2):81–7. doi: 10.1002/pd.5402.

Chen GX, et al. *Asian J Androl.* 2022;24(1):73–7. doi: 10.4103/aja202165.

Cocuzza M, et al. *Urology.* 2008;71(3):490–4. doi: 10.1016/j.urology.2007.11.041.

Colasante A, et al. *Arch Ital Urol Androl.* 2019;90(4):254–9. doi:10.4081/aiua.2018.4.254.

Condorelli RA, et al. *Front Endocrinol (Lausanne).* 2020;11:558374. doi: 10.3389/fendo.2020.558374.

Crow JF.*Nat Rev Genet.* 2000;1(1):40–7. doi: 10.1038/35049558.

D'Onofrio BM, et al. *JAMA Psychiatry.* 2014;71(4):432–8. doi: 10.1001/jamapsychiatry.2013.4525.

Dakouane M, et al. *Fertil Steril.* 2005;83(4):923–8. doi: 10.1016/j.fertnstert.2004.12.005.

De Kluiver H, et al. *Am J Med Genet B Neuropsychiatr Genet.* 2017;174(3):202–13. doi: 10.1002/ajmg.b.32508.

De La Rochebrochard E, et al. *J Androl.* 2003;24(4):459–65. doi: 10.1002/j.1939-4640.2003.tb02694.x.

de Mateo S, et al. *Proteomics.* 2011;11(13):2714–26. doi: 10.1002/pmic.201000799.

De Meyer T, et al. *Hum Mol Genet.* 2007;16(24):3097–102. doi: 10.1093/hmg/ddm271.

Duits FH, et al. *Fertil Steril.* 2010;94(4):1356–9. doi: 10.1016/j.fertnstert.2009.05.075.

Eisenberg DT, et al. *Proc Natl Acad Sci U S A.* 2012;109(26):10251–6. doi: 10.1073/pnas.1202092109.

Eisenberg ML, Meldrum D. *Fertil Steril.* 2017;107(2):301–4. doi: 10.1016/j.fertnstert.2016.12.018.

Feldman HA, et al. *J Clin Endocrinol Metab.* 2002;87(2):589–98. doi: 10.1210/jcem.87.2.8201.

Fernandez-Encinas A, et al. *Int J Mol Sci.* 2020;21(14):5046. doi: 10.3390/ijms21145046.

Ford WC, et al. *Hum Reprod.* 2000;15(8):1703–8. doi: 10.1093/humrep/15.8.1703.

Frattarelli JL, et al. *Fertil Steril.* 2008;89(5):1118–22. doi: 10.1016/j.fertnstert.2007.05.025.

García-Peiró A, et al. *Fertil Steril.* 2011;95(1):105–9. doi: 10.1016/j.fertnstert.2010.06.053.

George K, Kamath MS. *J Hum Reprod Sci.* 2010;3(3):121–3. doi: 10.4103/0974-1208.74152.

Giacomini E, et al. *Reprod Biomed Online.* 2015;30(5):522–31. doi: 10.1016/j.rbmo.2015.01.010.

Goriely A, Wilkie AO. *Am J Hum Genet.* 2012;90(2):175–200. doi: 10.1016/j.ajhg.2011.12.017.

Gunes S, et al. *J Assist Reprod Genet.* 2016;33(4):441–54. doi: 10.1007/s10815-016-0663-y.

Guo Y, et al. *Front Endocrinol (Lausanne).* 2023;13:1058250. doi: 10.3389/fendo.2022.1058250.

Guttenbach M, et al. *Biol Reprod.* 2000;63(6):1727–9. doi: 10.1095/biolreprod63.6.1727.

Haidl G, et al. *Hum Reprod.* 1996;11(3):558–60. doi: 10.1093/humrep/11.3.558.

Hamada A, et al. *Fertil Steril.* 2013;99(5):1216–26.e2. doi: 10.1016/j.fertnstert.2012.11.046.

Hammoud AO, et al. *Fertil Steril.* 2008;90(6):2222–5. doi: 10.1016/j.fertnstert.2007.10.011.

Hassan MA, Killick SR. *Fertil Steril.* 2003;79 Suppl3:1520–7. doi:10.1016/s0015-0282(03)00366-2.

Hassanin AM, et al. *Andrology.* 2018;6(5):654–61. doi: 10.1111/andr.12511.

Hassold T, Hunt P. *Nat Rev Genet.* 2001;2(4):280–91. doi: 10.1038/35066065.

Intasqui P, et al. *Fertil Steril.* 2015;104(2):292–301. doi: 10.1016/j.fertnstert.2015.04.037.

Jenkins TG, et al. *BMC Genomics.* 2018a;19(1):763. doi: 10.1186/s12864-018-5153-4.

Jenkins TG, et al. *Transl Androl Urol.* 2018b;7(Suppl 3):S328–35. doi: 10.21037/tau.2018.06.10.

Jenkins TG, et al. *PLoS Genet.* 2014;10(7):e1004458. doi: 10.1371/journal.pgen.1004458.

Johnson L, et al. *Biol Reprod.* 1987;37(3):739–47. doi: 10.1095/biolreprod37.3.739.

Johnson L, et al. *Anim Reprod Sci.* 2008;105(1-2):23–51. doi: 10.1016/j.anireprosci.2007.11.029.

Johnson SL, et al. *Ageing Res Rev.* 2015;19:22–33. doi: 10.1016/j.arr.2014.10.007.

Karlin NJ, et al. *Gerontol Geriatr Med.* 2016;2:2333721415623911. doi: 10.1177/2333721415623911.

Khandwala YS, et al. *Hum Reprod.* 2017;32(10):2110–6. doi: 10.1093/humrep/dex267.

Kimura M, et al. *PLoS Genet.* 2008;4(2):e37. doi: 10.1371/journal.pgen.0040037.

Klonoff-Cohen HS, Natarajan L. *Am J Obstet Gynecol.* 2004;191(2):507–14. doi: 10.1016/j.ajog.2004.01.035.

Koppers AJ, et al. *Free Radic Biol Med.* 2010;48(1):112-9. doi: 10.1016/j.freeradbiomed.2009.10.033.

Korbakis D, et al. *BMC Med.* 2017;15(1):60. doi: 10.1186/s12916-017-0817-5.

Kühnert B, Nieschlag E. *Hum Reprod Update.* 2004;10(4):327–39. doi: 10.1093/humupd/dmh030.

Légaré C, et al. *Fertil Steril.* 2013;100(5):1253–60. doi: 10.1016/j.fertnstert.2013.07.1984.

Lettieri G, et al. *Int J Mol Sci.* 2020;21(12):4198. doi: 10.3390/ijms21124198.

Liu FJ, et al. *Hum Reprod.* 2015;30(4):861–9. doi: 10.1093/humrep/dev003.

Liu K, Case A. *J Obstet Gynaecol Can.* 2011;33:1165–75. doi: 10.1016/S1701-2163(16)35087-3.

Liu W, et al. *Front Oncol.* 2022a;12:899861. doi: 10.3389/fonc.2022.899861.

Liu X, et al. *Mol Med Rep.* 2019;19(4):2471–8. doi: 10.3892/mmr.2019.9926.

Liu X, et al. *Andrologia.* 2022b;54(2):e14321. doi: 10.1111/and.14321.

Luetjens CM, et al. *Hum Reprod.* 2002;17(7):1826–32. doi: 10.1093/humrep/17.7.1826.

Luna M, et al. *Fertil Steril.* 2009;92(5):1772–5. doi: 10.1016/j.fertnstert.2009.05.036.

MacDonald AA, et al. *Hum Reprod Update.* 2010;16(3):293–311. doi: 10.1093/humupd/dmp047.

Mahmoud AM, et al. *J Clin Endocrinol Metab.* 2003;88(1):179–84. doi: 10.1210/jc.2002-020408.

Marques CJ, et al. *Lancet.* 2004;363(9422):1700–2. doi: 10.1016/S0140-6736(04)16256-9.

Martins AD, et al. *Sci Rep.* 2020;10(1):7539. doi: 10.1038/s41598-020-64434-1.

Martins da Silva S, Anderson RA. *Rev Endocr Metab Disord.* 2022;23(6):1109–21. doi: 10.1007/s11154-022-09759-0.

McInnes B, et al. *Hum Reprod.* 1998;13(9):2489–94. doi: 10.1093/humrep/13.9.2489.

Mitchell M, et al. *Fertil Steril.* 2011;95(4):1349–53. doi: 10.1016/j.fertnstert.2010.09.038.

Nikitaras V, et al. *Antioxidants (Basel).* 2021;10(7):1079. doi: 10.3390/antiox10071079.

Nixon B, et al. *J Cell Physiol.* 2011;226(10):2651–65. doi: 10.1002/jcp.22615.

Nybo Andersen AM, Urhoj SK. *Fertil Steril.* 2017;107(2):312–8. doi: 10.1016/j.fertnstert.2016.12.019.

O'Leary MP, et al. *Int J Impot Res.* 2003;15(3):185–91. doi: 10.1038/sj.ijir.3900996.

Oakes CC, et al. *Proc Natl Acad Sci U S A.* 2007;104(1):228–33. doi: 10.1073/pnas.0607521104.

Oakes CC, et al. *Proc Natl Acad Sci U S A.* 2003;100(4):1775–80. doi: 10.1073/pnas.0437971100.

Paick JS. *Int J Urol.* 2000;7 Suppl:S42–7. doi: 10.1046/j.1442-2042.2000.00170.x.

Panner Selvam MK, et al. *Genes (Basel).* 2019;10(7):522. doi: 10.3390/genes10070522.

Panner Selvam MK, et al. *Int J Mol Sci.* 2020;21(14):4817. doi: 10.3390/ijms21144817.

Pennings G, et al. *Hum Reprod.* 2021;36(4):833–9. doi: 10.1093/humrep/deaa373.

Pilch B, Mann M.*Genome Biol.* 2006;7(5):R40. doi: 10.1186/gb-2006-7-5-r40.

Pino V, et al. *JBRA Assist Reprod.* 2020;24(1):82–6. doi: 10.5935/1518-0557.20190058.

Plastira K, et al. *J Assist Reprod Genet.* 2007;24(10):437–43. doi: 10.1007/s10815-007-9162-5.

Robertshaw I, et al. *Reprod Sci.* 2014;21(5):590–3. doi: 10.1177/1933719113506497.

Rosiak-Gill A, et al. *Aging (Albany NY).* 2019;11(15):5399–411. doi: 10.18632/aging.102120.

Sampson N, et al. *J Pathol.* 2007;211(2):206–18. doi: 10.1002/path.2077.

Sartorelli EM, et al. *Fertil Steril.* 2001;76(6):1119–23. doi: 10.1016/s0015-0282(01)02894-1.

Sartorius GA, Nieschlag E. *Hum Reprod Update.* 2010;16(1):65–79. doi: 10.1093/humupd/dmp027.

Schmid TE, et al. *Hum Reprod.* 2013;28(1):274–82. doi: 10.1093/humrep/des321.

Sermondade N, et al. *Hum Reprod Update.* 2013;19(3):221–31. doi: 10.1093/humupd/dms050.

Setti AS, et al. *Andrologia.* 2022; 54(8):e14485. doi: 10.1111/and.14485.

Sharma R, et al. *Reprod Biol Endocrinol.* 2013a;11:48. doi: 10.1186/1477-7827-11-48.

Sharma R, et al. *Reprod Biol Endocrinol.* 2013b;11:38. doi: 10.1186/1477-7827-11-38.

Sharma R, et al. *Reprod Biol Endocrinol.* 2013c;11:85. doi: 10.1186/1477-7827-11-85.

Sharma R, et al. *Reprod Biol Endocrinol.* 2015;13:35. doi: 10.1186/s12958-015-0028-x.

Siva AB, et al. *Mol Hum Reprod.* 2010;16(7):452–62. doi: 10.1093/molehr/gaq009.

Slama R, et al. *Am J Epidemiol.* 2003;157(9):815–24. doi: 10.1093/aje/kwg056.

Sloter E, et al. *Fertil Steril.* 2004;81(4):925–43. doi: 10.1016/j.fertnstert.2003.07.043.

Smith KR. *J Med Ethics.* 2015;41(9):775–9. doi: 10.1136/medethics-2014-102405.

Takeshima T, et al. *Reprod Med Biol.* 2020;20(1):41–52. doi: 10.1002/rmb2.12353.

Verón GL, et al. *Fertil Steril.* 2018;110(1):68–75.e4. doi: 10.1016/j.fertnstert.2018.03.016.

Well D, et al. *Semin Nucl Med.* 2007;37(3):173–84. doi: 10.1053/j.semnuclmed.2007.01.004.

Wu S, et al. *Acta Psychiatr Scand.* 2017;135(1):29–41. doi: 10.1111/acps.12666.

Yang H, et al. *Mol Imaging Biol.* 2011;13(2):391–8. doi: 10.1007/s11307-010-0341-x.

Yatsenko AN, Turek PJ. *J Assist Reprod Genet.* 2018;35:933–41. doi: 10.1007/s10815-018-1148-y.

Yeste M, et al. *Sci Rep.* 2016;6:27543. doi: 10.1038/srep27543.

Zhang C, et al. *J Assist Reprod Genet.* 2022;39(9):1969–86. doi: 10.1007/s10815-022-02533-w.

Zhu QX, et al. *Fertil Steril.* 2011;96(3):572-6. doi: 10.1016/j.fertnstert.2011.06.058.

Chapter 9

Functionalized Nano Hydroxyapatite-Based Ceramic Scaffolds for Treating Bone Injuries

Ashok Kumar[1,2,3,4,*]

[1]*Department of Biological Sciences and Bioengineering, Indian Institute of Technology Kanpur, Kanpur, U.P., India*

[2]*Centre for Environmental Sciences and Engineering, Indian Institute of Technology Kanpur, Kanpur, U.P., India*

[3]*The Mehta Family Centre for Engineering in Medicine, Indian Institute of Technology Kanpur, Kanpur, U.P., India*

[4]*Centre of Excellence for Orthopaedics and Prosthetics, Gangwal School of Medical Sciences and Technology, Indian Institute of Technology Kanpur, Kanpur, U.P., India*

**Email: ashokkum@iitk.ac.in*

Bone injuries are caused by trauma, sports accidents, osteoporosis, and osteomyelitis which significantly impair the quality of life. In clinics, there are several treatment strategies to regenerate bone like autografts and allografts, but these techniques face several limitations including graft availability, the requirement of second surgery in case of autografts while allografts face issues of graft rejection, and risk of disease transmission. Bone substitutes provide a solution to these clinical problems and have immense potential to be utilized for tissue regeneration. These materials should be biocompatible, osteoconductive, osteoinductive, and mechanically stable.

Calcium phosphate (hydroxyapatite, HAP) and calcium sulfate (CS) based materials are utilized as bone fillers because of their property to be injected in bone voids. Hydroxyapatite is a natural component of the bone, but it has a slow resorption rate. So, to achieve a bone filler that has a porous structure for bone ingrowth and remodeling, HAP is used in combination with CS. It was also observed that this material could be utilized as a carrier for drugs, antibiotics, and several bioactive factors.

In order to better mimic the nano topography of bone, and to obtain a bone substitute that has improved integration with the native bone, nano-hydroxyapatite (nHAP) was synthesized. The combination of nHAP and CS hemihydrate was utilized in the ratio of 4:6 to form nano cement (NC), which showed the property to set in a period of 15 minutes which is clinically feasible. It has been observed that using nHAP in synthetic grafts for bone, the bioactivity is enhanced significantly in comparison to large-size HAP particles. So, nHAP provides an edge over the previous studies and has shown enhanced bone regeneration. Bioactive molecules like bone morphogenetic protein (BMP), and zoledronic acid (ZA) have been utilized in this study. BMPs show very strong osteoinductive potential while ZA is a third-generation bisphosphonate molecule that decreases the BMP-induced osteoclast activity, ultimately causing net increase in the remodeling of bone. BMP and ZA incorporated in the NC matrix can be co-delivered at the site of injection in the bone defect leading to a direct local effect on bone remodeling (Figure 1). This study was carried out to fill the critical size (8.5 mm) cranial defect in rats using biphasic NC loaded with different combinations of bioactive molecules (BMP and ZA). Micro-computed tomography (Micro-CT) proved that the NC+BMP+ZA group showed highest mineralized material volume which was followed by NC+ZA group at both 8- and 12-weeks' time point. The control group had the least amount of mineralized bone volume formed at defect site. So, due to the mechanical properties of NC, it has potential application to be utilized in cranioplasty because of its ease of handling, provide sufficient working time before it sets and can properly fill the bone defect. Even the NC showed controlled resorption and integration with the newly generated mineralized tissue as well.

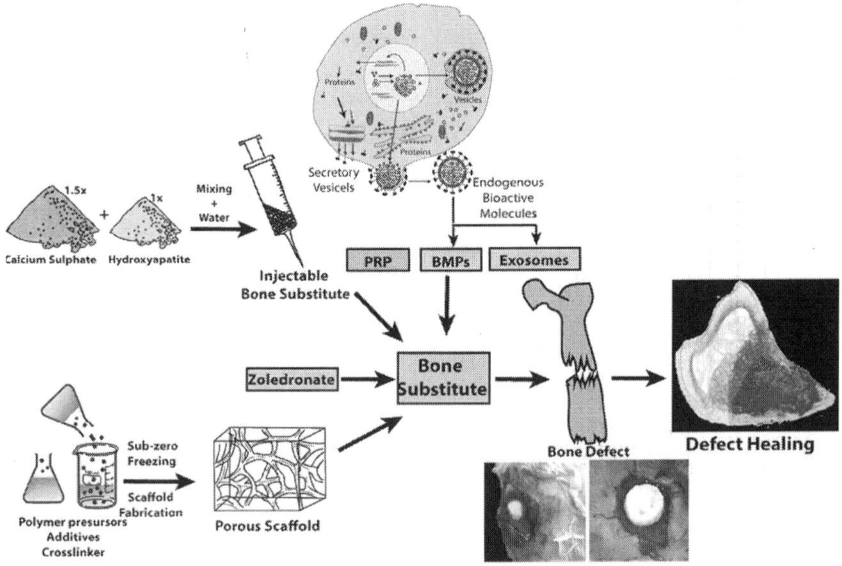

Figure 1: Schematic showing the use of injectable nano cement (NC), bioactive factors and porous scaffolds for bone defect healing [Reproduced with permission from the Ph.D thesis of Dr. Arun Kumar Teotia (Bioinspired functionalized bone substitutes for skeletal regenerative therapies), IIT Kanpur, 2018].

Stem cell therapy has been utilized to aid in bone regeneration which is mostly attributed to the paracrine-mediated suppression of secreted pro-inflammatory cytokines. The effect can be due to the extracellular vesicles (especially exosomes) which deliver the protein, DNA and RNA cargo to the recipient cells. Several miRNAs are involved in the osteogenic differentiation of mesenchymal stem cells (MSCs), and bone formation. Overexpression of miRNA-196a, miR-148, and miR-218 were observed to be involved in osteogenic pathways. So, a study was carried out where the potential of MSC derived exosomes has been evaluated in combination with the NC. The exosomes were isolated from MSCs cultured in normal media, or osteogenic media or exosomes isolated from osteoblasts. The treatment was checked in critical size (4 mm) defect in the tibia metaphysis of the rat. Micro-CT showed very high mean volume of mineralized tissue in groups where osteoblast and MSC exosomes has been delivered locally at the defect site using NC. Histological evaluation also conferred good bone formation and cell infiltration in the exosome groups showing the potential of exosomes in bone remodeling.

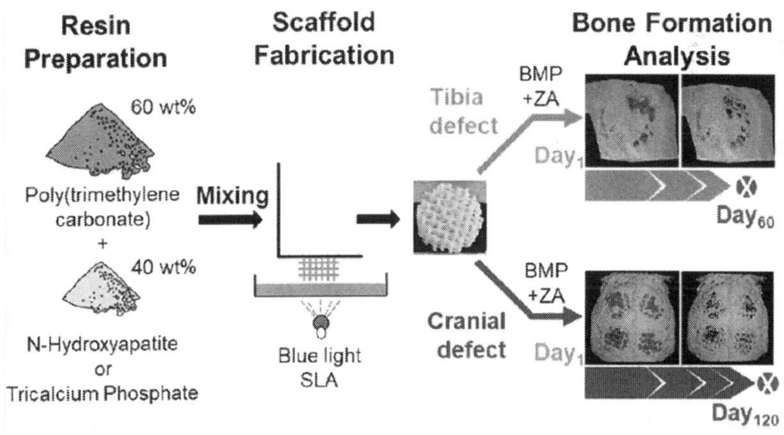

Figure 2: Schematic showing the use of poly (trimethylene carbonate) (PTMC) and nHAP/TCP for fabrication of 3D printed scaffold and its subsequent effect over bone regeneration. [Reprinted with permission from A.K. Teotia, et al., ACS Appl. Mater. Interfaces. 12 (2020) 48340–48356. Copyright 2020, American Chemical Society].

3D printing has gained immense attention due to its clinical relevance and bringing the research outcomes from bench to bedside of the patient. For diverse and complex anatomical shapes and sizes, engineering a suitable bone graft to fill the defect poses major challenges. Additive manufacturing can provide solution to this problem, where it enables layer-by-layer solidification of photo cross-linkable resins using stereolithography (SLA). A study was carried out to explore the potential of polymeric material poly (trimethylene carbonate) (PTMC) in combination with ceramic component i.e., nHAP or tricalcium phosphate (TCP) which was further functionalized with BMP and ZA in tibia and cranium [3]. Full thickness critical size (8 mm) defect was created in rabbit cranium and several combinations of treatment were evaluated comprising of PTMC, nHAP, TCP, BMP and ZA (Figure 2). The combination of PTMC+HAP+BMP+ZA showed higher amounts of mineralized tissue which infiltrated deep inside scaffold from the periphery side. The findings showed that SLA-fabricated scaffolds functionalized with bioactive molecules as the next generation of patient-specific bone substitutes.

A very interesting work was carried out to evaluate the nHAP based ceramic carrier i.e., NC for promotion of bone formation in femoral neck canal defect of osteoporotic rats [4]. The animals were first ovariectomized by bilateral removal of the ovaries to create osteoporosis condition. Then systemic and local treatment i.e., NC+ZA, NC+MSC derived exosomes+ ZA, NC+BMP +ZA were compared in femoral neck canal. The results showed that MSCs derived exosomes promoted bone formation in the same manner as BMP. It inferred that exosomes can be utilized as bioactive molecules for the replacement of BMP. Overall, the study established that NC can be utilized as a carrier for the delivery of drugs and bioactive molecules.

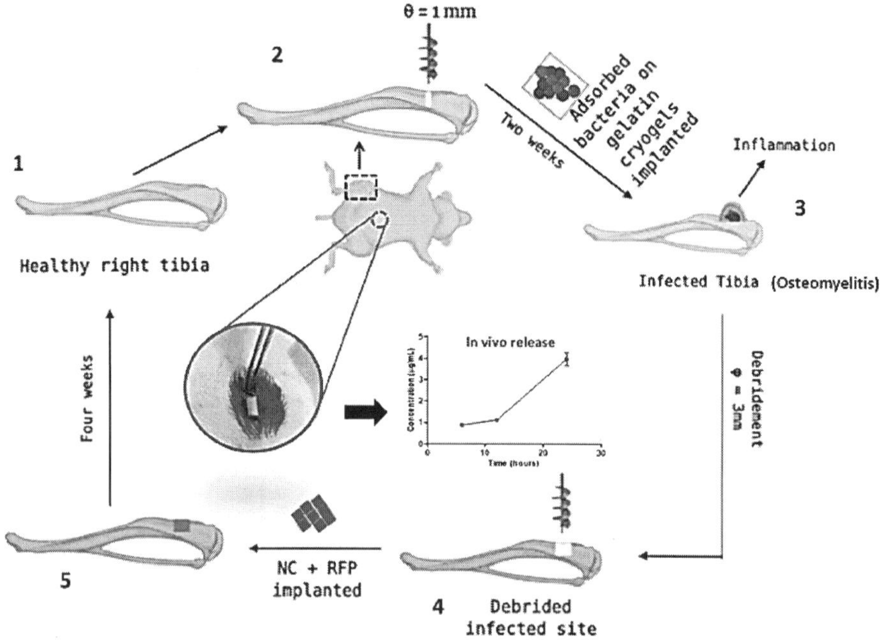

Figure 3: Graphical showing the surgical procedure where the bone defect was created infected with bacteria followed by treatment with nano cement (NC) loaded with rifampicin. [Reprinted with permission from I. Qayoom, et al., ACS Infect. Dis. 6 (2020) 2938–2949. Copyright 2020, American Chemical Society].

Another area of application of bone substitutes was to engineer periosteum mimicking tissue engineered scaffold where polyurethane ascorbic acid calcium peroxide (PUAOC) fibers were electro spun over collagen and collagen membrane (CM) to make a membrane. The tibia bone defect was filled using cryogel made up of gelatin, collagen, bioglass and nHAP which was then wrapped with PUAOCC. Bioactive molecules included combination of BMP, ZA and vascular endothelial growth factor (VEGF). The study concluded that using the membrane for periosteal regeneration in addition to a bone composite is an effective approach for repairing critical-size bone defects with damaged periosteum (Figure 4).

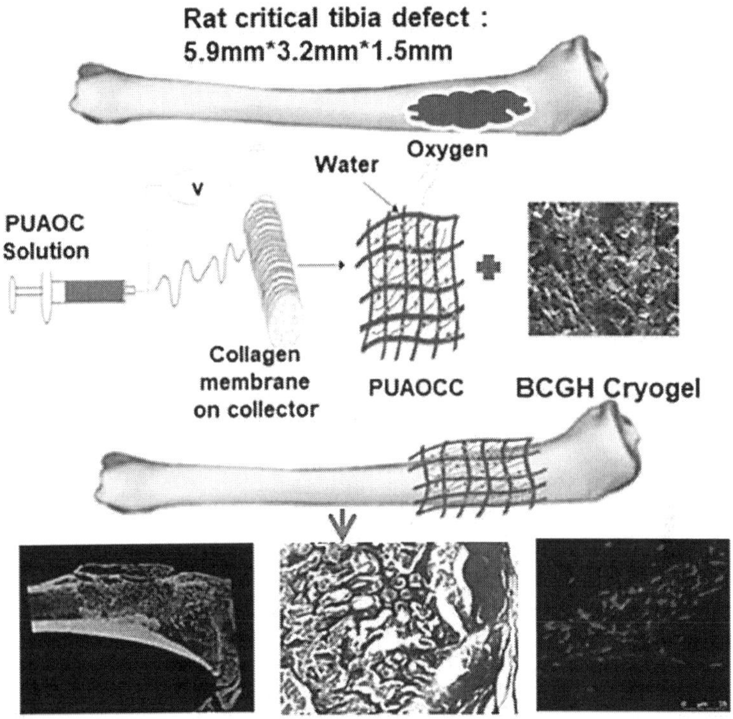

Figure 4: Schematic showing the use of cryogel and membrane for bone defect and periosteum regeneration. [Reprinted with permission from S. Gupta, et al., ACS Appl. Mater. Interfaces. 15 (2023) 8824–8839. Copyright 2023, American Chemical Society].

In another study, NC was loaded with exosome and doxorubicin and a herbal membrane was developed which was laden with Cissus quadrangularis (CQ) extract [8]. Further, osteosarcoma induced tumor model was developed with critical size bone defect. Interestingly, it was observed that even after 30 days of scaffold implantation, NC was able to release doxorubicin and was successful in killing tumor cells. Rat bone marrow-derived MSCs exosomes were able to enhance bone formation 2.6-fold in comparison to the empty group and periosteum development got assistance from the implanted herbal membrane. The work described a cell-free, biomaterial-based approach to regenerate bone in osteosarcoma.

To enhance the cellular interaction of the NC, gelatin was incorporated to form gelatin cement. The enhancement of osteoblast cell proliferation and differentiation of mouse myoblast cells was shown by an increase in the alkaline phosphatase activity [9]. This cement aided in enhancement in the bone biomarkers using polymerase chain reaction, which proved its osteoinductive potential. The gelatin cement was implanted in critical size (3.5 mm) tibial metaphysis defect in the wistar rat. BMP and ZA were also incorporated inside the gelatin cement to functionalize it. Cement resorbed slowly leaving the nHAP in the defect area where new bone remodeling occurred. Very efficient bone bridging was observed with high biocompatibility with maximum bone formation in groups having bioactive factors.

The nHAP has been utilized in the fabrication of the cryogels for the subchondral bone for the osteochondral tissue. nHAP and gelatin have been utilized to fabricate the bone part of the scaffold which showed enhanced pre-osteoblast proliferation and differentiation. nHAP particles were observed under scanning electron microscopy where particles were seen embedded on the pore walls of the cryogel. In another study, endogenous platelet-rich plasma (PRP) was utilized with composite collagen-nHAP bone filler. BMP and ZA have been utilized to functionalize the composite with different combinations with PRP. Polymer scaffold was fabricated using collagen, gelatin, and chitosan. The results showed that PRP aided in enhancing the osteoconductive property of scaffolds by enhancing cell adhesion and neovascularization. These scaffolds can be utilized efficiently and effectively as bone substitute biomaterials.

These results shed light on the advantages of using nHAP based bone substitutes for plethora of applications related to bone biomedical engineering. The promising results are highlighting the importance of NC based bone substitutes for carrying out bone remodeling and acting as an efficient carrier for local delivery of the bioactive molecules. BMP, ZA, and exosomes derived from the MSCs aided in enhancing the bone regeneration when delivered at the defect site locally. The scaffolds fabricated as NC, cryogels, and 3D printed scaffolds had nHAP as common component which was well established to show enhanced bone regeneration.

REFERENCES

A.K. Teotia, D.B. Raina, C. Singh, N. Sinha, H. Isaksson, M. Tägil, L. Lidgren, A. Kumar, Nano-hydroxyapatite bone substitute functionalized with bone active molecules for enhanced cranial bone regeneration, ACS Appl. Mater. Interfaces. 9 (2017) 6816–6828. https://doi.org/10.1021/acsami.6b14782.

A.K. Teotia, I. Qayoom, P. Singh, A. Mishra, D. Jaiman, J. Seppälä, L. Lidgren, A. Kumar, Exosome-Functionalized Ceramic Bone Substitute Promotes Critical-Sized Bone Defect Repair in Rats, ACS Appl. Bio Mater. 4 (2021) 3716–3726.

A.K. Teotia, K. Dienel, I. Qayoom, B. van Bochove, S. Gupta, J. Partanen, J. Seppälä, A. Kumar, Improved bone regeneration in rabbit bone defects using 3D printed composite scaffolds functionalized with osteoinductive factors, ACS Appl. Mater. Interfaces. 12 (2020) 48340–48356.

I. Qayoom, A.K. Teotia, A. Kumar, Nanohydroxyapatite based ceramic carrier promotes bone formation in a femoral neck canal defect in osteoporotic rats, Biomacromolecules. 21 (2019) 328–337.

I. Qayoom, A.K. Teotia, A. Panjla, S. Verma, A. Kumar, Local and sustained delivery of rifampicin from a bioactive ceramic carrier treats bone infection in rat tibia, ACS Infect. Dis. 6 (2020) 2938–2949.

I. Qayoom, E. Srivastava, A. Kumar, Anti-infective composite cryogel scaffold treats osteomyelitis and augments bone healing in rat femoral condyle, Biomater. Adv. 142 (2022) 213133.

S. Gupta, A.K. Teotia, I. Qayoom, P.A. Shiekh, S.M. Andrabi, A. Kumar, Periosteum-mimicking tissue-engineered composite for treating periosteum damage in critical-sized bone defects, Biomacromolecules. 22 (2021) 3237–3250.

S. Gupta, I. Qayoom, P. Gupta, A. Gupta, P. Singh, S. Singh, A. Kumar, Exosome-Functionalized, Drug-Laden Bone Substitute along with an Antioxidant Herbal Membrane for Bone and Periosteum Regeneration in Bone Sarcoma, ACS Appl. Mater. Interfaces. 15 (2023) 8824–8839.

A.K. Teotia, A. Gupta, D.B. Raina, L. Lidgren, A. Kumar, Gelatin-modified bone substitute with bioactive molecules enhance cellular interactions and bone regeneration, ACS Appl. Mater. Interfaces. 8 (2016) 10775–10787.

A. Nikhil, A. Kumar, Evaluating potential of tissue engineered cryogels and chondrocyte derived exosomes in articular cartilage repair, Biotechnol. Bioeng. 119 (2022) 605–625.

A.K. Teotia, I. Qayoom, A. Kumar, Endogenous platelet-rich plasma supplements/augments growth factors delivered via porous collagen-nanohydroxyapatite bone substitute for enhanced bone formation, Acs Biomater. Sci. Eng. 5 (2018) 56–69.

Chapter 10

Therapeutic Implications of Placental Derived MSCs in Neuronal Disorders

Fozia Shah, Mohammad Rayees Dar, Nowsheen Amin, Zahoor A. Pampori, Dilruba Hasin, Ovais Aarif, Aasif A. Sheikh, Sumeira Shafi, Uroos Ali, Suhail A. Khan and Safia Zahoor

Division of Veterinary Physiology, Faculty of Veterinary Sciences & Animal Husbandry, Shuhama, SKUAST-Kashmir

ABSTRACT

The mesenchymal stem cells (MSCs) are considered as a readily available source for tissue engineering. They have multipotent differentiation capacity and can be differentiated into various cell types. Regenerative treatments such as tissue engineering and cell transplantation have shown potential in clinical applications for degenerative diseases. The unique characteristics of mesenchymal stem cells (MSCs) make them among the most sought after cell sources. Researchers have extensively studied the modulatory properties of MSCs and their engineering, labeling, and delivery methods to the brain. Therefore, amnion and MSCs derived from amnion can be applied to cell therapy in neuro degeneration diseases. MSCs identified from amniotic membrane (AM-MSCs) and amniotic fluid (AF-MSCs) shows advantages for many reasons, including the possibility of non-invasive isolation, multipotency, self-renewal, low immunogenicity, anti-inflammatory, non tumorigenicity properties and minimal ethical problem. The AF-MSCs and AM-MSCs can be a source of mesenchymal stem cells for regenerative medicine, as an alternative to embryonic stem cells (ESCs). Cell-based therapy has emerged in clinical trials due to potential applications in regenerative medicine. Tissue engineering using stem cells has introduced a new field of repair in the treatment of degenerative tissues or diseases. Neural stem cells (NSCs) seemed to be an optimal choice for therapeutic intervention in the central nervous system; however, to date, the majority of studies report trophic and immuno modulatory effects rather than neuronal replacement as primary therapeutic mechanisms.

INTRODUCTION

Mesenchymal Stem cells (MSCs) are the multipotent stem cells that can develop into an array of lineages. MSCs are idyllic candidates for cell therapy because of their multipotent nature, ability to differentiate into mesodermal and non- mesodermal tissue and minimal ethical issue. These cells can be obtained from Umbilical cord, Amniotic fluid, Wharton's jelly, foetal liver, among other tissues and have notable regenerative properties. For stem cell-based therapy, MSCs possess many attractive properties: (i) they do not express major histocompatibility complex class II or co-stimulatory molecules and, thus, lack significant immunogenicity (ii) they regulate the inflammation of injured or diseased tissues toward tissue regeneration (iii) they produce a variety of bioactive factors to support the normal function of resident cells in hostile micro environments. The central nervous system (CNS) is typically an unrecoverable site, that is, it cannot be completely regenerated after damage (1). Therefore, most degenerative neurological diseases and mechanical and physical injuries remain incurable. To improve the treatment of neuro degenerative disorders, stem cell based regenerative therapy has been investigated. Types of stem cells include embryonic stem cells (ESCs), adult stem cells, mesenchymal stem cells (MSCs) and induced pluripotent stem (iPS) cells have been considered as possible sources of regenerative treatment. MSCs, generally from adult stem cells, are derived from the mesoderm and identified available in mammalian tissues, such as bone marrow, adipose, umbilical cord blood, olfactory bulb, amnion, and Wharton's jelly (2, 3). MSCs can be multipotent and differentiated into various cell types, not only mesenchymal lineage cells, such as chondrocytes, adipocytes, osteocytes, but also non mesodermal lineage, such as epithelial cells, hepatocyte cells, cardiomyocyte cells, insulin secreting pancreatic β-cells, and neuronal cells (4,9). In addition, MSCs have several advantages, including their non tumorigenicity and anti-immunogenic activity and minimal ethical problems compared with any other candidates for regenerative therapy. These facts suggest that MSCs are considered a readily available source for regenerative medicine. Stem cells' regenerative capacity, transplantation therapies of various stem cells have been tested in basic research and preclinical studies, and some have shown great promise. Previous work with NSCs indicates that long term survival and integration with host tissue are not observed, and therapeutic effects may be linked to the paracrine activity. With this evidence, the focus switched to mesenchymal stem cells (MSCs), known for their paracrine and immune-modulatory potential (Figure 1). They are readily obtainable from various sources such as bone marrow, adipose tissue, etc. [5]. MSC-based treatments have demonstrated beneficial effects in different animal models of neurological diseases in experimental studies. At the same time, significant progress has been made in developing clinically accepted delivery and monitoring protocols. Experimental studies for the treatment of central nervous system diseases; cell therapy using MSCs is currently one of the most dynamically developing branches of regenerative medicine.

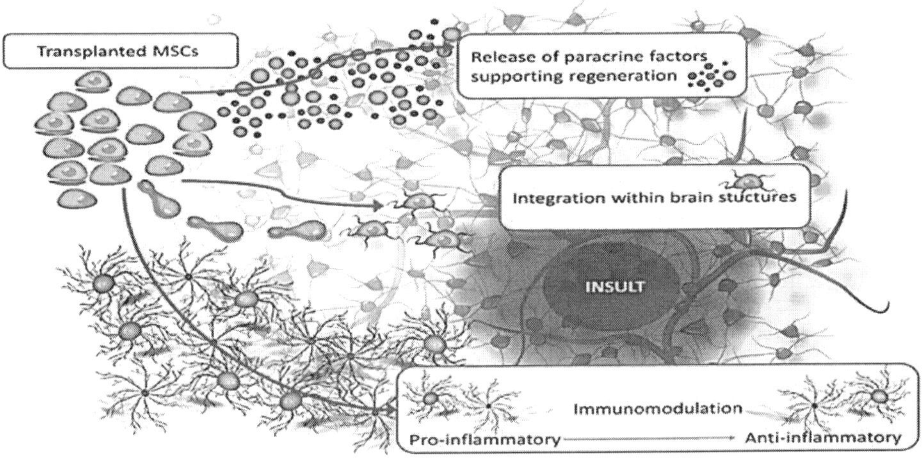

Figure 1

The simplicity of obtaining MSCs from various sources and their low immunogenicity and immune-modulatory abilities means that they can be transplanted in the auto and allogeneic system. Also, the anti-apoptotic, paracrine, and multi directional ability of MSCs to differentiate has driven their current evaluation in translational research and clinical trials for the treatment of the most common diseases, including neurological disorders involving CNS structures such as stroke, Alzheimer's disease (AD), amyotrophic lateral sclerosis (ALS), Huntington's and Parkinson's diseases (HD, PD), multiple sclerosis (MS), and spinal cord injury, The MSCs derived from amniotic membrane (AM-MSCs) and amniotic fluid (AF-MSCs) have been reported as a better new prospective field of regenerative medicine compared with other MSCs sources, because of their easily acquisition, reduced donor damage, multipotency, low immune response, and acceptable ethical issue (10). In this chapter, we will describe the potential of the AF-MSCs and AM-MSCs in tissue engineering and cell transplantation strategies for curing degenerative neuronal diseases.

MSCS-DERIVED FROM AMNIOTIC MEMBRANE

The amniotic membrane is a component of the placenta that originates in the extra-embryonic tissue and functions to protect the fetus during pregnancy with supplemental nutrients. The amniotic membrane is generally known as biomaterial for treatment scaffolds of burns, skin, and corneal transplantation, because it has the ability to scarring reduction and anti-inflammatory properties (17). The AM-MSCs can differentiate into all three germ layers for ectodermal lineage cells, mesodermal lineage cells, and endodermal lineage cells (18). They are positively expressed mesenchymal markers, such as CD105 and CD90, and negatively expressed hematopoietic markers, such as CD29, CD34, CD45, and CD105 (19). In addition, the amniotic membrane expresses anti angiogenic and anti-inflammatory proteins, and does not express human leukocyte antigen (HLA)-A, -B, and DR antigens (20). These results show that the AM-MSCs are very important for advanced regenerative medicine, because inflammatory and immunogenicity remain indispensable factors in successful transplantation. Moreover, despite the pluripotent marker expression of AM-MSCs, such as Oct-4, Nanog, TRA-1-60, and TRA-1-81, they do not form teratoma. In addition, the native amniotic membrane expresses many types of growth factors, and these growth factors reduce inflammation and prevent fibrosis induced by inflammation. Further, amniotic membrane has no blood vessels or nerves, and it enhances wound healing by inhibition of proteinase activity. Therefore, immunological rejection after transplantation does not occur in the amniotic membrane and the cells derived from it. For these reasons, amniotic membrane and AM-MSCs might be useful sources for transplantation for regenerative disease treatment.

MSCS DERIVED FROM AMNIOTIC FLUID

The amniotic fluid is formed at 2 weeks after fertilization in the amniotic cavity of early gestation. Amniotic fluid is important to keep the fetus safe, and it supports organ development. The first progenitor cells derived from amniotic fluid was reported in 1993 by Torricelli et al. The amniotic fluids incorporated a heterogeneous population of cells of fetal origin, and these cells maintained fetal-specific alleles without loss of the chromosomal telomere length in 250 doubling times. Many studies have identified amniotic fluid (AF) as a new source of MSCs, and these AF-MSCs express the pluripotent marker Oct-4 in almost 90% of the active condition, and they also have multiple differentiation capacity like the AM-MSCs. Further, AF is routinely used to perform the standard evaluation of karyotyping and they are genetic and molecular tested for diagnostic purposes. After prenatal diagnostic testing, AF cells can be used as a source of fetal progenitor cells or otherwise discarded. Use of these cells could minimize the ethical objections, have a high renewal activity, and maintain stability. The AF-MSCs enable the uses of autologous cells obtained from patients' tissues. They can be easily isolated. Moreover, they maintain genetic stability and offer advantages of non tumorigenicity, low immunogenic activity, and present minimal ethical issues. These findings show that AF-MSCs are being considered as potential sources of treatment by many researches and clinical application

USE OF MSCS IN MANAGEMENT OF NEUROLOGICAL DISEASES

Despite the inability to regenerate injured CNSs, research focused on repairing damage resulting from neuro degenerative diseases is a public interest. As research continues, the clinical trials of stem cell-mediated neuronal regeneration therapy are being announced. Many of MSC-type cell studies have reported that MSCs have the ability of differentiated into neural-like cells *in- vitro* and they have a long history as potential sources for neural differentiation studies. Recent research has confirmed that the MSCs can be remyelinated in models of demyelination that do not involved inflammation. The amniotic membrane and AF have been noted as new alternative sources of MSCs that would be useful for clinical applications. In the undifferentiated condition, AM-MSC and AF-MSC membrane and amniotic fluid cells possess characteristics primed for neural differentiation by expression of the neuron and neurotransmitter factors. Moreover, they are expressed neurotrophic factors, and these factors lead to bio delivery and enhance the protection and promote the regeneration of damaged tissue (35).The dopamine and tyrosine hydroxylase (TH) enzyme weakly express undifferentiated amnion, and they are ready for use as potential sources for the induction of functional dopaminergic neurons. Further, the therapeutic effects of AM-MSCs and AF-MSCs can significantly improve the motor functions of Parkinson's diseases models. Thus, amnion-derived stem cells have the potential to be differentiated into dopaminergic neurons. Thus AM-MSCs and AF-MSCs could be attractive engraft materials of differentiation neuronal-like cells and developing cell-based treatments for various neuronal degenerative disorders.

Neuro degeneration involves a progressive and irreversible loss of neurons. Alzheimer's, Parkinson's, and multiple sclerosis are some of the neuro degenerative syndromes. The neuromuscular disorder amyotrophic lateral sclerosis (ALS) is a degenerative process caused by motor neuron loss. Stem cells therapy arises as a therapeutic alternative based, either on the replacement of the lost neurons, or on a neuro protective action through release of neurotrophic factors. Placental mesenchymal stem cells (PMSC) are able to differentiate *in-vitro* into several neural lineages, including neurons, oligodendrocytes, glial cells, and dopaminergic neurons.

Alzheimer's disease (AD) is a chronic neurodegenerative disease that manifests itself as progressive dementia resulting in memory loss and cognitive impairments. Its pathogenesis is characterized by a deposition of β-amyloid peptide and hyper phosphorylation of tau causing loss of the synaptic and neuronal activities and neuroinflammation and histo-pathological picture of the brain in this disorder shows an accumulation of amyloid plaques and intracellular formation of neurofibrillary tangles that lead to loss of cholinergic neurons. Chronic accumulation activates microglia, which accelerates neuronal loss and cognitive decline [44]. The placental mesenchymal stem cells transplanted into an Alzheimer's disease mouse model, controlled the inflammatory response. Moreover, mice injected with these cells presented higher levels of β-amyloid degrading enzymes, decreased levels of pro-inflammatory cytokines, and increased levels of anti-inflammatory cytokines (TGF-β and IL-10). The effect of injection of these cells caused an improvement of memory function [45]. Among all treatment approaches, MSC-based therapy is ready to apply modality for this disease. Experimental studies of infusions of MSCs have been performed through intravenous and intra ventricular routes. Preclinical studies indicate that the infusion of MSC improves cognitive impairments in Alzheimer's disease recipients. Some reports have shown enhanced neurogenesis in the hippocampus of AD treated mice or rats transplanted with MSCs by enhancing cell proliferation and Nesting expression and diminishment of long term survival of newly generated neurons. It was shown to be accompanied by up regulation of the levels of neurotropic factors, i.e., brain-derived neurotropic factor (BDNF), nerve growth factor (NGF), and vascular endothelial growth factor (VEGF) in the brains of AD disorders receiving MSC graft that could protect neurons and neuronal integrity. Infusion of MSCs in the brain in an AD rat model increased the level of acetylcholine and the expression of choline acetyltransferase and acetylcholinesterase, which are the proof of functional improvement of hippocampus neurons. Cognitive impairment in AD is also related to synaptic loss. MSC treatment restored the levels of Synaptotagmin-1 (SYT1), Synaptophysin (SYP), and glutamic acid decarboxylase 65 synaptic markers in the hippocampus of the sporadic AD rat model, suggesting a protective role of MSCs against synaptic protein loss . Moreover, since it was shown that microglial processes have connections with neuronal synapses, prolonged activation of microglia related to AD induce synaptic toxicity, and accelerates neuronal loss. It has been revealed that MSC infusion can change the inflammatory effect in AD animal models. Significant reduction in microglial activation in mouse cortexes and decreased expression of pro inflammatory factors, i.e., TNF, IL-6, Macrophage chemotactic protein (MCP)-1, was observed in MSC recipients. Transplantation of MSCs has been shown to switch activated microglia from M1 phenotype producing pro inflammatory cytokines to M2 phenotype, which have an anti-inflammatory effect on AD and improve neuron survival. Numerous studies have shown that AD patients' treatment using different pharmaceuticals only relieves the symptoms without curing the disease. Recently, stem cell therapy, predominantly MSC transplantation, provides new potential in the treatment of AD. Based on preclinical research, MSCs have been shown to decrease amyloid plaque deposits and abnormal protein degradation, up regulate acetylcholine levels and increase neuronal survival, thereby improving spatial learning memory of AD animal models. Moreover, MSC transplantation enhances hippocampal neurogenesis and stabilizes synapses in rodents subjected to AD. Importantly, MSC infusion regulates neuroinflammation by adjusting microglia and astrocytes' activation in AD disorders' brains. The improvement of AD symptoms observed in experimental studies maintains excellent prospects for MSC therapy in AD patients. Single trials with stereotactic brain infusion of MSCs in AD patients demonstrated to be feasible and safe without serious complications.

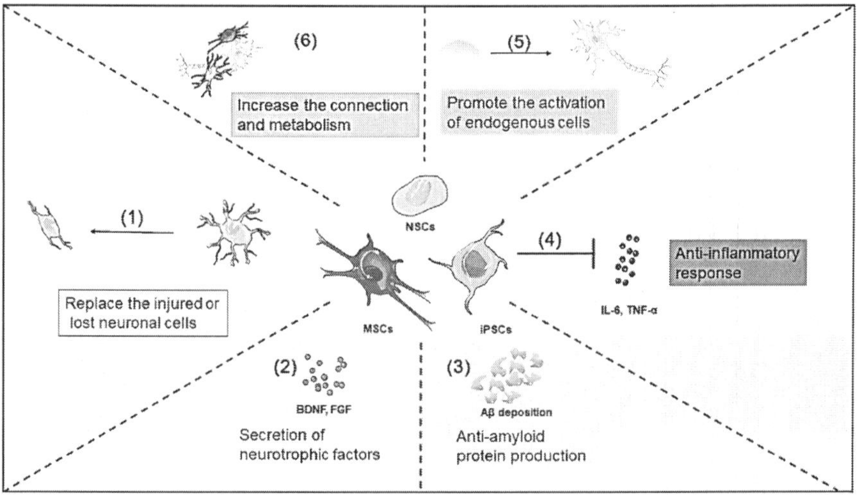

Figure 2

Parkinson's disease (PD) a progressive neuro degenerative disease associated with a specific loss of dopaminergic neurons in the substantia nigra and depletion of dopamine levels in the striatum. The main therapeutic objective in this disease is the recovery of dopaminergic neuro transmission in the striatum. Cellular replacement has been emerged as a suitable therapeutic strategy. First-trimester human placental mesenchymal stem cells differentiated to neural progenitors and transplanted into the striatum of a rat model of PD, underwent dopaminergic differentiation and showed an attenuation of the symptoms. Parkinson's disease motor pathology is also accompanied by other disabilities, such as, mood disorders, constipation, and hyposmia. It is expected that besides the regenerative effects of placental mesenchymal stem cells, the secretion of trophic factors, their anti-inflammatory and antiapoptotic effects, could also alleviate these nonmotor symptoms.

Amyotrophic lateral sclerosis (ALS) is a fatal neurodegenerative disease characterized by damage of nerve cells in the brain and spinal cord, leading to muscle weakness, paralysis, respiratory problems, and eventually, death. Multiple intravenous injections of placental mesenchymal stem cells in a mouse model of ALS, caused protection of motor neurons from inflammatory effectors delaying functional deterioration and increasing lifespan.

Multiple sclerosis (MS) is a chronic disease of the central nervous system characterized by demyelinated areas in the brain and spinal cord that heal forming a glial scar (sclerosis). This disease is caused by T cell-mediated autoimmune reaction against proteins of the myelin sheath inducing oligodendrocytes and neuronal loss. Most of the therapies in MS patients target the immune system or the inflammatory process. Since the pathogenic process of MS can be divided into inflammatory and degenerative phases, placental mesenchymal stem cell based therapy looks suitable since it may be able to specifically regulate immune responses and also induce neuronal regeneration. The experimental animal model that closely resembles with symptoms of multiple sclerosis is the experimental autoimmune encephalomyelitis (EAE) in mice where the myelin antigens were injected to the animals that initiate an immune response. In another study, intracerebroventricular (ICV) transplantation of placental mesenchymal stem cells at day 5 (pre-symptomatology) or day 14 (at the beginning of the disease) after immunization, reported that significant reduction of severity of the disease and prolonged survival without delaying the onset of the disease. Several intra-peritoneal injections of placental mesenchymal stem cells in EAE mice delayed the onset of the symptoms and declined disease incidence in the treated group respect to control, as well as inhibiting T cell proliferation and down regulating the production of pro-inflammatory factors while enhancing the production of anti-inflammatory cytokines. Likewise, ICV or intrathecal (ITH) injection of placental mesenchymal stem cells in EAE rats, also delayed the onset of motor symptoms, reduced inflammation, prevented axonal loss, and reduced severity of the disease.

The limitation of the regenerative properties of the CNS is that it can be seriously life-threatening. Total number of patients with the most common neurological disorder, Alzheimer's disease, is estimated at 36 million people worldwide, and Parkinson's disease affects 1% of the population above the age of 60 (58). Much more advanced approach of therapeutic research has suggested the possibility that stem cells may have therapeutic effects for various neurological diseases.

Stem cell based therapeutic strategies are showing potential in experimental studies. However, some problems of stem cells including safety and ethical issues have limited their clinical use. In addition, some MSCs also have safety problems and thus clinical application of treatment is engendered. Thus, the amniotic membrane and fluid are considered as noncontroversial sources because of the use of either heterologous ESCs or the less ethically disputed MSCs. Compared to other stem cells, amniotic cells can be easily collected during routine prenatal testing, and the amniotic membrane (AM) can also be obtained during cesarean section after birth. These isolation methods are noninvasive progress without destroying human embryos and thus alleviate the ethical controversy. A small amount of amniotic fluid (AF) obtained by amniocentesis and amniotic membrane samples could produce enough MSCs for applications of tissue engineering. Further, these MSCs secrete trophic factors that may be neuro-protection and may promote nerve regeneration after being transplanted into an injured neuron or neuronal site.

As needed, AM-MSCs and AF-MSCs could be stored and provided immediately for future autologous therapy. The autologous tissues made from patient-specific cells could be applied to non-rejected transplantation. Further, studies of AM-MSCs and AF-MSCs demonstrate the prospects of potential therapeutic uses for several CNS diseases. It is hoped that these beneficial effects of AM-MSCs and AF-MSCs will gradually be develop into therapeutic outcomes for neural regeneration.

REFERENCES

Ryu, H. H, Lim, J. H., Byeon, Y. E., Park, J. R., Seo, M. S., Lee, Y. W., Kim, W. H., Kang, K. S. and Kweon, O. K. (2009) Functional recovery and neural differentiation after transplantation of allogenic adipose-derived stem cells in a canine model of acute spinal cord injury. J. Vet. Sci. 10, 273-284. https://doi.org/10.4142/jvs.2009.10.4.273

Dar M. R., Gade N. E., Mishra O. P., Khan J. R., Kumar V. and Patyal A. (2015). In Vitro Cytotoxicity Assessment of Graphene Quantum Dots in Caprine Wharton's Jelly Derived Mesenchymal Stem Cells. Journal of Cell and Tissue Research, 15(1) 4703-4710.

Choi, S. A., Choi, H. S., Kim, K. J., Lee, D. S., Lee, J. H., Park, J. Y., Kim, E. Y., Li, X., Oh, H. Y., Lee, D. S. and Kim, M. K. (2013) Isolation of canine mesenchymal stem cells from amniotic fluid and differentiation into hepatocyte-like cells. In. Vitro. Cell Dev. Biol. Anim. 49, 42-51. https://doi.org/10.1007/s11626-012-9569-x

Barzilay, R., Kan, I., Ben-Zur, T., Bulvik, S., Melamed, E. and Offen, D. (2008) Induction of human mesenchymal stem cells into dopamine-producing cells with different differentiation protocols. Stem Cells and Development 17, 547-554. https://doi.org/10.10 89/scd.2007.0172

C. T. J. van Velthoven, F. Gonzalez, Z. S. Vexler, D. M. Ferriero,Front.Cell. Neurosci.2014,8, 207

Connell, J. P., Camci-Unal, G., Khademhosseini, A. and Jacot, J. G. (2013) Amniotic Fluid-Derived Stem Cells for Cardiovascular Tissue Engineering Applications. Tissue Engineering Part B-Reviews. 19, 368-379.

Sun, N. Z. and Ji, H. S. (2009) In vitro differentiation of human placenta-derived adherent cells into insulin-producing cells. J. Int. Med. Res. 37, 400-406. https://doi.org/10.1177/14 7323000903700215

Moussavou, G., Kwak, D. H., Lim, M. U., Kim, J. S., Kim, S. U., Chang, K. T. and Choo, Y. K. (2013) Role of gangliosides in the differentiation of human mesenchymal-derived stem cells into osteoblasts and neuronal cells. BMB Rep. 46, 527-532. https://doi. org/ 10.5483/BMBRep.2013.46.11.179

Li, R. D., Deng, Z. L., Hu, N., Liang, X., Liu, B., Luo, J., Chen, L., Yin, L., Luo, X., Shui, W., He, T. C. and Huang, W. (2012) Biphasic effects of TGFbeta1 on BMP9-induced osteogenic differentiation of mesenchymal stem cells. BMB Rep. 45, 509-514. https://doi. org/10.5483/BMBRep.2012.45.9.053

Toda, A., Okabe, M., Yoshida, T. and Nikaido, T. (2007) The potential of amniotic membrane/amnion-derived cells for regeneration of various tissues. J. Pharmacol. Sci. 105, 215-228. https://doi.org/10.1254/jphs.CR0070034

Evans, M. J. and Kaufman, M. H. (1981) Establishment in culture of pluripotential cells from mouse embryos. Nature 292, 154-156. https://doi.org/10.1038/292154a0

Thomson, J. A., Itskovitz-Eldor, J., Shapiro, S. S., Waknitz, M. A., Swiergiel, J. J., Marshall, V. S. and Jones, J. M. (1998) Embryonic stem cell lines derived from human blastocysts. Science 282, 1145-1147. https://doi.org/10.1126/science.282.5391.1145

Amit, M., Margulets, V., Segev, H., Shariki, K., Laevsky, I., Coleman, R. and Itskovitz-Eldor, J. (2003) Human feeder layers for human embryonic stem cells. Biol. Reprod. 68, 2150-2156. https://doi.org/10.1095/biolreprod.102.012583

Seminatore, C., Polentes, J., Ellman, D., Kozubenko, N., Itier, V., Tine, S., Tritschler, L., Brenot, M., Guidou, E., Blondeau, J., Lhuillier, M., Bugi, A., Aubry, L., Jendelova, P., Sykova, E., Perrier, A. L., Finsen, B. and Onteniente, B. (2010) The postischemic environment differentially impacts teratoma or tumor formation after transplantation of human embryonic stem cell-derived neural progenitors. Stroke 41, 153-159. https://doi.org/10.1161/STROKEAHA.109.563015

Abad, M., Mosteiro, L., Pantoja, C., Canamero, M., Rayon, T., Ors, I., Grana, O., Megias, D., Dominguez, O., Martinez, D., Manzanares, M., Ortega, S. and Serrano, M. (2013) Reprogramming in vivo produces teratomas and iPS cells with totipotency features. Nature 502, 340-345. https://doi.org/10.1038/nature12586

Medvedev, S. P., Shevchenko, A. I. and Zakian, S. M. (2010) Induced Pluripotent Stem Cells: Problems and Advantages when applying them in Regenerative Medicine. Acta. Naturae 2, 18-28.

Dua, H. S. and Azuara-Blanco, A. (1999) Amniotic membrane transplantation. Br. J. Ophthalmol. 83, 748-752. https://doi.org/10.1136/bjo.83.6.748

Tamagawa, T., Oi, S., Ishiwata, I., Ishikawa, H. and Nakamura, Y. (2007) Differentiation of mesenchymal cells derived from human amniotic membranes into hepatocyte-like cells in vitro. Hum. Cell 20, 77-84. https://doi.org/10.1111/j.1749-0774.2007.00032.x

Anker, P. S., Scherjon, S. A., Kleijburg-van der Keur, C., de Groot-Swings, G. M. J. S., Claas, F. H. J., Fibbe, W. E. and Kanhai, H. H. H. (2004) Isolation of mesenchymal stem cells of fetal or maternal origin from human placenta. Stem Cells 22, 1338-1345. https://doi.org/10.1634/stemcells.2004-0058

Adinolfi, M., Akle, C. A., McColl, I., Fensom, A. H., Tansley, L., Connolly, P., Hsi, B. L., Faulk, W. P., Travers, P. and Bodmer, W. F. (1982) Expression of HLA antigens, beta 2-microglobulin and enzymes by human amniotic epithelial cells. Nature 295, 325-327. https://doi.org/10.1038/295325a0

Miki, T., Lehmann, T., Cai, H., Stolz, D. B. and Strom, S. C. (2005) Stem cell characteristics of amniotic epithelial cells. Stem Cells 23, 1549-1559. https://doi.org/10. 1634/stemcells.2004-0357

Tseng, S. C., Li, D. Q. and Ma, X. (1999) Suppression of transforming growth factor-beta isoforms, TGF-beta receptor type II, and myofibroblast differentiation in cultured human corneal and limbal fibroblasts by amniotic membrane matrix. J. Cell Physiol. 179, 325-335. https://doi.org/10.1002/(SICI)1097-4652(199906)179

Kim, J. S., Kim, J. C., Na, B. K., Jeong, J. M. and Song, C. Y. (2000) Amniotic membrane patching promotes healing and inhibits proteinase activity on wound healing .

Torricelli, F., Brizzi, L., Bernabei, P. A., Gheri, G., Di Lollo, S., Nutini, L., Lisi, E., Di Tommaso, M. and Cariati, E. (1993) Identification of hematopoietic progenitor cells in human amniotic fluid before the 12th week of gestation. Ital. J. Anat. Embryol. 98, 119-126. 25.

Shay, J. W. and Wright, W. E. (2000) Hayflick, his limit, and cellular ageing. Nat. Rev. Mol. Cell Biol. 1, 72-76.

Tsai, M. S., Lee, J. L., Chang, Y. J. and Hwang, S. M. (2004) Isolation of human multipotent mesenchymal stem cells from second-trimester amniotic fluid using a novel two-stage culture protocol. Hum. Reprod. 19, 1450-1456. 27.

De Coppi, P., Bartsch, G. Jr., Siddiqui, M. M., Xu, T., Santos, C. C., Perin, L., Mostoslavsky, G., Serre, A. C., Snyder, E. Y., Yoo, J. J., Furth, M. E., Soker, S. and Atala, A. (2007) Isolation of amniotic stem cell lines with potential for therapy. Nat. Biotechnol. 25, 100-106.

Prusa, A. R. and Hengstschlager, M. (2002) Amniotic fluid cells and human stem cell research: a new connection. Med. Sci. Monit. 8, RA253-257.

Okano, H., Ogawa, Y., Nakamura, M., Kaneko, S., Iwanami, A. and Toyama, Y. (2003) Transplantation of neural stem cells into the spinal cord after injury. Semin. Cell Dev. Biol. 14, 191-198.

Tropel, P., Platet, N., Platel, J. C., Noel, D., Albrieux, M., Benabid, A. L. and Berger, F. (2006) Functional neuronal differentiation of bone marrow-derived mesenchymal stem cells. Stem Cells 24, 2868-2876.

Tio, M., Tan, K. H., Lee, W., Wang, T. T. and Udolph, G. (2010) Roles of db-cAMP, IBMX and RA in aspects of neural differentiation of cord blood derived mesenchymal-like stem cells. PLoS One 5, e9398.

Kim, E. Y., Lee, K. B., Yu, J., Lee, J. H., Kim, K. J., Han, K. W., Park, K. S., Lee, D. S. and Kim, M. K. (2013) Neuronal cell differentiation of mesenchymal stem cells originating from canine amniotic fluid. Hum. Cell 2013 Oct 29. [Epub ahead of print]

Tremblay, R. G., Sikorska, M., Sandhu, J. K., Lanthier, P., Ribecco-Lutkiewicz, M. and Bani-Yaghoub, M. (2010) Differentiation of mouse Neuro 2A cells into dopamine neurons. J. Neurosci. Methods 186, 60-67.

Uchida, S., Inanaga, Y., Kobayashi, M., Hurukawa, S., Araie, M. and Sakuragawa, N. (2000) Neurotrophic function of conditioned medium from human amniotic epithelial cells. J. Neurosci. Res. 62, 585-590.

Pan, H. C., Yang, D. Y., Chiu, Y. T., Lai, S. Z., Wang, Y. C., Chang, M. H. and Cheng, F. C. (2006) Enhanced regeneration in injured sciatic nerve by human amniotic mesenchymal stem cell. J. Clin. Neurosci. 13, 570-575.

Kakishita, K., Elwan, M. A., Nakao, N., Itakura, T. and Sakuragawa, N. (2000) Human amniotic epithelial cells produce dopamine and survive after implantation into the striatum of a rat model of Parkinson's disease: A potential source of donor for transplantation therapy. Experimental Neurology 165, 27-34.

Portmann-Lanz, C. B., Schoeberlein, A., Huber, A., Sager, R., Malek, A., Holzgreve, W. and Surbek, D. V. (2006) Placental mesenchymal stem cells as potential autologous graft for pre- and perinatal neuroregeneration. Am. J. Obstet. Gynecol. 194, 664-673.

A. M. Williams, I. S. Dennahy, U. F. Bhatti, I. Halaweish, Y. Xiong, P.Chang, V. C. Nikolian, K. Chtraklin, J. Brown, Y. Zhang, Z. G. Zhang,M. Chopp, B. Buller, H. B. Alam,J. Neurotrauma2019,36, 54.

M. Williams, Z. Wu, U. F. Bhatti, B. E. Biesterveld, M. T. Kemp, G.K. Wakam, C. A. Vercruysse, K. Chtraklin, A. Z. Siddiqui, Z. Pickell,S. E. Dekker, Y. Tian, B. Liu, Y. Li, B. Buller, H. B. Alam,J. TraumaAcute Care Surg.2020,89, 388.

Z.-X. Zhang, L.-X. Guan, K. Zhang, Q. Zhang, L.-J. Dai,Cytotherapy 2008,10, 134

M. Williams, Z. Wu, U. F. Bhatti, B. E. Biesterveld, M. T. Kemp, G.K. Wakam, C. A. Vercruysse, K. Chtraklin, A. Z. Siddiqui, Z. Pickell,S. E. Dekker, Y. Tian, B. Liu, Y. Li, B. Buller, H. B. Alam,J. TraumaAcute Care Surg.2020,89, 388.

Z.-X. Zhang, L.-X. Guan, K. Zhang, Q. Zhang, L.-J. Dai,Cytotherapy 2008,10, 134.

Bae, H. K. Jin, J. K. Lee, J. C. Richardson, J. E. Carter,Curr. Alzheimer Res.2013,10, 524.

Abshenas, T. Artimani, S. Shahidi, A. Ranjbar, A. Komaki, I. Salehi,I. Amiri, S. Soleimani Asl,Life Sci.2020,249, 117482.

T. Ma, K. Gong, Q. Ao, Y. Yan, B. Song, H. Huang, X. Zhang, Y. Gong,Cell Transplant.2013,22, 113.[82] L.-Y. Li, J.-T. Li, Q.-Y. Wu, J. Li, Z.-T. Feng, S. Liu, T.-H. Wang,J. Mol.Neurosci. MN2008,34, 157.

S. E. Park, N. K. Lee, D. L. Na, J. W. Chang,Histol. Histopathol.2018,33, 533.[84] F. Q. Hour, A. J. Moghadam, A. Shakeri-Zadeh, M. Bakhtiyari, R.Shabani, M. Mehdizadeh,J. Controlled Release2020,321, 430.

M. F. Zappa Villar, J. López Hanotte, J. Pardo, G. R. Morel, G. Maz-zolini, M. G. García, P. C. Reggiani,Mol. Neurobiol.2020,57, 600.

H. Wake, A. J. Moorhouse, S. Jinno, S. Kohsaka, J. Nabekura,J. Neu-rosci.2009,29, 3974.[87] H. J. Lee, J. K. Lee, H. Lee, J. E. Carter, J. W. Chang, W. Oh, Y. S. Yang,J.-G. Suh, B.-H. Lee, H. K. Jin, J.-S. Bae,Neurobiol. Aging2012,33,588.

Y. Naaldijk, C. Jäger, C. Fabian, C. Leovsky, A. Blüher, L. Rudolph, A.Hinze, A. Stolzing,Neuropathol. Appl. Neurobiol.2017,43, 299.[89] M. M. Varnum, T. Ikezu,Arch. Immunol. Ther. Exp.2012,60, 251.

A. Li, J. Zhao, C. Fan, L. Zhu, C. Huang, Q. Li, D. Gan, C. Wen, M.Chen, D. Lu,Neurobiol. Aging 2020,86, 81.

Chapter 11

Urine Based Pregnancy Diagnosis in Dairy Animal: Evaluation of Urinary Metabolic Signatures

Ashok Kumar Balhara* and Suman Sangwan
CAR-Central Institute for Research on Buffaloes, Hisar-125001
**Corresponding author: ashok.balhara@icar.gov.in*

Early pregnancy diagnosis is critical for adapting effective production. Identification of pregnancy biomarkers is critical for early diagnosis, disease classification, assessment of disease progression, and evaluation of diagnostic response. The current "omics" era has given a significant boost to the field of proteomics and metabolomics with significant advances in analytical platforms such as chromatographic or electrophoretic separation with integrated mass spectrometry (MS), fluorescence-based methods, and nuclear magnetic resonance spectroscopy (NMR) combined with state-of-the-art bioinformatics tools to achieve high sensitivity with reasonable precision. Metabolomics is an emerging branch of "omics," defined as the global analysis of small molecules (metabolites) that involves identification, characterization, and quantification in a biological sample such as a cell, tissue, biofluid, organ, or organism at a specific time point under specific genetic and environmental conditions (Oliver *et al*; 1998; German *et al*; 2005; Griffin and Vidal-Puig, 2008), and the set of metabolites considered in a given biological sample is referred to as the metabolome (Querengesser *et al*; 2007). Although metabolomics is a new field in clinical medicine, it was conceived nearly 80 years ago by Roger Williams based on individual variations and disease-specific "metabolic patterns" in the biological fluids of diseased individuals (Gates and Sweeley, 1978), while the term "metabolic profile" was coined in 1971 by Horning and co-workers based on quantitative metabolomics of urinary metabolites (Novotny *et al*; 2008).

A method for pregnancy diagnosis must be based on one or more of the changes in maternal physiology associated with the embryonic developmental profile. Accordingly, measurement of peripheral concentrations of progesterone, pregnancy-associated glycoproteins (PAGs), and early pregnancy factor are among the methods commonly used in cattle to detect pregnancy, with each method having its own advantages and limitations. In addition, in recent years, the possibility of using maternal/fetal metabolic traits to define new biomarkers and develop new methods for non-invasive pregnancy monitoring aimed at early pregnancy detection and prediction has been recognized.

Reproductive performance is the most important factor affecting the productivity of a dairy cattle. Late pregnancy detection means the loss of another period if the animal is not pregnant and oestrus synchronization is not performed. Again, late embryo loss causes serious economic losses because it is often detected too late to inseminate cows and increases the cost of artificial insemination. This also leads to extended calving intervals and a prolonged dry stall period, ultimately resulting in lower annual milk production and also lower net calf production.

METABOLOMICS ANALYTICAL PLATFORMS

The main analytical platforms for metabolomics are nuclear magnetic resonance spectroscopy (NMR) and mass spectrometry (MS). Of these, several MS modalities, including liquid chromatography- MS (LC - MS) and gas chromatography- MS (GC- MS), are the mainstay of current metabolomics analyses (Shao and Le, 2019). The applications of metabolomics analysis platforms are shown in Figure 1. The high applicability of LC - MS - NMR permeates the field of metabolomics due to its high spectral resolution and great metabolite identification capabilities (Walker *et al.*, 2016).

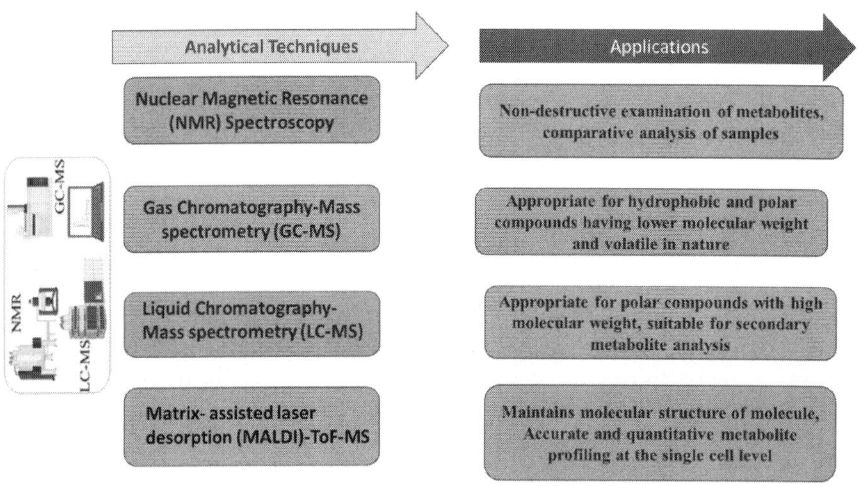

Figure 1: Analytical techniques and their applications in biomarker discovery

RESEARCH WORK IN THE PREGNANCY DIAGNOSIS FROM OUR LABORATORY STUDY

Laboratory studies in buffalo urine were initiated at ICAR-CIRB, first on proteomics and later on metabolomics platforms to decipher information on differential expression of metabolites depending on pregnancy status. Experiments were performed in which buffaloes were artificially inseminated and urine was collected in sterile collection containers. These urine samples were processed in the manner indicated:

- **Protein extraction** – Total protein in the urine was precipitated with ammonium sulphate/ trichloroacetic acid/ acetone. Alternatively, samples were concentrated by lyophilization followed by precipitation of proteins and peptides. These protein precipitates were analysed by 2DE - mass spectrometry-based proteomics (Bathla *et al*; 2015).

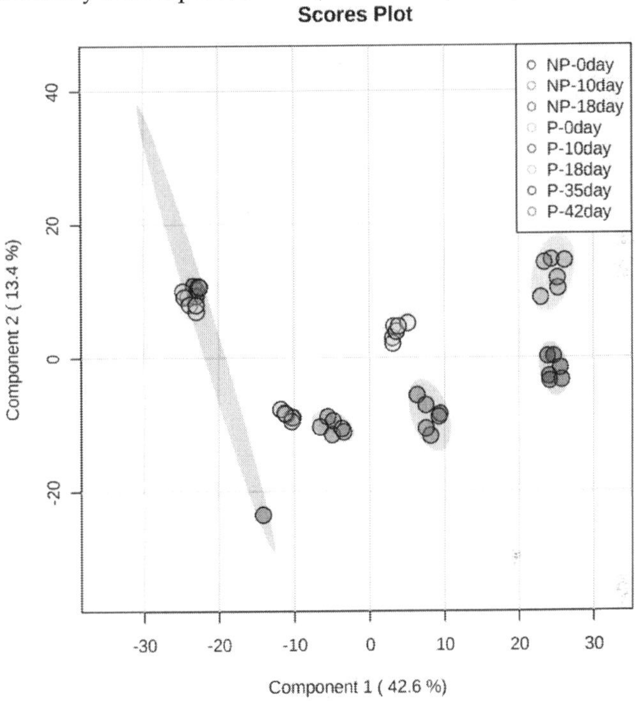

Figure 2: 2-D score plot of PLS-DA analysis of different groups in different days of early pregnancy

- **Extraction of metabolites** - Volatile, hydrophilic and hydrophobic compounds from buffalo urine samples were collected in appropriate polar and non-polar solvents. The as-prepared samples were analysed by deuterium (1H) NMR technique to study the difference in composition depending on the gestation status of the animals. Metabolite profiling and subsequent bioinformatics were performed using Chenomx and MestReNovo 6.0.2-5475 software programmes, and the Human Metabolome Database (HMDB) and Kyoto Encyclopaedia of Genes and Genomes (KEGG) online databases were used to identify metabolites. The selected identified metabolites were later validated by gas chromatography-mass spectrometry GC-MS, LC-MS, HPLC, infrared spectroscopy (IR Spectroscopy), thin layer chromatography (TLC) and colour tests. NMR studies of urine revealed that there are numerous metabolites that are present in good usable quality and have medical, agricultural, and industrial applications. In buffalo urine, amino acids (tyrosine, tryptophan, phenylalanine, 3-hydroxykunurenine, 5-hydroxytryptophan, anthranilate, histidine, tyramine, leucine, and lysine), chlorogenate, azelate, anthranilate, ethylene glycol, Hippurate, protocatechuate, 1,3-dihydroxyacetone, 1,6-anhydro-D-glucose, furoglycine, 3-indoxysulfate, butanone, imidazole, uracil, fumarate, glycolate, and tri-methylamine N-oxide metabolites were reported by (Sarangi *et al*; 2022). The 2D score plot of PLS-DA -analysis containing component 1 (42.6%) and component 2 (13.4%) shows conspicuous separate clusters of variation between groups and between days, except on day 0 (Fig.2)

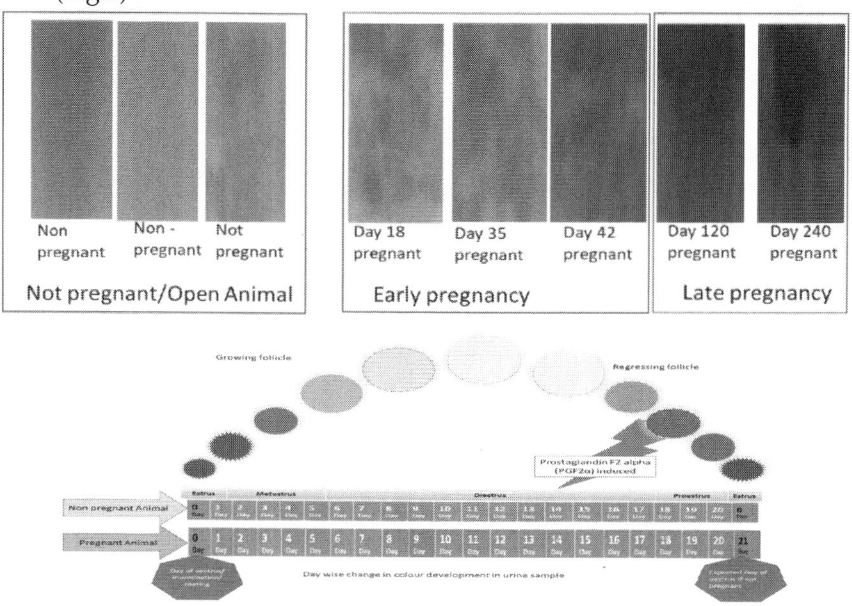

Figure 3: Colour variation with progression of pregnancy

◈ **Chemical Testing**: Chemical tests: the magic of chemistry can be observed in the test tube by applying some chemical reactions that give a certain color to certain functional groups in the animal fluid. The results, interpreted based on the above methods, specify some functional groups that are present in pregnant animals and absent in non-pregnant animals. The application of reagents to urine samples of animals and the specific color difference in the test tube can be an indication of the reproductive status of the animal. The color also has some precipitates that open a new way of improvement, such as a strip-based or sensor-based method that is farmer-friendly and easy to use. Figure 3 shows the color changes with the progress of gestation in animals. The institute has developed a prototype of a usable urine-based kit for pregnancy diagnosis in dairy animals, which has been filed for patent (Indian Patent Application No. 202011013074 dated 25/03/2020; published 10/01/2021).

URINARY METABOLIC SIGNATURES IN DAIRY ANIMAL PREGNANCY DIAGNOSIS:

Metabolomics-based studies of dairy cattle diseases are still evolving, although significant successes have been achieved recently (Table 1). In addition, animal models are commonly used for metabolomics studies of various physiological states that also occur in humans. However, there is currently little metabolomics literature evaluating and detecting biomarkers in dairy animals for pregnancy detection.

Table 1: Application of urine metabolomics in animal pregnancy diagnosis

Status	Species	Analytical Technique Used	Differentially regulated protein/metabolite	Reference
Early pregnancy	Buffalo	NMR	Tyrosine, tyramine, 3-hydroxykynurenine (3-HK), 5-hydroxytryptophan (5-HT) and anthranilate	Sarangi et al; 2022
Early pregnancy	Pig	UHPLC-MS/MS	A total of 269 urinary metabolites, including lipids and organic acids, Choline and PdG levels were consistently highly expressed in early phases	Zhou et al; 2022
Estrous, diestrus, and pre-estrous	Cow/ Buffalo	GC-MS/ MS, HPLC	Forty-two volatile compounds were identified from three phases of estrous cycle, more specifically 4-methyl phenol (p-cresol) and 9-octadecenoic acid (oleic acid) in estrus urine and evaluate a pheromone-based kit.	Muniasamy et al; 2017
Estrous	Buffalo	ELISA	Urinary Luteinizing Hormone (LH) concentration of buffaloes during estrus is higher in winter than summer and the range is higher for heifers than multiparous animals in both seasons	Ramu et al; 2018

Status	Species	Analytical Technique Used	Differentially regulated protein/metabolite	Reference
Heat stress	Goat	NMR	Hippurate and other phenylalanine derivatives are suggested as urinary biomarkers to identify heat-stressed animals.	Jodar et al; 2019
Early pregnancy	Mithun	NMR	A total of 270 urinary metabolites, including lipids and organic acids, kynurenine, anthranilate, chlorogenate levels were consistently highly expressed in early phases	Unpublished work
Early pregnancy	Cow	LCMS/MS	42-45 pregnancy specific dipeptides and tripeptides were enlisted for pregnancy specific markers e.g. ferritin	Bathla et al; 2015

Since the indicated metabolites mainly represent the tryptophan pathway, the phenylalanine-tyrosine-tryptophan pathway, the TCA cycle, the tyrosine pathway, and the glucose pathway play important roles in early pregnancy.

Conclusion and Future Prospective

Recent developments in urinary metabolites have opened new avenues for developing field usable diagnostics. Amino acids, organic acids, amino sugars, and nucleosides in urine are being tested as molecular biomarkers for early pregnancy. These metabolite signatures can be used for metabolomics mapping and monitoring to assess healthy pregnancies in animals. Efforts are underway to further miniaturize the sensor-based equipment so that it can be operated under all types of field conditions.

REFERENCES

Bathla, S., Rawat, P., Baithalu, R., Yadav, M. L., Naru, J., Tiwari, A., Balhara, A. K., ... & Mohanty, A. K. (2015). Profiling of urinary proteins in Karan Fries cows reveals more than 1550 proteins. *Journal of proteomics, 127*, 193-201.

Contreras-Jodar, A., Nayan, N. H., Hamzaoui, S., Caja, G., & Salama, A. A. (2019). Heat stress modifies the lactational performances and the urinary metabolomic profile related to gastrointestinal microbiota of dairy goats. *PLoS One, 14*(2), e0202457.

German, J. B., Hammock, B.D. and Watkins, S.M. (2005). Metabolomics: building on a century of biochemistry to guide human health. *Metabolomics*, 1 (1), 3 – 9.

Griffin, J.L. and Vidal- Puig, A. (2008). Current challenges in metabolomics for diabetes research: a vital functional genomic tool or just a ploy for gaining funding? *Physiological Genomics*, 34 (1), 1 – 5.

Muniasamy, S., Selvam, R. M., Rajanarayanan, S., Saravanakumar, V. R., & Archunan, G. (2017). p-cresol and oleic acid as reliable biomarkers of estrus: evidence from synchronized Murrah buffaloes. *Iranian Journal of Veterinary Research, 18*(2), 124.

Novotny, M.V., Soini, H.A. and Mechref, Y. (2008). Biochemical individuality reflected in chromatographic, electrophoretic and mass- spectrometric profiles. *Journal of Chromatography B: Analytical Technologies in the Biomedical and Life Sciences*, 866 (1– 2), 26 – 47.

Oliver, S.G., Winson, M.K., Kell, D.B. *et al.* (1998). Systematic functional analysis of the yeast genome. *Trends in Biotechnology*, 16 (9), 373 – 37 8.

Querengesser, L., Vogel, H.J., Sykes, B.D. *et al.* (2007). HMDB: The Human Metabolome Database. *Nucleic Acids Research*, 35 (suppl. 1), D521 – D526

Ramu, M. S., Onteru, S. K., Singh, D., & Govindaraju, A. Urinary Luteinizing Hormone: a tipoff for estrus detection in Murrah Buffalo (Bubalus bubalis) 2018.

Sarangi, A., Ghosh, M., Sangwan, S., Kumar, R., Balhara, S., Phulia, S. K., ... & Balhara, A. K. (2022). Exploration of urinary metabolite dynamicity for early detection of pregnancy in water buffaloes. *Scientific Reports, 12*(1), 16295.

Walker, L.R., Hoyt, D.W., Walker, S.M. II *et al.* (2016). Unambiguous metabolite identification in high through put metabolomics by hybrid 1D (1) H NMR/ ESI MS (1) approach. *Magnetic Resonance in Chemistry*, 54, 998 – 1003.

Zhou, C., Cai, G., Meng, F., Hu, Q., Liang, G., Gu, T., ... & Hong, L. (2022). Urinary metabolomics reveals the biological characteristics of early pregnancy in pigs. *Porcine Health Management, 8*(1), 1-12.

Chapter 12

Emerging Technologies in Livestock Production System for Food Security

Z.A. Pampori, D. Hasin, Aasif A Sheikh, O. Aarif, Fozia Shah, M. Rayees, S. Sumeira, A. Uroos & A. Nowsheen

Division of Veterinary Sciences & AH, SKUAST-Kashmir, Shuaham, Alusteng-190006, JK, India

ABSTRACT

The human population has significantly increased in last century and it expanded very rapidly from nineteen sixties. This increase in human population has lead to the significant increase in food production through application of mechanization, chemical fertilization and genetic selection in agriculture. However, the enormous production of food has posed lots of pressure on natural resources and were over utilized and degraded. Further these operations has increased the green house gas emissions several folds that resulted into global warming, the change that has challenged the life on earth planet, consequences of which are being observed in the form of floods, draughts, cloud bursts, melting of glaciers & sea ice, rising of sea level and loss of species. The world population by 2050 is anticipated to touch 9 billion that means an increase of 30% which will be demanding 70% increase in the food. Further the urbanization, improved economies and changed dietary preferences, the demand for food of animal origin is rising. Globally animal products provide 67% of the protein and the requirement for meat and milk by 2050 is expected to increase by 73% and 58% respectively 2050. Therefore, livestock production has to be augmented to have food and nutritional security of growing population but without compromising on conservation of natural resources and green environment. As such technology driven, precision, smart livestock farming is inevitable that must integrate all the techniques, skills, knowledge and innovations to produce safe, sufficient, affordable, accessible and sustainable animal food with minimum environmental impacts.

INTRODUCTION

The world human population was 1 billion in 1804 that doubled in a century and was 2 billion in 1927. It reached 3 billion just in a span of 32 years in 1960 and 4 billion in just 14 years in 1974. Thereafter, human population growth curve illustrates a spike and we have in 2021global human population of 7.2 billion that is projected to be 9.6 billion by 2050(FAO,*2009)*.The biggest challenge was food security of such an ever-rising human population and it led to the exploitation of natural resources viz land & water, use of chemical fertilizers, pesticides, of course accompanied with genetically improved, high yielding varieties of grains and farm mechanization to bridge the gap between demand & production of food for human consumption. This non-eco-friendly and unsustainable approach of food production resulted into emission of enormous quantities of green house gases that subsequently lead to climate change and global warming. Livestock has always remained an integral part of farming agriculture and has served as protein security and economic buffer against crop farming failures. Livestock has been providing meat, milk, eggs, wool, pelts since its domestication. Urbanization, dietary changes and increased income has increased demand for agri-foods, particularly the foods of animal origin (Nelson *et al.*, 2010). The demand for agriculture products is expected to increase by 70% by 2050. The demand for meat and milk in 2050 is projected to grow by 73% and 58%, respectively especially in developing countries and emerging economies.

Livestock sector globally supports the livelihood of over 1 billion poorest people, employs 1.1 billion people, accounts for 40% of global agricultural gross domestic product, and provides over 33% of the world's protein intake and 7% of global kilocalorie consumption*(The World Bank, 2022)*. The livestock sector is one of the most important sectors in global food security. Livestock can play a vital role in improving the lives of millions by providing the sufficient and reliable supplies of meat, milk, eggs and dairy products, diversifying food basket with animal-source foods; helping to generate income and creating employment and strengthening the rural household assets. Livestock production can also help improve children's cognitive and physical development as well as school attendance and performance, empower rural women, improve natural resource-use and support sustainable economic growth *(*Pampori, *2021)*.

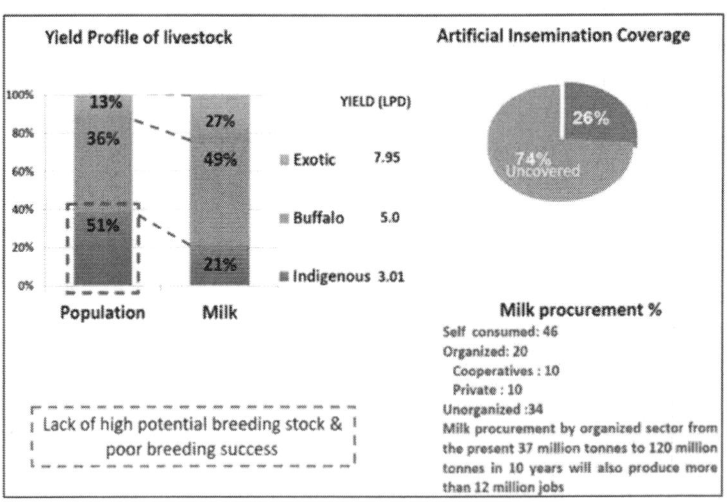

Figure 1

FiThe increasing population and demands for food warrants sustainability and efficiency in production systems in milieu of climate change and natural resource depletion.

LIVESTOCK SCENARIO IN INDIA

India has a huge livestock population of 535.8 million (20th Livestock Census) and ranks number one in cattle & buffalo population in the world. India although stands largest producer of milk, makes up to 23% of the world's milk annually yet the per animal milk production is too less as compared to developed countries. Because of this huge livestock population in India with low average production per animal, Indian livestock sector is considered as the main contributor to the global climate change. The livestock sector is often associated with negative environmental impacts such as land degradation, air and water pollution, GHG production and biodiversity destruction (Bellarby *et al.*, 2013). It is well realised that the livestock production system in India is not much efficient, as it has a high proportion of low yielding indigenous livestock. 51 % of the cattle in India are non-descript with an average milk production of 3 kg per day, contributing only 21% of total milk pool (Fig.1). The average age at first calving is 60 months and long calving interval of 20 to 24 months are the indicators of not having an efficient system of livestock production. The exotic blood although very limited 13% of population yet contributes 27% to the milk pool. Increases in livestock production are expected to originate from a declining natural resource base, which will cause further environmental damage without proper natural resource management. Climate change affect livestock production through competition for natural resources, quantity and quality of feeds & forage, emerging & re-emerging livestock diseases, heat stress, high mortality and biodiversity loss (Steinfeld *et al.*, 2006). In year 2000, 16% of livestock breeds (ass, water buffalo, cattle, goat, pig, sheep, and horse) were lost (TWB, 2022). In addition, the FAO, 2007, has stated that from 7,616 livestock breeds reported, 20% were at risk, and almost one breed per month was being lost. Animal genetic diversity is a precious and irreplaceable resource that needs to be conserved and used as it serves a great choice for the farmers to have climate resilient and disease resistant livestock species. Conservation and sustainable use of genetic resources will be critical for the development of smart livestock farming (FAO, 2007).

An efficient system of livestock production is inevitable wherein livestock products are produced with low carbon foot prints, wherein inputs are efficiently utilized by the animal to produce optimum with low GHG emissions. Sustainable livestock production will mean sustainable increase inclean, nutritious, safe productivity, its judicious consumption with minimal losses at farm or table. The smart livestock production system will require efficiencies in various operations, plans and activities common to all systems of livestock production. The efficiency in production system can be achieved through use of emerging technologies.

KNOWLEDGE & SKILL-BASED LIVESTOCK PRODUCTIVITY

Livestock productivity is measured as the ratio of outputs to inputs. Efficient livestock productivity will lead to both improved food security, improved farm income and reduced GHG emissions. Knowledge and skill-based livestock farming shall be aimed at increasing number of animals born and raised per breeding animal per year, increasing growth rates and market weights of animals anticipated for slaughter, or increasing number of livestock products per animal per year at minimum carbon foot prints per unit of livestock product. In Netherlands, milk production per cow increased from 6270 kg/yr in Kyoto base in year 1990 to 8350 kg / yr in 2008, with a concomitant decrease in CH_4 production from 17.6 to 15.4 g/ kg milk, respectively (Bannink et al.2011). Flachowsky (2011) estimated that a dairy cow producing 40 kg milk/d would produce 50% lower CO_2–equivalent (CO_2e) emissions per kilogram of edible protein than a cow yielding 10 kg/d. Similarly, GHG emissions would be about 70% lower from beef cattle gaining 1.5 vs. 1.0 kg/d, 40% lower from a growing or fattening pig gaining 900 vs. 500 g/d, and 60% lower from a laying hen with 90 vs. 50% laying performance. Proficient way of increasing livestock productivity is to employ all the available technologies, skills, strategies as per the production system to augment productivity.

1. Breeding Management

It will involve selection & breeding of more productive animals through well-designed selection and culling strategies, cross-breeding programmes, marker assisted selection for productive traits, fecundity genes and artificial insemination programmes. Breeding management is a key strategy to increase livestock productivity by improving traits such as live weight gain, milk yield, disease resistance or fertility. (Hare *et al.*, 2006; Norman *et al.*, 2009).Animal biotechnology provides new and quick opportunities for genetic improvement in the production of farm animals. It can be used in promoting growth, increasing growth rates, improving nutrient intake efficiency, augmenting milk production, fecundity, hair, and fiber, reducing environmental impacts, imparting disease resistance and augmenting reproductive performance (Nguyen &Ly, 2018). Cutting edge technologies of gene editing, cloning, embryo transfer technology, embryo splitting, cryopreservation, transgression, transgenesis, can be employed to increase productivity. Artificial insemination technology though a very old technology to enhance progenies of high merit with reduced number of breeding males, yet has not achieved its full potential because of being highly professional or skilled task. While AI exploits male genetics, embryo transfer technology exploits female genetics also with production of high genetic merit embryos and transferring them in surrogates (Wheeler,2013; Murray and Maga, 2016).Semen sexing technology has opened a one more window to produce progeny of the desired sex, either male or female. DNA polymorphisms evaluation through restriction fragment length polymorphisms (RFLP) and randomly amplified polymorphic DNA (RAPD) are reliable techniques to estimate the genetic uniqueness of populations that can be exploited for increasing genetic makeup of livestock for production traits, disease resistance etc. (Yadav *et al.*, 2017).

2. Feeding Management

It is an established fact that livestock farming consumes 70% of inputs in feeding only. Improving diets so that animals produce more protein with less feed and lower emissions should be the goal in feeding management. Balanced feed ration is of upmost importance to improve, growth, reproduction and reproductive life. Waghorn and Hegarty (2011) reported that good quality pastures/ fodders reduce methane emissions and calculated that 20% increase in ME of fodders can reduce methane emissions by 50%. Therefore, improving the quality of feed, formulating appropriate feed rations with high-quality feed ingredients will be important strategy. Other strategies like (i) enhancing forage digestibility through, chopping, soaking, urea treatment, enzyme treatments or silage and hay preparation (ii) target feeding/ strategic feeding with energy and nutrients as per the type of animal, species, age, production and its physiological state(Makkar, 2013) (iii) selecting better feed resources, including alternative feed products and feed additives along with supplementation of small amounts of concentrate feed and multinutrient blocks (mineral/urea/molasses) in diets to improve feed conversion (iv)produce concentrate by strategically mixing agro-industrial by-products that are rich in energy or proteins (Makkar, 2013) (v)introduction of insect-based feed products as a source of protein in animal feed rations like Black soldier flies, common housefly maggots, silkworms, locusts/grasshoppers/crickets and yellow mealworms (Harinder *et al.*, 2014) should be employed to have efficient livestock production. Use of herbal products in animal feed has also yielded good results in augmenting milk production and reproductive health of livestock. Hasin et al. (2021) used fenugreek in lactating goats and reported significant increase in milk production, similarly Ovais et al. (2020) reported 10% increase in milk production in lactating cows during chilly winter in which otherwise there is sharp decrease in production with feeding of fenugreek blended with Jaggery (2:1) as a "winter chocolate". They further reported improved body condition score and increased levels of prolactin, growth hormone and decreased level of cortisol in fed animals as compared to control animals.

3. Manure Management

Livestock manure management is of utmost importance because of its impact on water and air quality through carbon dioxide, methane, nitrites and phosphorus released from manure (van Dijk *et al.*, 2016; Web *et al.*, 2012). Manure management refers to manure accumulation, its collection, storage, processing and application to crops (Hristov *et al.*, 2013). Globally, livestock manure supplies up to 12 % of gross nitrogen input for cropping and up to 23% in mixed crop-livestock systems in developing countries (FAO, 2019).The total nutrients from livestock manure exceed nutrients from synthetic fertilizers. Animal manure contains most of the essential micro- and macro-elements required for plant growth and represents a valid alternative to other fertilizers that release GHG emissions. Most methane emissions from manure derive from swine, poultry and beef cattle feedlots where production is carried out on a large scale and manure is stored under anaerobic conditions. Manure is linked to both CH4 and N2O emissions. Most of the nitrous oxide emissions come from the manure of pigs and poultry (Fig). Most of the manure-related CH4 emissions are produced under anaerobic conditions during storage and very little following land application. Manure from grazing ruminants does not produce significant quantities of CH4 because it remains largely aerobic. Solid manure is mainly stored in field heaps, very little in covered storages and slurry is spread over fields.

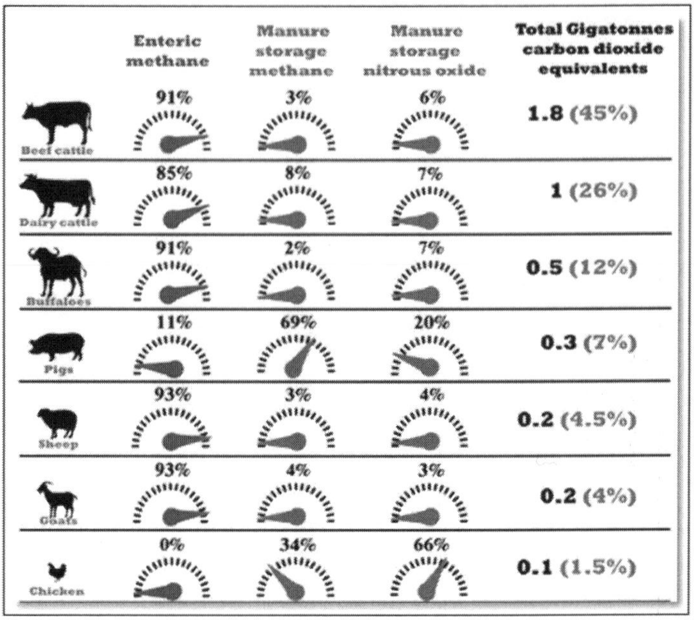

Figure 2

Many technological solutions are available for reducing environmental impacts of manure which include; (I) manure shall not be stored or spread in the vicinity of water resources and a minimum of 100 meter distance should be maintained (ii) farmers must have adequate storage capacity to enable storage for a minimum period (45 days) before land spreading (iii) land spreading should be forbidden on certain lands like bare soil, sloping ground, saturated land, frozen ground that otherwise lead to environmental impact via run off or by leaching (iv) ammonia production from the manure is also n important source of air pollution that can be reduced by acidification of manure during storage or field application,treatment with urease inhibiting enzymes and covering manure. (v) solid–liquid manure separation allows for wastewater to be used in flushing feed alleys and for irrigating fields, whereas the solids can be used as animal bedding, composted or air dried for application to the field(vi) anaerobic digestion and activated sludge have been developed to recycle and reuse organic wastes,capturing and transforming the CH_4 in biogas systems to generate renewable energy that can be used to run electric generators, milking machines, farm heating or lighting systems.(vii) Vermicomposting has proved to be a successful strategy to produce wealth from waste.

4. Herd Management

Improving animal health services, including disease prevention and management, has a strong impact on the efficiency of livestock systems, food security and adaptation to climate change (Place & Mitloehner, 2010). Decreasing dry period, increasing lactation days can reduce the GHG emissions significantly. Improving animal health and reducing morbidity and mortality to improve efficiency of the livestock production system offer opportunities to reduce both CH_4 and N_2O from enteric fermentation and animal manure. In large herd size and increased animal productivity, the focus is more on subclinical disease and systematic health management (LeBlanc et al., 2006).Establishing strong animal health institutions, formulating dedicated policies and initiating research programmes focused on changing conditions are essential to improve livestock efficiency and increase the preparedness against new risks of emerging & re-emerging diseases as a result of close herding and climate change. Proper animal health services will also lead to an increased lifetime productive performance. For effective herd health management various emerging techniques can be employed for clear productivity that will include; (I) animal disease surveillance, tracking, early warning and rapid response (ii) door services for health and insemination using mobile vans (iii) use of advanced techniques like telemedicine, livestock health mobile Apps (iv) careful management of transition period in dairy cows that involves careful attention to the metabolic status of cows in the pre- and postpartum period(v) day light length management during lactation and dry period (vi) provision of adequate access to shade and water, minimizing transport or herding of animals over long distances (vi) use of biotechnological tools and techniques in pathogen detection and characterization in infected hosts for early detection of diseases and their effective control (vii) recombinant DNA technology in the production of effective vaccines and the diagnosis of infectious diseases and their prevention (Nascimento and Leite, 2012) (viii) recombinant technology and protein engineering to develop novel enzymes with modified structures for thermal stability, substrate specificity, or the ability to work under extreme conditions(Gurung et al., 2013) (ix) use of metabolic engineering, an important biotechnological tool, to produce valuable metabolites or natural secondary compounds in large amounts that are otherwise difficult to extract and purify from their natural sources, production of antibiotics, vaccines, vitamins, enzymes, and other useful bioactive products that improve the animal health and consequently their production (Tang and Zhao, 2009).

5. Waste to Wealth – Solid Waste Management

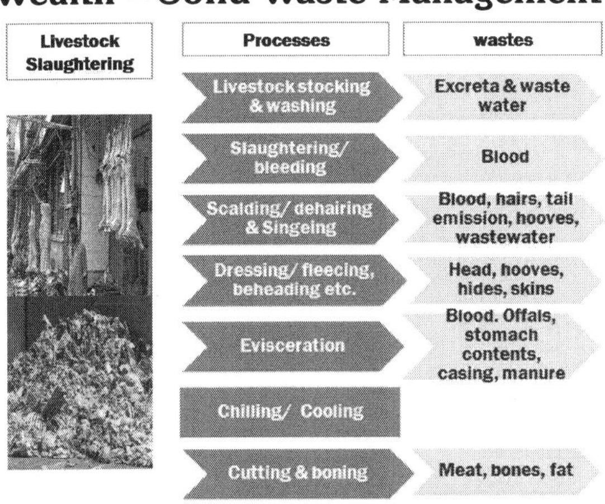

Figure 3: Livestock slaughter processes & waste

A large volume of livestock products is wasted even before reaching the consumer. Food wastage from production to consumer is estimated to be 1/3rd of produce. In developing countries most of the wastage is at production source and little with consumer, however, in developed countries the wastage is more at table and little at production source. If the loss of food in value chain in India is reduces it can eliminate the hunger from the country alone (Pampori, 2021). Waste reduction can substantially contribute to improving resource use efficiency such as land, water, energy, as well as other inputs such as nutrients. The energy embedded in global annual food losses is thought to be around 38 % of the total final energy consumed by the whole food chain (FAO, 2017). Similarly efficient use of food waste and converting it into products to improve farm returns can be a strong strategy to reduce environmental issues and poverty. The waste to wealth can be achieved through use of various technologies and mitigation strategies that include; (I) ensuring proper sanitation at all stages of the value chain (ii) mechanized and hygienic processing units (iii) appropriate processing, labelling and packaging, distribution, transportation and storage of livestock products (iv) cold sterilization (v) use of apeel (a natural ingredients obtained from plants)as a preservative instead of chemical preservatives (vi) slaughter house solid waste disposal{a tremendous pressure on the environment and public health creating several environmental (water, air, and soil pollution) and health issues (waterborne diseases and respiratory illness)} (Tahir et al., 2015).Slaughterhouse wastes are animal by-products that remain unutilized after slaughtering and it has been estimated that about 30% to 50% of the total weight of slaughtered animal remains as slaughterhouse waste in livestock and poultry industry (Adhikari et al., 2018; Meeker, 2009) and are recognized drivers of GHGs.The slaughterhouse waste is majorly comprised of rumen (80%), dung/manure (12%), blood (5%), and others (3%) by weight (Fig.) Further rising population and increased liking for animal foods is going to increase the abattoir waste especially in urban areas in coming years, thus becomes a huge challenge Segregation of organic wastes collected from slaughterhouses or abattoir shops or centralized markets from other inorganic waste fractions is the main issue with solid waste disposal. As such mechanized slaughter houses with modern, hygienic processing units and efficient mechanism of slaughterhouse material collection, segregation, utilization and disposal is priority. Slaughterhouse and abattoir waste has a huge potential for energy and product recoveries like protein hydrolysate synthesis, enzymes, and lipids. Anaerobic digestion of the waste is eco-friendly and more valuable as it produces renewable energy. Innovative technologies to convert livestock waste to wealth should be employed viz, Biodiesel production (derived from animal fat, plant and vegetable oils through transesterification of long chain fatty acids producing methyl, ethyl or propyl esters). Pyrolysis (process of thermal decomposition of organic wastes in absence of oxygen in a controlled environmentto stable solid carbon residue called as bio-char, liquid bio-oil and gaseous products). Hydrothermal carbonization for wet waste (thermo-chemical treatment process to produce a value-added carbon-rich hydrochar material besides gaseous and water-soluble products through hydrolysis, dehydration and decarboxylation processes). Extraction of keratin/protein(a natural structural fibrous protein found in vertebrates making up scales, hair, nails, feathers, wool, horns, claws and hoovesand outer layer of skin in mammals, birds and reptiles). Keratin hydrolysate has been used in shampoos, applications in pharmaceutical, biomedical, food, and cosmetic industries (Li, 2019). Fibreboard production (an engineered wool product from mixed waste poultry feathers and wood residues (Safari et al., 2020). Bioplastic sheet production (Slaughterhouse/poultry wastes are one renewable sources of protein that can be used for the fabricationof bioplastic films).

6. Weather Information, Warning System, Disease Surveillance and Livestock Insurance

The use of weather information to predict health and production risks and assist in risk management is a potentially effective option for efficient, smart livestock farming system. Use of weather data to provide advisories and early warnings to the livestock farmers for better management of livestock. Disease surveillance and assessment of association of different environmental conditions with different diseases can be a better tool to risk management in livestock farming. Livestock insurance schemes that are weather indexed can be run by the private sector. Public-private partnership approaches to index-based livestock insurance in situations where risks are unacceptably high need to be practiced.

7. Information, Digital and Smart Phone Technologies in Livestock Production System

Technology required for efficient livestock production system depends on country, physical environment, infrastructure, climate, culture, literacy, economic conditions and governance. Artificial intelligence (AI), internet of things (IoT) and machine learning (ML) have been inviting the attention of agriculturalists and livestock managers to make a breakthrough in livestock management.

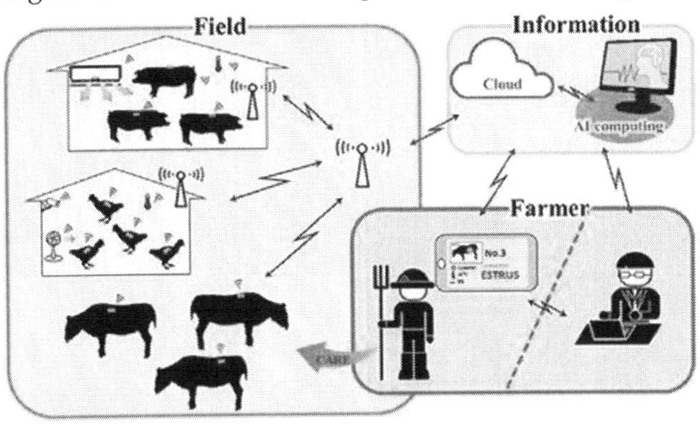

Figure 4: IoT & AI driven livestock farm model

The technology involves connecting of biological and environmental information of livestock obtained by IoT sensors, storing the data in cloud, analysing, diagnosing and changing it into simple and valuable information through artificial intelligence, making informed decisions and subsequently relayed to the farmers or automatically controlled system for effective implementation (Fig.). Biosensors have been developed that record the physiological parameters of every single animal and through application of artificial intelligence possibility of disease occurrence is accordingly relayed to the farmers, and farmers can take timely necessary care of the livestock. It will equip the farmer with forecasting skills of the highest grade for prompt prediction of disease outbreaks, timing of various livestock practices - "Smart cow-house".Use of information & digital technology will improve production efficiency and reduce physical labour and labour cost. Through use of IoT &AI technology, farmers can formulate rations depending upon the production, functional state, weather, behavior of livestock and available resources. IoT-AI-ML technology can be used for intelligent marketing in prediction of customer preferences, precise prediction of shelf life of products to reduce the post-harvest losses. Similarly block-chain technology ensures and guarantees traceability of animal products from farm to fork, thus providing a dynamic system of disease outbreak monitoring and consequently preventing the related economic losses and food-related health pandemics. Use of robotic milking machines, automatic calf feeders in dairy farms can make farming smart, efficient, more profitable, sustainable and green. Remote sensing technology, global positioning system (GPS), geographic information system (GIS), satellites can now be integrated and used in assessing the needs of livestock thus can help in efficient & sustainable utilization of resources, reducing the input costs with efficient production. The cleaning technology will reduce disease occurrence and shall creates a cleaner environment for the animal besides minimising the contact of farmers with the waste. Use of smart phone technology can be effectively used in livestock production system through integrating and monitoring various farm activities remotely not even being physically present in the farm.

REFERENCES

Adhikari, B.B., Chae, M. and Bressler, D.C. (2018). Utilization of slaughterhouse waste in value-added applications: recent advances in the development of wood adhesives. Polymers10:176.

Alonge, D.O. (2005).Textbook of meat and milk hygiene. Farmcoe Press, Ibadan, Nigeria, pp 77–86

Bannink, A., Van Schijndel, M. W., Dijkstra, J. (2011). A model of enteric fermentation in dairy cows to estimate methane emission for the Dutch National Inventory Report using the IPCC Tier 3 approach. Animal Feed Science Technology. 166: 603–618.

Bellarby, J., Tirado, R., Leip, A., Weiss, F., Lesschen, J. P., Smith, P. (2013). Livestock greenhouse gas emissions and mitigation potential in Europe. Global Change Biology. 19(1), 3-18.

Dickie, A., Streck, C., Roe, S., Zurek, M., Haupt, F.,Dolginow, A. (2014). "Strategies for Mitigating Climate Change in Agriculture: Recommendations for Philanthropy." Climate Focus and California Environmental Associates, prepared with the support of the Climate and Land Use Alliance. Report and supplementary materials available at: www. Agricultural mitigation.org

FAO. (2007). The State of Food and Agriculture: Paying Farmers for Environmental Services. Agricultural Development Economics Division (ESA), FAO, Rome. www.fao.org/docrep/010/a1200e/a1200e00.htm

FAO. (2009). 'How to feed the World in 2050', Food and Agriculture Organization of the United Nations, paper prepared for How to feed the World in 2050: High-level expert forum, 12–13 October 2009, Rome

FAO. (2016) http://www.fao.org/news/story/en/item/421871/icode/

FAO. (2017). The future of food and agriculture – Trends and challenges. Rome. https://www.fao.org/3/i6583e/i6583e.pdf

FAO. (2019). Sustainable Livestock and Animal-Sourced Food in Sustainable Food and Agriculture. 225–232. Academic Press. doi:10.1016/B978-0-12-812134-4.00022-4

FAO. (2022). Global Report on Food Crises: acute food insecurity hits new highs.

Firdous, A. Sheikh. (2021). Achieving zero hunger target: innovative solutions through science and technology. In "Achieving Zero Hunger" by Z.A. Pampori. Astral International Publications, New Delhi.

Flachowsky, G. (2011). Carbon-footprints for food of animal origin, reduction potentials and research need. Journal of Applied Animal Research. 39: 2–14.

Fleming, E., Payne, J., Sweet, W., Craghan,M., Haines, J., Hart, J.F., Stiller,H., Sutton-Grier, A. (2018). *Coastal effects.* In: *Impacts, risks, and adaptation in the United States: Fourth national climate assessment, volume II* (Reidmiller,et al.(Edn.). U.S. Global Change Research Program, Washington, DC. pp. 322–352.

Gerber, P., Vellinga,T., Opio, C., Steinfeld, H. (2011). Productivity gains and greenhouse gas emissions intensity in dairy systems. Livestock Science. 139: 100–108.

Gerber, P.J., Steinfeld, H., Henderson, B., Mottet, A., Opio, C., Dijkman, J., Falcucci, A.,Tempio, G. (2013). Tackling climate change through livestock – A global assessment of emissions and mitigation opportunities. Food and Agriculture Organization of the United Nations (FAO), Rome.

Global Report on Food Crises. (2021). WFP-2021. https://www.wfp.org/publications/global-report-food-crises-2021

Global Report on food crises. (2022). FSIN and Global Network Against Food Crises. https://www.fao.org/documents/card/en/c/cb9997en/

Hare, E., Norman, H. D., Wright, J. R. (2006). Survival rates and productive herd life of dairy cattle in the United States. J. Dairy Science.89: 3713–3720

Harinder, M., Gilles, T., Valérie, H., Philippe, A. (2014).State-of-the-art on use of insects as animal feed. Animal Feed Science and Technology. 197: 1-33

Hasin. D., Z. A. Pampori., O. Aarif.,A. A. Sheikh. and I.A.Bhat.Milk production and hormonal profile as affected by fenugreek supplementation in lactating goats of Kashmir Valley.Biological Rhythm Research.52 (7): 986-993

Hristov, A. N., Oh, J., Firkins,J., Dijkstra, J., Kebreab,E., Waghorn, G., Adesogan,A., Yang,W., Tricarico,J., Lee, C., Gerber,P. J., Henderson, B., Makkar, H. P. S. (2013). Mitigation of methane and nitrous oxide emissions from animal operations: I. A review of enteric methane mitigation options. Journal of Animal Science.91:5045–5069.

LeBlanc, S. J., Lissemore,K. D., Kelton,D. F., Duffield, T. F., Leslie, K. E. (2006). Major advances in disease prevention in dairy cattle. Journal of Dairy Science.89:1267–1279.

Makkar, H. P. S. (2013). Feed and fodder challenges for Asia and the Pacific. In: Asian livestock: Challenges, opportunities and response. Proc. International policy forum, Bangkok. Thailand. www.fao.org/ docrep/017/i3166e/i3166e00.

Meeker, D.L. 2009. North American rendering-processing high quality protein and fats for feed. R Bras Zootec. 38:432–440.

Murray, J.D. and Maga, E.A. (2016). Genetically engineered livestock for agriculture: a generation after the first transgenic animal research conference. Transgenic Res. 25(3): 321-7.

Nelson, G., Rosegrant, M., Palazzo, A., Gray, I., Ingersoll, C., Robertson, R., Tokgoz, S., Zhu, T., Sulser, T., Ringler, C., Msangi, S., You, L. (2010). Food security, farming and climate change to 2050: Scenarios, results, policy options, Washington DC, www.ifpri.org/sites/default/files/publications/rr172.

Nguyen, Duc, Bach and Ly ThiBich Thuy. (2018). Current research, challenges, and perspectives of biotechnology: An Overview. VJAS. 1(2): 187-199.

Norman, H. D., Wright, J. R., Hubbard, S. M., Miller, R. H., Hutchison, J. L. (2009). Reproductive status of Holstein and Jersey cows in the United States. Journal of Dairy Science. 92:3517–3528.

OvaisAarif, Z.A. Pampori , DilrubaHasin, Aasif A Sheikh, Irfan A Bhat and J.D. ParraAccessing drop in milk production in cattle due to cold climate and subsequent nutrient amelioration in temperate Kashmir.Indian Journal of Animal Research. 54: 143-148 DOI: 10.18805/ijar.B-3760

Pampori, Z.A. (2021). Saga of Hunger in India- Challenges, Chances and Resolutions:AReview. Asian Journal of Dairy and Food Research. 40 (4): 398-407

Pampori, Z.A. (2021). Saga of hunger in India: challenges, chances and resolutions. Asian Journal of Dairy and Food Research. 40: 398-407.

Pampori, Z.A. (2022). Battle of hunger in India in "Achieving zero hunger" by by Z. A. Pampori. Astral International Publications, New Delhi.pp235-55

Pingali, P.L., Aiyar. A. and Abraham, M. (2019). Transforming food systems for rising India.Springer Nature. https://doi.org/10.1007/978-3-030-14409-8.

Prakash, B. S. (2021). Role of livestock in alleviating burden of hunger by 2030. In "Achieving Zero Huger" by Z. A. Pampori. Astral International Publications, New Delhi.

Safari,C. R., Zemlji,C. L.F., Novak, M., Dugonik, B., Bratina, B., Gubeljak, N., Bolka, S. and Strnad, S. (2020). Preparation and characterisation of waste poultry feathers composite fibreboards. Materials13:4964. Overview of child health & nutrition programme in India. pp- 95-102

Sila Deb. (2022). Overview of child health and nutrition programme in India. In "Achieving Zero Huger" by Z. A. Pampori. Astral International Publications, New Delhi.pp 95-102

Snir, A., Nadel, D., Groman-Yaroslavski, I., Melamed, Y., Sternberg, M., Bar-Yosef, O. and Weiss, E. (2015). "The Origin of Cultivation and Proto-Weeds, Long Before Neolithic Farming". PLOS ONE. 10 (7): e0131422.

Steeneveld, W., Van Der Gaag, L.C., Ouweltjes, W., Mollenhorst, H. and Hogeveen, H. (2010). Discriminating between true-positive and false-positive clinical mastitis alerts from automatic milking systems.J. Dairy Sci. 93: 2559-2568.

Steinfeld, H., Gerber, P., Wassenaar, T. D., Castel, V., Rosales, M.,de Haan, C. (2006). Livestock's long shadow: environmental issues and options. FAO.

Stephens, L., Fuller, D., Boivin, N., Rick, T., Gauthier, N., Kay, A., Marwick, B., Armstrong, C. G. and Barton, C. M. (2019). "Archaeological assessment reveals Earth's early transformation through land use". Science. 365 (6456): 897-902.

Stevenson, G. C. (1971). Plant agriculture selected and introduced by Janick Jules and others San Francisco: Freeman (1970), Cambridge University Press. pp. 246

Tahir, H. U., Sarfraz, R. A., Ashraf, A., & Adil, S. (2016). Chemical composition and antidiabetic activity of essential oils obtained from two spices (Syzygiumaromaticum and Cuminum cyminum). International journal of food properties, 19(10), 2156-2164.

Tahir, M., Hussain, T., Behaylu, A. and Tilahun, A. (2015). Scenario of present and future of solid waste generation in metro cities of India. J. Environ. Earth Sci. 5:164–170.

Tang, W.L. and Zhao, H. (2009). Industrial biotechnology: Tools and applications. Biotechnol. J. 4: 1725–1739.

The Word Bank. (2022). Moving Towards Sustainability: The Livestock Sector and the World Bank.

UN Environment Programme Data. (2021). https:// www. unenvironment. org/ explo re- topics/ resource- efficiency/ what- we- do/cities/ solid- waste-management.

van Dijk, K. C., Lesschen, J. P., Oenema, O. (2016). Phosphorus flows and balances of the European Union Member States. Science of the Total Environment. 542:1078–1093.

Vora, R. and Vishwanath, K. (2020). Say cheese, says the organised dairy sector. In "The Hindu- Bussinessline" newspaper. September-21.

Waghorn, G. C. and Hegarty, R. S. (2011). Lowering ruminant methane emissions through improved feed conversion efficiency. Animal Feed Science &. Technology. 166: 291–301.

Webb, J., Sommer, S., Kupper, T., Groenestein, K., Hutchings, N.,Eurich-Menden, B. (2012). Emissions of ammonia, nitrous oxide and methane during the management of solid manures. In Agroecology and Strategies for Climate Change, (Edn E. Lichtfouse). Springer. pp.67–107.

Wheeler, M.B. (2013).Transgenic Animals in Agriculture. Nature Education knowledge. 4(11):1

Yadav, A.K., Tomar, S. S., Amit, K.J. and Jitendra, S. (2017). Importance of molecular markers in livestock improvement: a review. International Journal of Agriculture Innovations and Research.5 (4): 2319-1473.

Zong, Y., When, Z., Innes, J. B., Chen, C.,Wang, Z. and Wang, H. (2007). "Fire and flood management of coastal swamp enabled first rice paddy cultivation in east China". Nature. 449 (7161): 459–462.

Chapter 13

"Improvement of Livestock Reproductive Health Through Manipulation of Estrous Induction/ Synchronization Protocol Under Exemplar Swing of Climate Change"

Kajal Sankar Roy

**Principal Scientist, ICAR-National Institute of Animal Nutrition and Physiology, Adugodi, Bangalore- 560 030, Karnataka, India. (*E-mail:ksroy123star@gmail.com)*

INTRODUCTION

It is well proven now that reproductive biotechnology is one of the most important tools, which can play a major role in tremendous progress of modern day livestock sector. These are estrus synchronization, artificial insemination (AI), in vitro fertilization, embryo transfer (ET), cloning, transgenesis etc. These reproductive biotechnologies have an impressive effect on the farmer's livelihood through the improvement of livestock production, preventing diseases, facilitate transportation, advancement of germplasm, conserving endangered animals and reducing economic loss. Artificial insemination in animals was originally developed to control the spread of disease, avoiding the transport of animals with potential pathogens to other animal units for mating and avoiding physical contact between individuals. The use of semen extenders containing antibiotics also helped to prevent the transmission of bacterial diseases. India has numerous world's best livestock species and breeds that provides superior germplasm throughout the world; like buffalo, indigenous cows, sheep, goat etc. In spite of being about one third in numbers compared to the cattle population, buffaloes contribute more than 50 percent of total milk production in India. India possesses about 56 % of the world buffalo population. However, a large population of buffaloes and cows remains unproductive during their productive life due to sub-estrus/anoestrus condition. The buffalo however, has certain inherent limitations which are contributing to its poor fertility. Among limitations, which are responsible for poor fertility in buffaloes include – (a) late maturity (b) poor estrus expressivity or silent estrus (c) poor conception rates (d) long post partum calving period and (e) summer infertility due to heat stress in the buffalo inhabiting areas during hot summer months, are the factors most responsible for reduced reproductive efficiency in buffaloes (Kanai and Shimizu, 1983; Prakash, 2002; Paul and Prakash,2005; Roy and Prakash,2009a,b). Various reasons have been ascribed for these limitations but no long lasting solutions have been found to solve these problems except the presently acclaimed 'Synch Protocols along with TAI'; and here we will discuss topic in details.

MAJOR PREDICAMENT IN BUFFALOES AND COWS

An accurate detection of estrus is essential in any breeding program using artificial insemination (AI) to capitalize on efficient utilization of superior sires available. As the estrus signs in buffaloes are less obvious than in cattle (Hafez, 1954; El-Sheikh and El-Fouly, 1971; Kanai and Shimizu, 1982, 1983), the accuracy of estrus detection is one of the major problems, hence limiting the use of AI in this species. Though the use of vasectomized bull (teaser) for estrus detection has solved the problem of weak estrus symptoms, but it requires labour, frequent parading of bull and its upkeep as well as time for proper heat detection. One of the main problems for improvement of buffalo production is the low reproductive efficiency. Among other factors influencing the reproductive performance, poor heat expression and seasonal breeding are the important contributory factors (Madan, 1988). Drost *et al.* (1985) reported that the estrus behaviour of buffaloes differs from that of domestic cattle in the putative lack of expression of homosexual behaviour and the secretion of copious amounts of clear estrus mucus. Swelling of the vulva, increased frequency of urination, restlessness and repeated vocalization are suggestive, though not reliable indicators of estrus. As noted by Jainudeen (1986), it has been commonly believed that 'silent estrus' (ovulation unaccompanied by estrus) is a major problem in buffalo breeding. Prakash (2002) evaluated the incidence of silent heat occurrences in buffaloes by milk progesterone monitoring of Murrah buffaloes throughout the year with an objective to study the influence of changing environmental temperatures on heat occurrences. Out of total 292 estruses recorded by milk progesterone monitoring, 108 estruses (37%) went unobserved. The incidence of silent heat was lowest in December (10.5%) while the peak was seen in April (70%). Due to the high incidence of silent heat large numbers of buffaloes are left un-bred and substantially contribute to a prolonged service period in this animal. Determination of when a buffalo is in estrus is difficult because often the animal shows few external signs of "heat". This increases the chances of missing a cycle, especially for artificial insemination. The usual weak symptoms of estrus in the normal breeding season (October to February in India) become still weaker during the hot months of summer (Prakash, 2002; Roy and Prakash, 2007a, b). Therefore, to reduce the time of estrus detection, a few estrus synchronization protocols have been devised both in cattle (Pursley, 1995; 1997a, b) as well as in buffaloes (Odde, 1990; Singh *et al.*, 2000, Paul and Prakash, 2005; Roy and Prakash, 2009a, b).

PROGRESS OF 'SYNCHRONIZATION PROTOCOL AND TIMED ARTIFICIAL INSEMINATION (TAI)' ACROSS THE WORLD

"Synchronization of estrus has been defined by Roberts (1971) as regulation of estrous cycle at will". The use of pharmacological agents to regulate the estrous cycle has helped to synchronize animals in estrus, and to allow a short period of time to study intensively the behavioral symptoms of heat among the herd.

As in many domestic species of animals, including buffaloes, the duration of estrous cycle is controlled by the life span of corpus luteum (CL) in each cycle (Odde, 1990; Singh and Madan, 1991; Singh *et al.*, 2000). Progesterone secreted by the CL imposes a block for the estrus and ovulation. Therefore, if estrus and ovulations are desired the luteal function must be terminated. With this objective, various methods for regression of CL and induction of estrus have been developed but were beset with their own advantages and disadvantages. Ideally, an estrus synchronization system should elicit a fertile, tightly synchronized estrus response in a high percentage of treated females. Methods of evaluating synchronization systems include estrus response (percentage of females showing estrus), synchronized conception rate (percentage of females conceiving) and pregnancy rates during different seasons. Enhanced precision of estrus depends on controlling the life of CL and follicular development (Fogwell *et al.*, 1986). An increase in the basic understanding as well as the development of treatment regimes to manipulate ovarian follicular growth and corpus luteum regulation over the last two decades have resulted in development of novel Ovsynch protocol (Pursley *et al.* 1995) for estrus synchronization which is based on elimination of the dominant follicle and initiation of new follicular wave followed by synchronization of ovulation and fixed-time artificial insemination. The technique has also been successfully applied for estrus synchronization and timed A.I. in lactating buffaloes and repeat breeding heifers (Paul and Prakash, 2005; Roy and Prakash, 2009a, b). Ovsynch protocol successfully produces pregnancy rates equal to those after detected estrus (cows 37.8% and heifers 35.1%, Pursley *et al.* 1997). Reproduction in buffaloes is influenced by season and fertility and is reduced in the period of the year increasing day light hours (Baruselli *et al.*, 2001;2003) due to an environmental effects on the activity of hypothalamo-hypophyseal axis (Perera, 2011). However, various studies indicated that the majority of acyclic buffaloes display variable degree of ovarian activity, characterized by follicular turn over in one or both ovaries and associated to absence of estrus signs. To rescue acyclic animals, several hormonal protocols have been employed (Saini *et al.*, 1986; Rao *et al.*, 1985; Chohan *et al.*, 1995). The estrous cycle in buffaloes can vary from 16 to 28 days (Campanile et.al, 2010) and the duration of estrus is typically 8 to 20 hours (Mohan et.al, 2010). They show waves of ovarian follicular development during estrous cycles similar to cattle, and the number of follicular waves during an estrous cycle can vary from 1 to 3, with 2 waves being the most common (Campanile et.al,2010). Ultrasonic imaging of buffalo ovaries indicates mature follicles range in size from 13 to 16 mm in diameter (Campanile et.al, 2010; Baruseli et.al, 1997, 2003; Perera, 2011; Yindee et.al., 2010). As the reproductive efficiency of buffalo is hampered by poor estrus expression, prolonged calving intervals, and delayed maturity

(Madan and Prakash,2007), understanding the expression of estrus behaviors and their relationship with the hormonal injections and associated endocrine changes that control estrus are also fundamental for the creation of strategies aimed at improving the detection of estrus and fertility improvement. It has been reported that estrogen acts as a key regulator of the endocrine and behavioral events associated with the natural estrous cycle and induces estrus behavior, the release of GnRH, an LH surge, and finally ovulation (Hafez and Hafez,2000). In India, currently, anestrous is one of the major causes of economic losses in both dairy and beef industries. To enhance the reproductive efficiency of buffaloes, during the last two decades several researchers were trying to develop the biotechniques through studying their reproductive endocrinology and ovarian function. For instance, after the development of Ovsynch and Heatsynch protocols in cattle (Pursely, et.al. 1995; Pancarci et.al., 2002; Paul and Prakash, 2005; Roy and Prakash, 2009a, b) and Mohan, et al. (2009) successfully performed the Ovsynch and Heatsynch programs in Murrah buffaloes for synchronization of ovulation and timed artificial insemination (TAI) with a range of success in pregnancy rates from 30% to 40%. Further, Cirit, et al. (2007) developed a new synchronization protocol (Doublesynch) by administration of an additional prostaglandin F2 (PGF2) 48 hour before the Ovsynch program. It has been reported that estradiol benzoate (EB) has some advantages compared with GnRH (*i.e.* cheaper hormone price, easier scheduling and implementation for injection and insemination, greater uterine tone, ease of insemination, and occurrence of estrus as has been recorded using the Heatsynch protocol (Mohan, et al., 2009; Mohan, et al.,2010; Thatcher et.al., 2002). Later, Öztürk, et al. (2010) confirmed the success of pregnancy rates (43% units more in relation to Ovsynch) of Doublesynch protocol in both cyclic and anestrus cows. The Doublesynch and Estra-Double synch protocol in both cycling and anestrus Murrah buffaloes has also been successfully performed (Mirmahmoudi and Prakash, 2012; 2014). It has been found an increase in the pregnancy rate after TAI using the Doublesynch and Estra-double synch protocol compared with AI after the spontaneous detection of estrus. This higher pregnancy rate to the high rates of ovulation detected after both the first and second GnRH treatments, that itself was owing to the high release of LH after both GnRH injections(Mirmahmoudi and Prakash,2012; 2014). Presently, in an ICAR sponsored "All India Coordinated Research Project on Nutritional and Physiological interventions for enhancing reproductive performance in animals", we are performing these 'Synch Protocols with TAI' on cows and buffaloes at twelve different centers across India. The different methods of estrus synchronization protocols utilized here are represented in schematic diagram as follows:

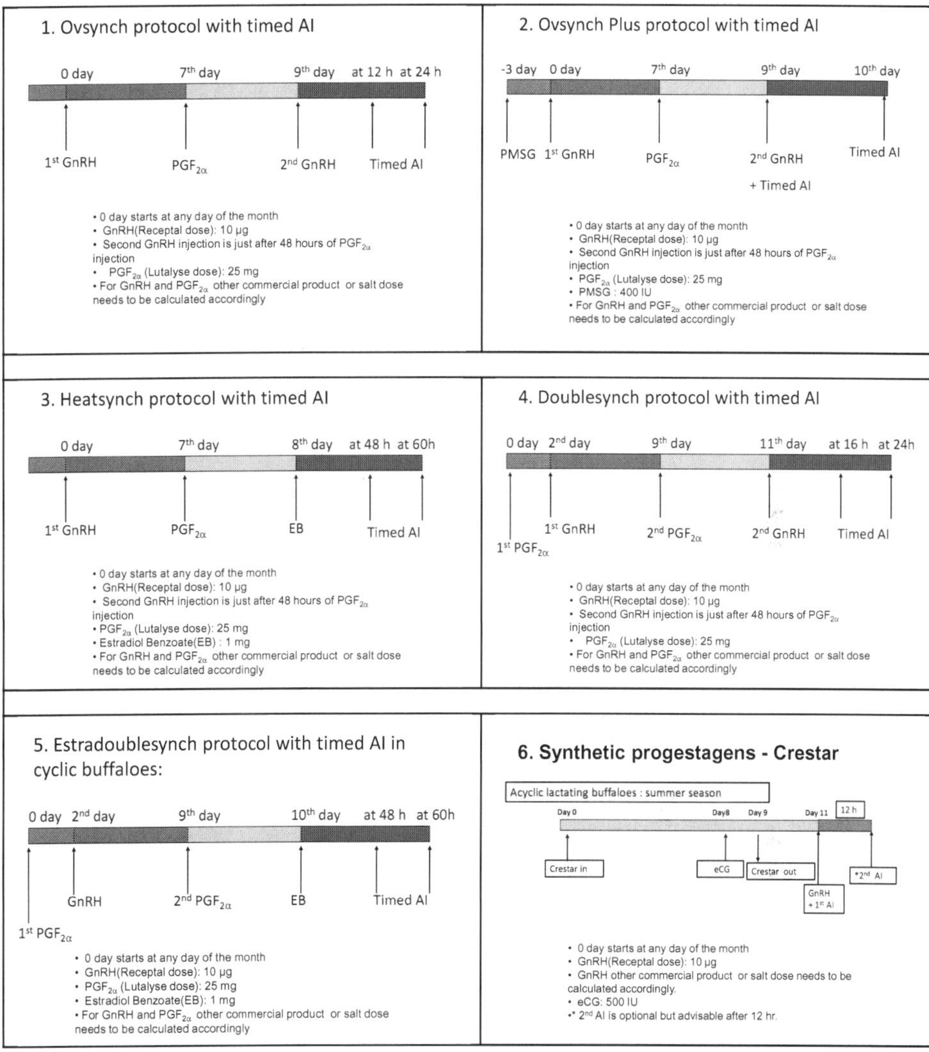

Figure : Different Synchronization Protocol presented in tabular form as ready reckoner

Development of 'Reprovardhak®' Along with 'ProKisAna Protocol' for Induction/ Synchronization of Estrous in Recent Time

The recent studies have clearly demonstrated involvement of the KISS1/ GPR54 system in the physiology and pathophysiology of the HPG axis. In our continuous study at NIANP, Bangalore, we have observed that the Kisspeptin is a very potent stimulator of GnRH secretion and mediates through negative and positive feedback mechanism of sex steroids on the brain. It is known that the two major populations of KISS1-expressing neurons located at the POA and ARC have been detected in the mammalian hypothalamus. Kisspeptin has been implicated in the regulation of puberty onset, ovarian function, fertility regulation, parturition etc. Thus, it may offer a potential treatment for reproductive disorders, characterized by low or high gonadotropins etc. The treatments for female infertility disorders often include hormone replacement (estrogen, progestin, FSH, and LH etc.) to help menstrual/estrous regulation and ovulation and/or in vitro fertilization etc. With our uninterrupted effort and hard work at our lab, a new therapeutic agent (Reprovardhak®) along with a new protocol (ProKisAna) has been developed recently with potential promise for induction of estrus in animals (Roy et al. 2021, 2022) as follows:

For small ruminants

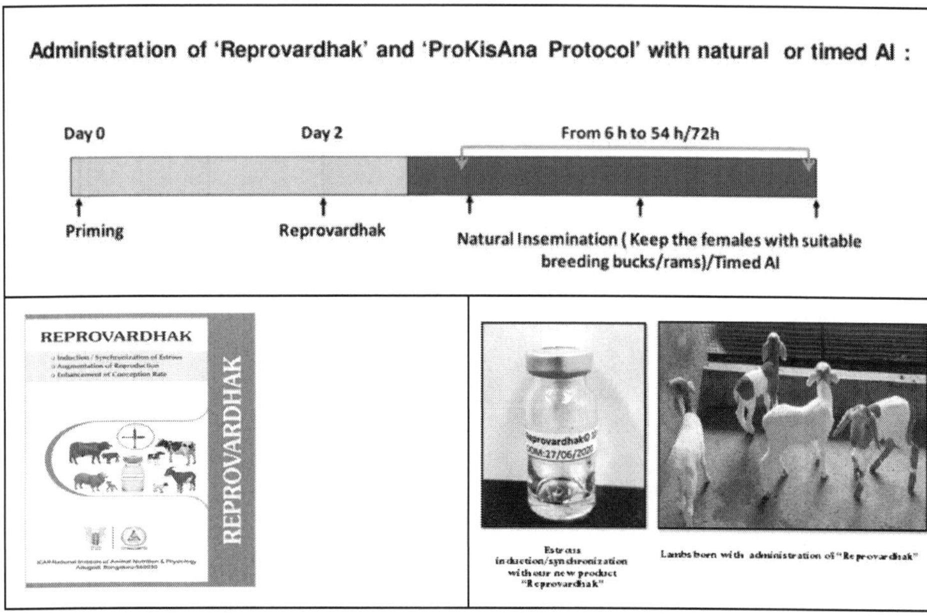

Figure 2

CONCLUSIONS

The above stated estrous synchronization protocols have been established as most effective and useful tool for reproductive management in buffalo, cattle and livestock species during different seasons across the country. However, if proper levels of nutrition, body condition and health are not maintained, the program may not be highly successful. So, necessary improvements in amenities and management may be essential before implementing an estrous synchronization program. This in turn can bring considerable and significant economic return to the dairy farmers. Further, the recently developed synthetic Kisspeptin analogue like Reprovardhak® can acts as potential therapeutic agent for induction of estrous in different animals over the existing 'Synch protocols'. However, further research is required of these newer peptides towards augmentation of reproduction and treatment of reproductive disorders.

Suggested Readings/References: Can be obtained from the author on request.

Chapter 14

Conservation, Conflict and Captivity of Wild Life in India: Role of an Animal Physiologist

[1]G. Girish Varma and [2]K. Raji

[1]*Vice Chairman, Bioengine Synergies Industries Private Ltd. & Former Faculty Dean (Dairy Science), Faculty Dean (Poultry Science), Kerala Veterinary & Animal Sciences University*

[2]*Assistant Professor, Kerala Veterinary & Animal Sciences University*

"Everyone knew there were wolves in the mountains, but they seldom came near the village - the modern wolves were the offspring of ancestors that had survived because they had learned that human meat had sharp edges."

INTRODUCTION

Human beings live in this planet earth with more than eight million other species of plants and animals. Obviously, the responsibility of protecting the globe and its environment for the future generations is largely vested in humans. Conservation of plant and animal species forms part of such a responsibility. Conservation entails *in situ* methods in all possible instances; other options such as rehabilitative and captive methods are minimal in principle and practice. Shift in priority for conservation can result from explosion of human population and shift in expansion/constriction of other flora and fauna. Interestingly, major threats such as illegal wildlife trade, habitat destruction, invasive species, pollution and climate change have serious deleterious effects on wildlife. The illegal wildlife trade ranks the fourth largest criminal industry in the world, after drugs, arms, and human trafficking.

However, the major focus of this paper confines to 'animal welfare' involved in conservation, conflict and captivity of wildlife. Recent media reports portray escalating frequency of man-animal conflict in India leading to loss of property, livelihood, and even life. Blind retaliation to check the menace would even cause extinction of the species in question. Further, increasing conflict between human and animal populations on 'physical' attributes, other than the zoonotic threat falling due to microbial etiology, poses special concern to animal scientists. Since 'function' defines an organism at its most basic level, animal physiologist, who traverses the 'function' of animals takes the first bit of the concern. Ultimately, the aim of scientists is to apply 'science' to analyze the situation, to integrate the remedies and thus to improve the protection of humans and animals through mutual benefits of coexistence.

PHYSIOLOGY OF ANIMAL ADAPTATION, THE BASIS OF ANIMAL WELFARE

Ethical concerns over the quality of life of animals compel research on animal welfare, but the paradigms and inferences of experiments vary widely (Duncan & Fraser 1997). Both empirical 'values' and operational issues may contribute to the difference.

Quality of life of animals include: (1) natural adaptations and capabilities of animals (2) experiencing normal pleasure with freedom from prolonged and intense negative feelings such as fear and pain and (3) normal bodily functions such as sound health, growth and physiological and behavioural status. However, the 'subjective' pleasure/pain aspects find little place in research because of the intrinsic limitations and the presumption of its reflections in 'measurable' parameters.

The degree of animal adaptation is challenged at three (overlapping) levels: (1) unpleasant experience that may not affect the biological function, (2) functional alterations without subjective 'feelings' (emotion, behaviour), and (3) inadequate adaptations leading to unpleasant behaviour with impairment of physiological function.

'Natural-Living' Based Concerns

Brambell (1965) and Duncan & Fraser (1997) argue that animals should have full freedom to lead its 'natural' life, even without tethering, housing, and man-induced management. On the other hand, Rollin (1993) proposed the concept of 'telos' (defined as the inherent, genetically encoded 'nature' of a species and advocated that welfare ensured when an animal be allowed to live in accordance with its telos.

'Feelings-Based' Boncerns

'Feelings-based' concerns emphasises the affective experience of the animal. Animals should experience comfort, contentment and pleasure avoiding prolonged or intense pain, fear, hunger and other negative states.

'Functioning-Based' Boncerns

This view has been propagated by farmers and veterinarians, allowing special importance to health and the 'normal' functioning of the animal's biological systems. Thus, Sainsbury (1986) promoted protection of animal health as a duty and Taylor (1972) argued for shelter, nutrition and health care as advantages that would compensate for keeping animals in confinement.

Resource-Based and Animal-Based Indicators in Issues of Animal Welfare

There are different approaches in assessing animal welfare and resolving them. Resource-based approach focuses on the environment (such as water, food, shelter, space) of the animal for diagnosis of welfare breach. In animal-based methods tha major attention is given to the animal as an individual or in its group or cluster. In fact, both are mutually complementary in nature.

ROLE OF ANIMAL BEHAVIOR AND MANAGEMENT

Animal behaviour is all about how the animal interacts with itself and its environment. Genes influence animal morphology, physiology and behaviour. Genes will also influence animals' learning, and thus its ability to cope with new challenges. Animals have evolved to perform definite repertoire of behaviours that help them cope and thrive in specific environments. This is called behavioural adaptation.

In practical point of view, behaviour study offers the first line of evaluation of animal welfare. Emotional state of the animal will affect its reaction and behaves in any situation. Social situations will also impact animal behaviour. Frustrated/ depressed animals react and respond differently to those experiencing feelings of contentment or pleasure. Animal behaviour is also influenced by its motivational state. Encouraging natural and normal behaviour is vital for both good physical and mental health of animals. Good behavioural management is providing with the space, environment and resources and giving animals' choice so that they can feel in control of their own environment.

The environment, and especially the perinatal environment, can influence animal development, physiology and health and have long-term impacts on animal behaviour. Different species will be genetically designed in accordance with their characteristic telos. These behaviours will persist, even in a captive setting.

PHYSIOLOGICAL INDICATORS

Physiological measures can also provide useful information on the welfare of animals. The most commonly used physiological indicators are those that measure the hypothalamic-pituitary-adrenal (HPA) axis activity, because the stress response involves the activation of the HPA axis, which in turn results in an increased secretion of glucocorticoids. Concentration of cortisol, corticosterone or its metabolites is used to measure the stress response and, therefore, to assess animal welfare. The concentration of glucocorticoids can be measured in various biological samples, plasma, saliva, faeces and hair or feather being the most commonly samples used in zoo animals. Other physiological measures such as oxytocin concentration, telomere length, heterophil:lymphocyte ratio and acute phase proteins are also used as welfare indicators. Prolactin also has been implicated in affective emotions and orientation of animals.

WELFARE OF CAPTIVE WILDLIFE

Major Steps

Association of Zoos and Aquariums (AZA), has worked to create species-specific animal care manuals that describe best practices for keeping various species of wild animals in captivity.

Captive breeding programs and the Species Survival Plan are used to help assure perpetuation of species, especially endangered species. Some species have successfully been reintroduced into protected environment. Other species may never be able to be reintroduced safely into their original habitat.

Environmental enrichment is helping animals fully express species-specific behavioural repertoire, thereby providing environmental stimuli necessary for optimal physical and emotional wellbeing. It can encourage natural behaviours by providing them the power and perception of choice. It is not a substitute for poor management or enclosure design or substandard care.

Indigenous/traditional knowledge systems (of tribal/aboriginal people) can be relied for understanding (wild) animal welfare, managing them including treatment for ailments.

Rehabilitation of totally wild or captive wild animals may be attempted as individual animals, or in appropriate groups (1) pair - sexual partners, social partners, etc. (2) family (3) complementary - mutualistic, comensalistic, competitive and parasitic (4) comprehensive - several species together.

Resource mapping, Resource assurance/ simulations (real and virtual) are certain other measures to be considered.

CONCLUSION

Captive animal husbandry and welfare practice require more realistic research at gross and micro levels, under discrete and integrated paradigms, and with legislative and judiciary implications. Just for instance, positive effects of enrichment on the welfare of animals, not limited to captive wildlife, have to be explored.

REFERENCES

Brambell F W R 1965 Report of the Technical Committee to Enquire into the Welfare of Animals kept under Intensive Livestock Husbandry Systems. Her Majesty's Stationery Office: London, UK

Duncan I J H and Fraser D 1997 Understanding animal welfare. In: Appleby M C and Hughes B O (eds) Animal Welfare pp 19-31. CAB International: Wallingford, UK

Fraser, D., Weary, D.M., Pajor, E.A. and Milligan, B.N. (1997) A Scientific Conception of Animal Welfare that Reflects Ethical Concerns. Animal welfare, 6, 187-205

Rollin B E 1993 Animal welfare, science, and value. Journal of Agricultural and Environmental Ethics 6. Supplement 2: 44-50

Sainsbury D 1986 Farm Animal Welfare. Cattle, Pigs and Poultry. Collins: London, UK

Taylor G B 1972 One man's philosophy of welfare. Veterinary Record 91: 426-428

Chapter 15

Technological Interventions Employed in the Poultry Farms for Increased Production

Azmat Alam Khan and Henna Hamadani
Sher-e-Kashmir University of Agricultural Sciences and Technology of Kashmir, Srinagar, Jammu and Kashmir

INTRODUCTION

Poultry sector is growing at a tremendous pace both nationally as well globally. It plays an important role in national economy. The revenue of the poultry industry in India has increased over 30% to Rs. 2,500 billion in FY 2022-23. In six years ending 2020-21, egg production grew by 7.6% CAGR. Poultry sector is expected to grow at a CAGR of over 8 per cent to reach $35 billion in the next five years. This growth is predicted to be driven by demographics, changing food habits and increasing urban incomes. With increased growth, the industry is getting more and more organised.

Factors like growing population along with rise in per capita income and fall in real poultry prices are further expanding this industry. Both egg and meat industries have registered significant growth. The poultry sector has undergone a paradigm shift in structure and operation over the years with sizeable investments in selection, breeding, hatching, rearing and processing technologies.

Indian poultry is self-sufficient, supported by a broad and strong genetic base. India ranks third in egg production and fifth in meat production. The population has increased from 729.2 million in 2012 as per the 19th Livestock Census to 851.81 million in 2019 according to the 20th Livestock Census, thereby showing an increase of 16.8% over the previous census.

The annual egg production is 94.2 billion eggs approximately with an average growth rate of 6% and the annual poultry meat production is reported to be 3.78 million tons with a growth rate of 8-10% according to the Basic Animal Husbandry

Statistics. In India, the annual per capita availability of egg is only 74 eggs and meat is only 2.8 kg which is far less than in developed countries where the per capita availability of eggs is 240 eggs and that of meat is 20 Kg indicating a huge gap and the need for further improvement of poultry production. There is a need to improve the efficiency of production, quality of eggs and meat and the health and welfare of poultry.

Many economically important traits like egg-production, livability, growth-rate, feed-efficiency, disease resistance, and meat and egg quality have been improved by employing modern technologies. Improvements have been seen in the layer and broiler components of poultry industry. The technologies used are such that they promote higher rate and persistency of egg production, better egg size, feed efficiency, egg quality (external as well as internal) and livability in layers and enhanced muscle mass, growth rate, carcass quality, livability and feed efficiency in broilers. Value addition and easy traceability are some additional advantages of integrating technology in poultry industry. New technologies used in different areas of poultry production are discussed in this chapter.

AUTOMATIC ENVIRONMENT CONTROL

It is necessary to monitor and maintain the environment inside the poultry sheds. The sheds in which the poultry birds are living should have the right temperature and relative humidity so they feel comfortable. An optimum environmental condition inside the sheds improves the growth and health of birds. With the increasing availability of advanced automation systems, farmers can achieve the right climate inside their poultry sheds. Having the right measuring instruments in the sheds is crucial for creating the optimum climatic conditions. The automatic systems need to balance heating, cooling and ventilation. This can be done on the basis of temperature, relative-humidity and negative pressure inside the poultry houses. As the house temperature fluctuates, the automatic controller switches the brooders or fans on as per the requirement. Now-a-days the level of carbon dioxide and ammonia inside the poultry farm can also be monitored with the help of specially designed equipment for the same. In environmentally controlled houses a monitoring and control system should provide easy-to-use scheduling of lights. A system than can pre-program lighting schedules over the life of the flock is very useful for management. It is also important to provide the desired intensity of light. The controller operates brooders, fans, inlet machines, curtain machines, evaporative cooling systems and lights. Many controllers also allow house conditions to be monitored remotely as well with the help of internet.

Full genetic potential of broilers cannot be achieved unless the proper environment is maintained in the broiler house. The fast growing, modern broiler lines are more dependent on proper environmental conditions than birds from lines raised just a few years ago. Maintaining proper temperature to promote efficient growth is key to profitable broiler production. Chicks are not able to completely maintain their body temperature until approximately 14 days of age. During this time, it is crucial that room temperature is maintained between 85-90 degrees F with minimum variation.

For controlled-environment housing of layers, multi-tier cage systems are common. Most large-scale commercial farms use controlled-environment systems to provide the ideal thermal environment for the birds. The performance of poultry birds in controlled-environment sheds is reported to be generally superior to those reared in naturally ventilated houses, as the conditions can be maintained in the birds' thermal comfort zone. Achieving the ideal environment for birds depends on appropriate management of the poultry house. It has been reported that although the investment cost per bird is higher in EC housing system but the returns are also higher due to higher standards of production and lower mortality.

Fire Detection and Control System

There can be sometime an outbreak of fire in the poultry farms due to power failure or any other thing which can lead to huge losses to the farmer. In order to control such incidents, fire and smoke detectors can be employed in the farms. Smoke detectors can detect alarms and alert the farmers via siren, bell or even a message. Fire detectors can activate the fire extinguishers in extreme situations.

Odour Control System

Intelligent systems have been developed for measuring odours in the poultry farms. The system consists of gas humidity and temperature sensor. The gas sensors were specifically selected for detecting odours in the poultry farms. Once odours are detected in the farm, necessary control measures like activation of exhaust fans and other things are taken.

AUTOMATIC FEEDING AND WATERING

With a decrease in the availability of labour and a rise in labour costs, automatic feeding is the need of the hour since feeding operation is a routine task at farms which cannot be delayed or avoided at any cost. This especially needed for large farms with the capacity of more than 4000 birds. Automatic feeding system are used both in broiler and breeder farms. Such systems focus on high feed conversion ratio & negligible feed wastage in broiler farms and in the breeder farms they target accurate feeding & ease of use for the farmers. Automatic feed control developed by various companies consists of a silo weighing system which automatically sends the right amount of feed from the silo to the hoppers in the poultry house. The amount of feed is determined based on the number of grams per animal per day. To accurately determine the amount of feed in the silo, weighing cells are used under the silo. This gives an insight of the daily feed consumption by birds and the status of the remaining feed in store.

Alarm System

Modern poultry rearing can be automatized to increasing efficiency and optimize performance, but this is entirely dependent on electricity and the proper operation of modern equipment. It is difficult for a poultry farmer to be present all the time at the farm. Therefore, it is important to have an alarm system installed to alert the farmer of the power failure or any other problem at the farm. While the system may not rectify the problem on its own, its main purpose is to get someone into the farm for assessing and addressing the problem. Alarms are used to notify if there is loss of power or if the house internal temperature gets too high or too low in relation to the desired temperature. The alarm system can either activate a bell, located at the facility, to alert anyone close by or send a message to the farm manager's cell phone if he is away from the farm. In the case of power shutdowns, emergency generators or backups systems can be activated automatically for ventilation, feeding and watering systems to prevent losses. The emergency generator should have the capability of automatic power switch-over and be capable of delivering service for extended periods of time to operate the systems mentioned above.

Chapter 16

Herbal Galactogogues-A Way to Ameliorate Milk Production in Dairy Animals

O Aarif, D Hasin, Z A Pampori, F Shah, A A Sheikh, M R Dar, U Ali, N Amin and S Shafi

Division of Veterinary Physiology, Sher-e-Kashmir University of Agricultural Sciences and Technology, Srinagar, India

INTRODUCTION

Optimal milk production is the key requirement in the management of dairy economics. The demand for the supply of milk and milk products is growing at a much faster rate than the supply. Milk production per animal in developing countries is still very low as compared to world's average. This lower productivity might be attributed to many factors including the genetic and environmental factors such as non-availability of good quality feed resources, poor husbandry management practices and the small-scale dairy production units.

Galactogogues are substances used to induce, maintain, and increase milk production in animal dairy industry. Phyto-pharmacological research on natural products can show a ray of hope for the discovery of new active compounds with novel structure which have potential to serve as a natural lead compound for development of new galactogogues. Majority of these herbal preparations have however not been scientifically, systematically and thoroughly evaluated, but their traditional use suggests some safety and efficacy.

PHARMACOLOGICAL OVERVIEW OF GALACTOGOGUES

Galactogogues elicit pharmacological effects, resulting in increased prolactin concentration through interactions with dopamine receptors and thereby augmenting milk supply. Commercially available synthetic drugs induce adverse effect on the neuro-endocrine axis of lactation physiology. Their prolonged uses have caused toxicity which opens a detrimental platform to normal health status of both human and animals. So the researchers have developed a keen interest in traditional herbs, because these are easily available, cheap and with a hope that they may not leave any toxic residues in milk. Phytopharmacological research on natural products can contribute for the discovery of new active compounds with novel structures which may serve as a lead for the development of new galactogogues. Although majority of these herbal preparations have not been evaluated their traditional use suggests that they are safe and effective.

As many herbal plants contain large number of chemical active principles, having galactogenic properties; can be used as herbal medicine for letting-down of milk in milch animals. Among these, Fenugreek (Trigonellafoenumgraecum), Fennel (Foeniculumvulgare), Raspberry leaf/Red Raspberry (Rubusidaeus), Nettle (Urticadioica), and Nettle leaf (Utica urens), Blessed thistle (Cnicusbenedictus), Chaste berry (Vitexagnus-castus), Alfalfa (Medicago sativa), Black cohosh (Cimicifugaresebosa), Dil (Anethumgraveolens), Goat's Rue (Galegaofficianalis), Milk thistle (Silybummarianum), Giant Cane (Arundodonax), Abuta or LaghuPatha (Cissampelospareira), and extracts of Bhringraj or false daisy (Eclipta alba), Ashwagandha and Shatavari (Asparagus racemosus) plant ingredients have been emphasized in Ayurveda to induce lactogenesis and lactation. So, a thorough, critical and scientific evaluation is necessary to include theses herbs as potent herbal galactogogues.

An effective nutritional regimen and use of herbal galactogogues act synergistically to enhance milk yield which would prompt a good augmentation in productivity of dairy herd. Herbal galactogogues act through interactions with dopamine receptors by exerting an influence through adreno-hypothalamo-hypophysealgonadal axis resulting in enhanced prolactin concentration and thereby augmenting milk production.

There exists a further need to deepen the horizon of research on the phytochemical composition of the herbs, their mode of action, and furthermore to assess the lethal dose as well as explain how further studies might be conducted to bridge the gap between common uses and lack of studies on the safety and effectiveness of these herbs in lactation. Hence, an optimal standardization and dosing recommendations of these herbal galactogogues by an explicit clarification in pre-clinical and clinical studies through in-vitro and in-vivo experimentations is needed before they are being harvested as a potential new drug in the market.

PHYSIOLOGY BEHIND HERBAL GALACTOGOGUES

Galactogogues are medications that aid in initiating, maintaining, and augmenting of adequate milk production. The term galactogogue refers to substances that augment established lactation, whereas the term galactopoietic is used independently to describe the hormone preparations which enhance milk production in an animal already in lactation (Asimo and Krouze, 1991).

Galactogogues may be synthetic, plant-derived or endogenous products. They act through exerting an influence on adreno-hypothalamo-hypophyseal-gonadal axis by blocking hypothalamic dopaminergic receptors or by inhibiting dopamine producing neurons. These medications increase prolactin secretion by antagonizing dopamine receptors (Gabay, 2002).

Herbs and their preparations have multiple diverse useful actions on the human and animal health. The advantages of herbal medicines are due to constituent chemicals developed as a result of co-evolution between flora and fauna and their enzyme driven synthesis leading to development of optically pure chiral molecules with specific reactions in the mammalian body (Behera et al., 2013)

Milk production (lactogenesis), which is a consequence of neuro-endocrine event, is a complex neurophysiological process that involves interaction of a number of physical and emotional factors along with action of multiple hormones, mainly prolactin. During parturition and expulsion of the placenta, progesterone concentration reduced resulting in initiation of full milk supply (Neville et al., 2001). Dopamine agonists and antagonists regulate prolactin synthesis and secretion through interaction with the hypothalamus and anterior pituitary and thereby control milk production (Behera et al., 2013). Thereafter, prolactin levels gradually decrease but milk supply is maintained or increased by local feedback mechanisms (Lawrence and Lawrence, 1999).

FEEDING TRIAL OF FENUGREEK IN GOATS

Hasin et al., 2019 conducted a feeding trial on lactating goats in Mountain Research Centre for Sheep and Goat (MRCSG), SKUAST Kashmir during the winter season. The lactating Bakarwal goats with uniform body weight and milk production were divided into two groups, namely, control and treatment. The goats in the treatment group were offered 30 g of fenugreek daily in addition to the normal feed ingredients. The blood and milk samples were collected weekly up to 6 weeks, and the data were presented as an average. There was a significant ($p < 0.05$) decrease in plasma cortisol concentration in treatment (18.64 ± 1.72 ng/ml) as compared to control (22.58 ± 1.25 ng/ml) group. Thyroid stimulating hormone (TSH) showed a non significant increase in the treatment group (0.45 ± 0.03 µIU/ml) as compared to the control group (0.39 ± 0.05 µIU/ml). Prolactin was significantly ($p < 0.05$) higher in the supplemented group (3.94 ± 0.03 ng/ml) than the control group (2.72 ± 0.02 ng/ml). Blood glucose was significantly ($p < 0.05$) higher in control (57.30 ± 3.40 mg/dl) than the treatment (53.52 ± 2.79 mg/dl) group. Milk components like fat, protein, lactose, solids not fat (SNF) and total solids showed a non significant change after fenugreek supplementation. Finally, there was a drastic increase in the milk production of the supplemented group (559.00 ± 17.29 ml/day) than their counterparts (407.00 ± 23.59 ml/day). From the study, it could be concluded that fenugreek supplementation alters the hormone profile, enhances feed intake and thereby increases the milk production in lactating goats.

EFFECT OF HERBAL GALACTOGOGUE ON MILK PRODUCTION

Fenugreek supplementation leads to an increase in milk fat and proteins and a decrease in milk SNF, total solids and lactose. Ovais et al. (2019) observed that fenugreek supplementation (200 gms/day/cow) increased milk production from (4.48±0.21 kg/cow) in to (6.41±0.53 kg/cow). Shah and Mir (2004) reported that feeding fenugreek seeds improved the profile of functional fatty acids in the milk and could be tried in dairy animals to improve milk characteristics. Kholif and Abd El (2001) reported a non significant effect of fenugreek feeding on milk lactose. Tanwar et al. (2008), Baig and Bhagwat (2009) and Patel et al. (2013) showed a non significant effect of herbal supplementation on milk composition in dairy animals. Balgees et al. (2013), showed a decline in milk fat after incorporation of 10% and 15% fenugreek seeds in the ration of Nubian goats. Increase in the milk yield might be due to prolactin release from adenohypophysis (Balgees et al. 2013). The rise in prolactin hormone represents a possible endocrine mechanism for the galactopoietic action of fenugreek, the release of which may be due to phytoestrogens in the herb. Sayed et al. (2005) found a chemical compound, Diosgenin, similar to estrogen which promotes mammary gland development and improves milk flow. There is still further research needed to unravel the mechanism by which fenugreek exerts its effect on milk production.

Olivo et al. (2005) in agro-forestry production systems reported an increase of 9 to 11.5 kg of milk with the utilization of plant extract herbals. This may be related to the essential oils present in the herbal mixture used. In order to restore the animal productivity and to optimize the milk production in individual animals for better profits, various drugs, herbal preparations, hormones, mineral supplements and feed additives have been tried with variable results (Ramesh et al., 2000). Singhal (1995) observed 30.1% increase in milk yield of Payapro fed cows. Qureshi (1999) not only observed an increase in milk yield but also an increase in the fat percentage of milk in dairy cows fed with Lectovet (a herbal combination). Galactin a non-hormonal herbal preparation significantly enhanced the milk production in dairy cows and ultimately improved the dairy economics (Kumari & Akbar, 2006). Herbal preparations have also been shown to relieve the heat stress in dairy cows and ultimately improve their productivity (Zhang et al., 2007). Kolte et al. (2008) reported that indigenous herbal preparations effectively restored the altered milk constituents and increased the milk production in cows with sub-clinical mastitis.

EFFECT OF HERBAL GALACTOGOGUE ON BODY WEIGHT

Nallathambi et al. (2016) reported that supplementation of fenugreek seed at 10 g/day to lactating ewes resulted in a better growth rate of lambs. The higher body weight is more likely due to an increase in the feed intake. Similar trends were observed in poultry fed different herbal extracts (Tamara et al. 2009). Fenugreek seeds contain an active principal trigonelline which is a potent appetite stimulant, which increases feed intake and consequently the body weight (Kamel 2008). Feeding fenugreek seeds promotes appetite and feed intake (Attalmanan et al. 2013). Similarly, Srinivasan (2005) reported that fenugreek enhances the synthesis of bile acids in the liver and their excretion in the bile, which improves digestion and absorption of fats. This may increase feed intake and the body weight. An increase in body weight due to fenugreek supplementation may be attributed to a growth hormone (GH) secretagogue, Diocin, structurally similar to estrogen which stimulates GH secretion by binding to pituitary cell receptors that recognize GH-RH (releasing hormone) and thus, in turn, results in an increase in body weight and milk production (Graham et al. 2008). Fenugreek-induced feed intake is related to its ability to increase insulin sensitivity by interfering with intestinal glucose absorption.

EFFECT OF HERBAL GALACTOGOGUE ON HORMONE AND METABOLIC PROFILE

A decline in cortisol indicates an alleviation of lactation-induced stress in the fenugreek supplemented dairy goats. It reflects that hypothalamic pituitary adrenal (HPA) axis is not stimulated to an extent that leads to a sharp increase in adrenocorticotropic hormone (ACTH) and hence the plasma cortisol. The herbs help to increase the resistance of the animals' different stress factors, causing a decline in cortisol and increase in the absorption of essential nutrients, thus improving the growth of the animals (Windisch et al. 2008). Ovais et al. (2019) observed that fenugreek supplementation increased prolactin and Growth hormone whereas cortisol concentration decreased in lactating dairy cows. A rise in TSH in fenugreek supplemented goats may be due to a decrease in plasma T3. Lower T3 levels are due to inhibition of the peripheral conversion of T4 to T3 in the extra thyroidal tissues in the fenugreek supplemented group (Panda et al. 1999). With respect to the blood glucose, Al-Janabi and Ahmed (2012) reported a decline in the blood glucose in the fenugreek fed goats. Interestingly, streptozocin-induced diabetic rats showed decreased serum glucose when fed with fenugreek seeds (Eidi et al. 2007). On the other hand, some studies showed a rise in blood glucose in fenugreek fed buffaloes (Abo El-Nor et al. 2007). A decline in blood glucose can be attributed to enhance glucose partitioning towards the mammary gland to fulfill the demand of higher milk production. Fenugreek supplementation stimulates the release of insulin which leads to the uptake of glucose by the cells and hence the hypoglycemia (Baquer et al. 2009). Fenugreek seeds contain an amino acid called 4-hydroxy isoleucine, which acts on pancreatic beta cells to enhance insulin production. Contrary to this, some studies reveal that fenugreek seeds delay gastric emptying and suppress glucose transport due to higher pectin content in them. The reduced gastric emptying decelerates carbohydrate absorption (Gupta et al. 2001) and hence hypoglycemia. Further, a decline in glucose level is due to a modulation of glucose-metabolizing enzymes that control gluconeogenesis processes (Devi et al. 2003).

CONCLUSION

Herbal galactogogues have potential to increase milk production in dairy animals and are in veterinary practice since decades. There is a need to deepen the horizon of research on the phytochemical composition of the herbs, their mode of action, and furthermore to assess the lethal dose so that there will not be any health issues after their use in dairy animals.

REFERENCES

Abo El-Nor SAH, Khattab HM, Al-Alamy HA, Salem FA, Abdou MM. 2007. Effect of some medicinal plants seeds in the rations on the productive performance of lactating buffaloes. Intern J Dairy Sci. 2(4):348–355.

Al-Janabi AK, Ahmed F. 2012. Feeding effects of fenugreek seeds (Tringonella foenum-graceum) on lactation performance, some serum constituents and prolactin hormone level in Damascus crossbred goats. Diyala Agric Sci J. 4(1):1–8

Asimov, D. and Krouze, H. (1991) Composition and somatic cell count of milk in conventional and agro-ecological farm, Brazil. *Livest.Res.RuralDev.* 17: 1734-1740

Attalmanan BA, Jame MN, Rahamatalla AS, Amasaib E, Mahala GA. 2013. Effect of fenugreek (Trigonella foenum graecum) seeds supplementaion on feed intake, some metabolic hormones profile and milk yield of Nubian goats. J Anim Sci. 7:1–5.

Baig MI, Bhagwat VG. 2009. Study of the efficacy of Galactin Vet Bolus on milk yield in dairy cows. Vet World. 2(4):140–142

Balgees A, Atta E, Nuha MJ, Ramhatalla SA, Amasiab EO, Mahala AG. 2013. Effect of fenugreek (Tringonella foenum graecum) seeds supplementation on feed intake, some metabolic hormones profile, milk yield and milk composition of Nubian goat. Res J Anim Sci. 7(1):1–5

Baquer NZ, Taha A, Kumar P, McLean P, Cowsik SM, Kale RK, Singh R, Sharma D. 2009. A metabolic and functional overview of brain aging linked to neurological disorders. Biogerontology. 10:377–413

Behera, P. C., Tripathy, D. P. and Parija, S. C. (2013) Shatavari: Potentials for galactogogue in dairy cows. *Indian J.Tradit.Know.* 12(1): 9-17.

Devi BA, Kamalakkannan N, Prince PS. 2003. Supplementation of fenugreek leaves to diabetic ratseffect on carbohydrate metabolic enzymes in diabetic liver and kidney. Phytother Res. 17:1231– 1233. doi:10.1002/ptr.1357

Dilruba Hasin, Zahoor Ahmad Pampori, Aasif Ahmad Sheikh, Ovais Aarif, Irfan Ahmad Bhat & Muzamil Abdullah. 2019. Milk production and hormonal profile as affected by Fenugreek supplementation in lactating goats of Kashmir valley. Biological rhythm research https://doi.org/10.1080/09291016.2019.1608732

Eidi A, Eidi M, Sokhteh M. 2007. Effect of fenugreek (Trigonella foenum-graecum) seeds on serum parameters in normal and streptozotocin-induced diabetic rats. Nutrition Res. 27:728–733

Gabay, M. P. (2002) Galactagogues: medication that induce lactation. *J.Hum.Lact.* 18: 274–279.

Graham MR, Baker JS, Evans P, Kicman A, Cowan D, Hullin D, Thomas N, Davies B. 2008. Physical effects of short-term recombinant human growth hormone administration in abstinent steroid dependency. Horm Res Paediatr. 69:343–354.

Gupta A, Gupta K, Lai B. 2001. Effect of Trigonella foenum-graecum (fenugreek) seeds on glycemic control and insulin resistance in type 2 diabetes mellitus: a double blind placebo controlled study. J Assoc Physicians India. 49:1057–1061

Kamel C. 2008. Natural plant extracts: classical medies bring modern animal production solutions. Geneva (Switzerland): CIHEAM, Cahiers Options Mediterranéennes. http://ressources.ciheam. org/om/pdf/c54/01600008.

Kholif AM, Abd El G. 2001. Medical plant seeds supplementation of lactating goats' diets and its effect on milk and cheese quantity and quality. Egypt J Dairy sci. 29:139–150.

Lawrence, R.A. and Lawrence, R. M. (1999) Breast feeding: A guide for medical profession, 5th edition. St. Louis, Osby. p 62-64

Nallathambi B, Purushothaman MR, Nagarajan M, Natarajan A. 2016. Supplementation of fenugreek seeds to lactating ewes and effect on growth performance of pre-weaned twin lambs. J Anim Res. 6(3):543–545

Neville, Mc., Morton, J. and Unemura, S. (2001) Lactogenesis Transition from pregnancy to lactation. *Ped. Clin.North.* Am. 48: 45-52.

Ovais Aarif, Z.A. Pampori, Dilruba Hasin, Aasif A Sheikh, Irfan A Bhat and J.D. Parra. 2018. Accessing drop in milk production in cattle due to cold climate and subsequent nutrient amelioration in temperate Kashmir. Indian J. Anim. Res, DOI: 10.18805/ijar.B-3760

Panda S, Tahiliani PKA. 1999. Inhibition of triiodothyronine production by fenugreek seed extract in mice and rats. Pharmacol Res. 40:405–409. doi:10.1006/phrs.1999.0510

Patel MD, Tyagi KK, Sorathiya LM, Fulsoundar AB. 2013. Effect of polyherbal galactogogues supplementation on milk yield and quality as well as general health of Surti buffaloes of south Gujarat. Vet World. 6(4):214–218

Sayed MAM, Azoz AA, El-Mahdy AA, Adel-Khalek AM. 2005. Some performance aspects of doe rabbits fed diets supplemented with fenugreek seed and aniseed. Dokki (Egypt): Animal production Research Institute

Shah MA, Mir PS. 2004. Effect of dietary fenugreek seed on dairy cow performance and milk characteristics. Can J Anim Sci. 84:725–729

Srinivasan K. 2005. Spices as influencers of body metabolism: an overview of three decades of research. Food Res Int. 38:77–86.

Tamara F, Mojca V, Janez S, Vida R. 2009. Use of herbs and spices and their extracts in animal nutrition. Acta Agri Slovenica. 94(2):95–102.

Tanwar PS, Rathore SS, Yogendra K. 2008. Effect of shatavari (Asparagus recemosus) on milk production in dairy animals. Indian J Anim Res. 42(3):232–233.

Windisch W, Schedle K, Plitzner C, Kroismayer A. 2008. Use of phytogenetic products as feed additives for swine and poultry. J Ani Sc. 86:E140–E148.

Chapter 17

Insulin Resistance in Dairy Ruminants: Mechanism, Assessment and Amelioration

Sandhya S Chaudhary and Virendra Kumar Singh
Department of Veterinary Physiology and Biochemistry College of Veterinary Science and A.H., Kamdhenu University, Navsari (Gujarat)
sandhyachaudhary@kamdhenuuni.edu.in, virendrasingh@kamdhenuuni.edu.in

As per the data by Animal Husbandry Statistics (AHS) Division of Department of Animal Husbandry & Dairying (DAHD) released on 15th March 2023, total milk production registered an annual growth rate of 5.29% in the country from 209.96 (2020-21) to 221.06 million tones (2021-22). Per capita availability of milk in India has risen by 33.33% from 333 gm/day (2015-16) to 444 gm/day (2021-22). The gross value addition from milk at current basic prices at 931969 crores (2020-21) that is much higher (184.33%) than that of 327767 crores (2011-12). The number of milch animals has also increased 8.47% from 180155 (2012) to 195406 (2019) (Basic Animal Husbandry Statistics-2022). These statistics hint towards the increasing demand for milk production and indirectly highlights the need and urge of optimizing the dairy livestock health that are utilized for milk production.

TRANSITION PERIOD LEADING TO INSULIN RESISTANCE

Major milch species comprise different breeds of cattle breed (Indian, exotic, cross-bred), buffaloes and goats. Physiologically it is important for cyclic processes of reproduction and production to continue optimally to maximize milk production performance. However, the period spanning parturition (pregnancy to lactation) is referred as transition period (-3 weeks to +3 weeks of parturition) is the most critical to be taken care of as it is they are quite stressful and difficult to cope with. This mainly is due to advanced gestation when high demand exists by developing fetus prepartum and during early lactation in postpartum phase where in high demand is from milk biosynthesis that is featured by reduced feed (DMI) intake, high energy demand, stress of parturition and increasing milk yield (during early lactation). Metabolic derangements during this period directly and indirectly affect milk production. Direct losses may be observed in immediate lactation cycle with lowered milk yield and indirect losses may manifest as vulnerability of female animals to increased incidences of metabolic diseases like ketosis, infectious diseases like mastitis and long-term problems that may arise during future productive life span. To prevent this gravid uterus with developing fetus and lactating mammary gland are privileged for diversion of maternal energy towards themselves through preferential energy partitioning. This is physiologically-accomplished by reducing insulin-mediated uptake in body tissues and making glucose available for insulin mediated uptake in mammary gland. Thus, the need arises for development of insulin resistance.

INSULIN AND ITS MAJOR PHYSIOLOGICAL EFFECTS

Insulin hormone is a polypeptide containing 51 amino acids arranged in 2 chains (A&B). Chain A contains 21 amino acids and chain B has 30 amino acids that are linked by disulphide bonds. Biosynthesis of insulin occurs as pre-proinsulin that is converted to proinsulin and finally it is converted to insulin and C-peptide that gets stored in secretary granules which is released as and when it is required.

De Koster and Opsomer (2013) have reviewed the studies on major effects of insulin that comprise of stimulation of glycogenesis, synthesis of triglycerides and proteins, glycolysis, as well as suppression of gluconeogenesis, glycogenolysis, ketogenesis, degradation of proteins in liver; stimulation of glucose uptake, ketone body utilization, synthesis of protein, glycogenesis, glycolysis as well as suppression of degradation of protein, glycogenolysis in skeletal muscle; stimulation of uptake of glucose, lipogenesis as well as suppression of lipolysis in adipose tissue.

Underlying Processes of Insulin Resistance

Action of insulin through signaling pathway is intricate. Signaling of insulin is mediated by receptor tyrosine kinases. The binding of insulin hormone to insulin receptor alpha-subunit leading to self-phosphorylation of tyrosine residues and finally activation of insulin receptor beta-subunit. This triggers the cascade involving recruitment and activation of insulin receptor substrates followed by activation of Pl-3-kinase and phosphorylation of PI 4, 5-bisphosphate. These series of events activates protein kinase B (Akt) enabling GLUT translocation to plasma membrane. Peroxisome proliferator- activated receptor gamma (PPAR-γ) and adiponectin play a pivotal role in adipose tissue biology. PPAR-γ referred as insulin sensitizer can activate adipocyte-specific genes expression and stimulate its differentiation and is also known as an insulin sensitizer (Mann *et al.*, 2016). Adiponectin, a type of adipokine in plasma is released from adipose tissue also acts as insulin-sensitizing hormone that increases insulin sensitivity via activation of AMP protein kinase signaling (Yamauchi *et al.*, 2001). During insulin resistance in human and rodents, PPAR-γ has been attributed to raise adiponectin levels (Maeda *et al.*, 2001). Role of PPAR-γ in insulin sensitivity has been also established in dairy cows (Schoenberg *et al.*, 2011; Smith *et al.*, 2009). During IR it could be that lower PPAR-γ expression will have lower adiponectin levels. Blood levels of adiponectin levels during the dry period have been found to be positively correlated to insulin responsiveness of body tissues for glucose and fatty acid in dairy cows (De Koster *et al.*, 2017).

Insulin resistance can be defined as a state where normal concentrations of insulin elicit a reduced biological response (Kahn, 1978). However, spectrum of IR can be characterized into 2 distinct entities i.e. reduced insulin sensitivity and/ or insulin responsiveness. Reduction in insulin sensitivity refers to requirement of greater insulin concentration to elicit a normal biological response without any change in maximal response, whereas reduced insulin responsiveness refers to decrease in maximal biological response. Both IR and IS decreases during late gestation and early lactation in ruminants (De Koster and Opsomer, 2013). IR during transition is essential for mammary gland (an insulin dependent organ) for supply of energy for initiation. During lactation, expression of insulin independent transporters is 3 times greater than that in dry period. Peripartum period involving transition carries the burden of inflammatory processes which may not only be of infectious origin but also systemic and general in nature experienced by all transition cows (Bradford *et al.*, 2015). Metabolic responses to inflammation have been reviewed by Baumgard *et al.* (2017) to highlight that nutrient partitioning diverts glucose towards immune system under influence of decreased intake, increased insulin levels with increased insulin resistance. The glucose siphoning towards immune system is so strong in severe cases that even milk biosynthesis is reduced to spare glucose and make it available for immune system. Kushibiki *et al.* (2001) showed increase in IR with increased proinflammatory cytokine such as TNF-α that led to low blood glucose clearance even after insulin being administered IV.

Energy Homeorhesis and Endocrine Regulation of Insulin Resistance

Piantoni and VandeHaar (2022) have exhaustively reviewed impact of nutrients on partitioning of energy in lactating animals. Metabolism during physiological states like pregnancy or lactation is under homeorhetic regulation (Bauman and Currie, 1980) that along with associated hormonal variations is critical for partitioning of nutrients between developing fetus, mammary milk biosynthesis as well as body condition. This is mainly due to interplay of insulin as well as growth hormone (GH, somatotropin) vis-à-vis responsiveness of body tissues (Tucker, 2000; Baumgard *et al.*, 2017).

Pituitary gland is key regulator for development of mammary gland and milk production wherein under the influence of growth hormone mediated by increased IGF-I there are cellular proliferations and anabolic effects that have been attributed with galactopoietic activity (Tucker, 2000). This is one of the major events during transition phase in dairy animals. GH stimulates hepatic IGF-1 that exerts negative feedback on GH release. GH also directly decreases insulin sensitivity of tissues. Increase in lipolysis during negative energy balance and decrease in lipogenesis during positive energy balance occurs under influence of GH. It also reduces glucose transporter 4 (GLUT4) translocation leading to reduction in insulin dependent glucose uptake in adipose tissue.

Increased intake of feed is not the only factor that affects pancreatic secretion of insulin as implied by responses to glucose (Hove, 1978) some amino acids (Hertelendy et al., 1970) as well as butyrate and propionate (Manns et al., 1967;

Manns and Boda, 1967). Relative intake with respect to requirements also affects the insulin levels in blood. As glucose is diverted towards mammary gland (insulin independent) during peripartum, the amount of glucose to the adipose tissues and muscle decreases leading to IR. In such situation of higher requirement and even without any increase in intake, existing actual intake relatively acts as lower intake causing the reduction of insulin levels that has also been reported by Bradford and Allen (2007). Similar explanation seems to be valid as reason for low insulin concentration in high milk yielders as compared to low milk producing cows (Lucy et al., 2009; Zinicola and Bicalho, 2019).

Insulin seems to possess effects antagonistic to that of growth hormone as under influence of insulin, GLUT4 translocation to cell membrane occurs and leads to increased uptake of glucose by muscle and adipose tissue, and it inhibits protein degradation in muscle, lipolysis in adipose, and gluconeogenesis in liver (De Koster and Opsomer, 2013).

Apart from GH concentration, hormones like leptin (Muller et al., 1997) and proinflammatory cytokines such as TNF-alpha (Kushibiki et al., 2001) can reduce tissue sensitivity towards insulin. With low GH and high insulin, energy will more be diverted towards body reserves and away from milk production or developing fetus and vice versa.

Metabolic and hormonal adaptation in dairy cows during peripartum favor mobilization of body reserves towards fetal growth during advanced gestation and milk production. As the phase of lactation advances, there is increase in feed intake lowering the dependency for mobilization of body reserves. During late lactation milk yield decreases but development of fetus in pregnant females is quite rapid that justifies the need for drying off 2 months prior to parturition to facilitate replenishment of body reserves. This is further supported by increased GLUT 4 expression in muscle and adipose tissue (De Koster and Opsomer, 2013).Rapid fetal growth and mammary gland involution from previous state to remodeling for next stage (mammogenesis to lactogenesis) especially during advanced gestation necessitates the sparing of blood glucose (Bell, 1995; Bell and Ehrhardt, 2000).

During prepartum period, insulin resistance increases in the body tissues other than liver (Bell, 1995; Zachut et al., 2013). About 21 days before parturition hormone insulin and IGF-1 decline followed by rise in NEFA at 1 week prepartum (VandeHaar et al., 1999; Doepel et al., 2002). As compared to heifers, this effect is more prominent in cows especially the ones that are on diets low in energy (VandeHaar et al., 1999). During advanced gestation stage, levels of GH is low that begins to rise 1 week prepartum (Simmons et al., 1994). Prepartum insulin resistance of extra hepatic tissues, low insulin and high GH levels mobilize NEFA from adipose, selected amino acids from muscle and promote hepatic ketogenesis to be used as alternate sources of energy resulting in glucose uptake by fetus for development as well as mammary gland for mammogenesis and lactogenesis. In spite of normal circulating levels of GH in blood, around parturition hepatic expression of GH receptor 1A is downregulated along with decrease in biosynthesis as well as release of IGF-I (Lucy et al., 2001). This occurs due to uncoupling of somatotropic axis comprising GH, GH receptor, and IGF-I (Lucy et al., 2001). Lowered IGF-1 removes negative feedback on pituitary thus promoting release of GH in blood. This is pronounced in cows under severe NEB (Lucy et al., 2009).

In the initial phase of early lactation until 14-21 days after parturition, there is increased glucose utilization and production owing to increase in mammary cell number as well as activity, size of liver as well as gluconeogenic capacity (Bauman, 2000). Plasma insulin concentration remains low (Doepel et al., 2002), and insulin resistance of extra hepatic tissues (Bell, 1995) as well as GH concentration are high (Doepel et al., 2002), favoring partitioning of nutrients away from body reserves towards mammary gland for milk production. Under low insulin levels postpartum, liver is key for gluconeogenesis to cater for lactose biosynthesis and milk production so unlike extra hepatic tissues it is not insulin resistant (Zachut et al., 2013).

FATE OF NEFA AND REGULATION OF INTAKE

Adipose tissue is sensitive to insulin (major antilipolytic hormone) under normal circumstances but during negative energy balance and insulin resistance refractoriness to insulin reduces lipogenesis. Further, under influence of insulin resistance, they are mobilized for lipid catabolism resulting in release of NEFA along with glycerol. Adipose triglyceride lipase initiates lipolysis followed by the actions of hormone sensitive lipase on diacylglycerol and monoglyceride lipase on 2-monoacylglycerol. Insulin resistance especially lowered insulin sensitivity is key regulator for fat mobilization. (De Koster, 2013). The tilt of adipose tissue dynamics towards more lipolysis and less lipogenesis is pivotal to NEFA increase in circulation.

The beneficial effects of NEFA in terms of acting as source of energy for tissues including mammary gland and precursors for milk fat synthesis are outweighed when in excess they are attributed to many negative effects by increasing tendencies for IR (Pires *et al.*, 2007), hepatic fat (Bobe *et al.*, 2004), oxidative stress (Bradford, 2011), hepatic ketogenesis (Cadorniga *et al.*, 1997), displaced abomasum (Ospina *et al.*,2010), chronic inflammation (Sordillo, 2013) along with decrease in hepatic gluconeogenesis (Li *et al.*,2012), immune function (Scalia, 2006) and DMI (Allen *et al.*, 2009).

Circulating NEFA in liver has 3 fates i.e. either is exported or stored as triglycerides after esterification, converted into ketone bodies or completely oxidized for energy. NEFA is used for oxidative phosphorylation for energy as well as formation of BHBA. Excess mobilization of fatty acids leads to its accumulation in liver, increased ketogenesis and enhanced synthesis of BHBA with the help of enzyme NADH-dependent -hydroxybutyrate dehydrogenase (Grabacka et al., 2016). BHBA along with acetate also serves as precursor for biosynthesis of fatty acid by mammary epithelial cells.

Even though triglycerides contribute to production of milk fat on being exported, it may also cause hepatic steatosis on being stored. Ketone bodies that are formed and exported from liver may also serve as energy source or acts as precursor of milk fat. Oxidation of NEFA in liver leads to accumulation of acetyl CoA in hepatic tissues whose quantity during post-calving is inversely related to feed intake (Stocks and Allen, 2012). Intakes lower relative to higher requirement maintains low insulin levels leading to absence of insulin actions (inhibition of body reserve mobilization) resulting in higher NEFA and finally higher acetyl CoA. However, it is striking to note acetyl CoA production in liver, oxidation of NEFA or other nutrients have lesser control on intake as compared to hepatic energy charge represented by ([ATP]+0.5[ADP])/([ATP] + [ADP]+[AMP]) (Allen *et al.*, 2009; Allen and Piantoni, 2013; Allen, 2020) suggesting increase of intake if hepatic energy charge is less.

Feeding increases hepatic influx of gluconeogenic precursors like propionate, amino acids (glucogenic), glycerol and lactate, activates Kreb's cycle, promotes oxidation of acetyl CoA thus increasing hepatic energy charge followed by end of feeding (Allen and Piantoni, 2013; Allen, 2020). Feeding stimulates insulin increase that inhibits lipolysis and reduces NEFA in circulation which has been established to have positive and linear relationship in cows after calving (Piantoni *et al.* 2015). Speculated reasons also held increased insulin sensitivity responsible to reach higher intakes immediately after postpartum.

NUTRIENT PARTITIONING THROUGHOUT LACTATION CYCLE

During early phase of lactation (approx. 21 to 100 days), the nutrient partitioning even though is towards milk production it gradually starts sparing the body reserves. Capacities of mammary gland for milk biosynthesis and of liver for gluconeogenesis are high that sees simultaneous rising of insulin sensitivity and insulin concentration. As soon as the cow gets rid of NEB and enters the positive energy balance there is reversal of uncoupling of somatotropic axis (Sharma *et al.*, 1994; Kobayashi *et al.*, 1999), a reversal that seems to be positively affected by insulin concentrations (Butler *et al.*, 2003) which leads to lowering of GH (Koprowski and Tucker, 1973), increased IGF-I, upregulation of GLUT4 in muscle and adipose tissue. At this stage despite higher mammary biosynthesis of milk, partitioning of nutrients does not occur at the cost of mobilization of body reserves owing to increased insulin sensitivity and DMI. During mid (approx. 100-200 days) and late (after 200 days) lactation, the focus of nutrient partitioning gradually shifts more towards body reserves than towards milk production under the influence of high insulin level, low GH, high extra hepatic insulin sensitivity and high GLUT4 expression in adipose and muscle tissues.

ASSESSMENT OF INSULIN RESISTANCE (DIRECT AND INDIRECT MEASUREMENTS)

Hyperinsulinemic-Euglycemic Clamp (Direct Measurement) : This technique has been considered as gold standard that requires to administer insulin and glucose (using constant infusion IV clamps) to increase and maintain levels at steady state (insulin at higher than normal levels and glucose at normal fasting level) with simultaneous monitoring for blood glucose levels. Requirement of higher steady-state glucose infusion rate hints at high insulin-stimulated glucose uptake by peripheral tissues (De Koster and Opsomer, 2013). Is =SSIC/SSGIR (Mitrakou *et al.*, 1992) or SI clamp = M/(G) (Muniyappa *et al.*, 2008) can be used to assess insulin sensitivity (SSIC-steady-state insulin concentration, SSGIR -steady-state glucose infusion rate, M- glucose disposal rate, G - steady-state blood glucose concentrations, is the difference between fasting and steady-state blood insulin concentrations). Higher SI clamp indicates higher insulin sensitivity. Major limitation of this technique is that it costly, requires some skill, takes long time to perform and is labour intensive.

Glucose Tolerance Testing (Direct Measurement): This test can be done to assess systemic insulin sensitivity in dairy cows (De Koster and Opsomer, 2013). In this test blood levels of insulin, free fatty acid and glucose are measured at regular intervals after challenging the cows with I/V glucose at dose about 3-10 times higher than normal levels. Variations in glucose levels reflect hepatic and extra hepatic utilization as well excretion whereas insulin levels depend on pancreatic release and hepatic uptake. With respect to glucose lowered clearance rate, area under the curve (AUC) and increased time to attain basal concentrations are indicative of IR (De Koster and Opsomer, 2013).

Insulin Tolerance Testing (Direct Measurement): This test is based on challenging the cows with IV administration of insulin hormone followed by measurement of insulin and glucose at regular intervals. After insulin administration, lower clearance rate and area under curve for glucose as well as lower values of insulin-stimulated reduction of blood glucose levels from measurements made in the basal state are indicative of Insulin resistance (De Koster and Opsomer, 2013). However, the risk of hypoglycemic shock associated with IV administration of insulin along with cost consideration of this test acts as a disadvantage for this test.

Insulin Sensitivity Indices (Indirect measurement): Due to cost considerations, laborious nature and longer duration for assessment and attaining fasting state in pregnant or early lactating animals direct tests are less preferred and redundant in routine practice. Indirect tests comprise several surrogate indices that rely on measured blood parameters (glucose, insulin, NEFA and BHBA) such as QUICKI=1/[log insulin(µU/mL)+log glucose(mg/dL)] (Katz *et al.*, 2000), homeostasis model assessment of insulin resistance(HOMA-IR)=[glucose(mmol/L) insulin (µU/mL)/22.5] (Muniyappa *et al.*, 2008), $RQUICKI_{NEFA}$=1/[log glucose(mg/dL)+log insulin(µU/mL)+log NEFA (mmol/L)] (Perseghin *et al.*, 2001) and $RQUICKI_{BHBA}$=1/[log glucose (mg/dL)+log insulin(µU/mL)+log FFA(mmol/L)+logBHBA(mmol/L)] (Balogh *et al.*, 2008). Higher insulin resistance is indicated by lower QUICKI, higher HOMA-IR lower $RQUICKI_{NEFA}$ and lower $RQUICKI_{BHBA}$ and vice versa. Other indices which are more often calculated in humans for insulin sensitivity/resistance are McAuley index, Matsuda index, Belfiore index, Avignon index, Stumvoll index.

Other techniques for assessment: As ruminant animals have completely different metabolic milieu than humans, some other techniques despite being invasive can be attempted to develop greater insight into IR of dairy animals. Some examples include determining insulin response of hindlimb muscles through arteriovenous glucose difference in hindlimb of lactating and non-lactating sheep (Vernon *et al.*, 1990), studying muscle biopsies during HEC test for activation of the intracellular insulin signaling cascade to identify the signaling molecule that is responsible for inducing insulin resistance (Kruszynska *et al.*, 2002), in vivo and in vitro research of biopsies, short-term in vitro adipose tissue cultures for studying insulin response of the lipolytic and lipogenic pathways (Green and Newsholme, 1979; Arner, 1997)

CONSIDERATIONS FOR IR MEASUREMENT IN RUMINANT ANIMAL

There are some important aspects to be pondered upon while studying or performing tests of insulin resistance/sensitivity in pregnant (dry) animals as well as lactating animals. The difference also may exists for high and low yielders. Most of the direct tests rely on glucose disappearance phenomenon presuming it to be result of insulin mediated peripheral utilization. However in case of dry cows that are pregnant and lactating cows the insulin-independent glucose uptake accounts for 84% -92% owing to gravid uterus with developing fetus or lactating mammary gland. Moreover, uptake in mammary gland uptake is much higher than uptake by gravid uterus as it has been noticed that this uptake is 3 times higher in lactating goats than dry goats and 2 times higher in lactating cows than dry cows. Further, it is important to note that hepatic and renal gluconeogenesis in ruminants is predominant source of glucose that can be suppressed with administration of insulin as insulin has been known to inhibit gluconeogenesis. Therefore, glucose being infused during testing is likely to be partitioned for all the avenues including those that were served earlier by physiologically normal gluconeogenesis. All these tend to overestimate the insulin sensitivity in the animals being tested upon. Furthermore, over dependency on surrogate indices is marred by their accuracy of predicting IR/IS owing to variation in correlation with other gold standard techniques or key biomarkers of IR. In addition to these, there is severe dearth of studies that could have been of help to establish reference interval specific to species as well as physiological stage.

AMELIORATION OF INSULIN RESISTANCE

Development of insulin resistance is considered physiological event that primarily occurs to support preferential energy partitioning mainly during late pregnancy and early lactation. However, due to drastic changes in metabolism the IR and NEB creates a sustained vicious cycle that leads to problems like fatty liver, ketosis, vulnerability to other disorders of infectious as well as non-infectious origin. As sensitive and specific biomarkers of IR have not been well established in dairy ruminants, the indicators of NEB are generally used to assess such situations and use suitable ameliorative strategies. There are numerous studies on NEB but very few on IR. Studies underpinning the mechanism of development and severity of IR are gradually being undertaken but existing problem of IR can still be tackled to some extent based on our understanding of negative energy balance. The amelioration measures may comprise of following strategies alone or in combination: prevention of NEB by manipulating energy intake during transition, maintaining low BCS, increase insulin secretion, increase insulin sensitivity or responsiveness, provision of alternate energy source to reduce NEB and preventing fat accumulation in liver.

Some aspects for curtailing negative energy balance in dairy cows have been well reviewed by Mekuriaw (2023). He has highlighted and presented several studies for strategies of controlling NEB during transition period. Among them dry period management and nutrition is very important. Early phase of dry period can comprise of diets low in energy with increased energy ratio in 14-21 days prepartum (Janovick et al., 2011, Overton and Waldron, 2004, Contreras et al., 2004). Nutrients such as methionine, choline and some fatty acids if supplemented during peripartum period may also be useful to improve NEB (Overton and Waldron, 2004; Rulquin and Delaby, 1997; Folno i et al., 2019; uri i et al., 2020). Optimum fibre length as well as concentrate to roughage ratio also plays role in mitigating NEB (Zebeli et al., 2010) however rumen protection forms should be considered while planning such dietary inclusions. Rumen protected forms of fat (Shelke et al., 2012; Zenobi et al., 2018), glucogenic precursors (Patton et al., 2004) and direct-fed microbials/ probiotics (Sretenovi et al., 2008) have been proven to be useful. Insulinogeneic diets that comprises of starch along with high levels of insulin have also shown to increase reproductive performance (Gong, 2002) negating the NEB effects but negative effects of longer duration of insulinogenic diets compels its benefit only if given for a shorter duration. Attempts for increasing propionate levels in rumen by adding propylene glycol as also yield results indicating insulin stimulation along with reduced lipolysis and ketogenesis and improving energy status (Zhang et al., 2020). The excess burden on liver for metabolizing can be tackled by providing hepatic proteceting supplements in diet (García et al., 2011) but such studies are less. One such substance silymarin has been reportedly used to protect liver in dairy cows during transition period (Tedesco et al., 2004). Ketosis can be prevented by including niacin with precursors of glycogen such as propylene glycol and propionate-sodium (Overton and Waldron, 2004; Weiss and Gonzalo, 2006).

Some reports for reducing insulin resistance in dairy animals exist but the number of studies as well as success rate is not adequate to devise a precise as well as comprehensive ameliorative measures. Supplementation of rumen protected niacin may show benefits owing to its insulin sensitizing and anti-lipolytic effects. Supplementation of substances like berberine have been reported to modulate somatotropic axis as well as response of glucose and insulin to IVGTT and also resulted in improvement of glucose and insulin status in dairy goats (Ghavipanje *et al.*, 2022). Supplementation of berberine (at least 2 gram/day) has been reported to ameliorate insulin resistance (IR) and disorders of fat metabolism related to NEB of transition dairy goats (Ghavipanje, *et al.*, 2021). Other nutrients that may also ameliorate insulin resistance can be chromium and magnesium. Insulin sensitizers like Thiazolidinedione (rosiglitazone, pioglitazone) than can increase insulin sensitivity in adipose and muscle, potent insulin-sensitizing agonists of the nuclear receptor PPARG (Hosseini *et al.*, 2015).

Future strategies for prevention and treatment of insulin resistance in dairy animals may also explore the options that are used for treating diabetes in case of human beings for example use of insulin secretagogues, insulin sensitizers etc.

Work done at Department of Veterinary Physiology and Biochemistry, Veterinary College, Navsari, Kamdhenu University, Gujarat

Some studies with the aim of understanding insulin resistance and its amelioration have been conducted as well as being undertaken at our department.

One of the doctoral research from our department has been conducted to observe ameliorative effects of rumen protected niacin (RPN) supplementation on insulin resistance as well as other physio-biochemical parameters during transition in Surti goats wherein it was concluded that RPN supplementation during transition period showed potential in decreasing insulin resistance, reduced stress, decreased negative energy balance, decreased oxidative stress, enhanced body condition, improved hepatic function, improved milk composition and showed potential of increased milk yield, improved hematological parameters and immune status and had no adverse effect on physiological parameters.

One of the ongoing doctoral research is presently focusing on insulin resistance during different stages of lactation in Surti buffaloes and another departmental project has also been proposed to observe such effect of rumen protected niacin supplementation on physio-biochemical and milk production parameters in peripartum Surti Buffaloes during transition period.

Some other studies were undertaken at our department that were not directly related to studying insulin resistance but their results do point towards ameliorative potential in tackling insulin resistance in dairy ruminants especially by enhancing hepatic functioning. Few such studies included study of physio-biochemical changes and growth performance in young Surti goats supplemented with rumen protected choline, to study physiological and biochemical changes on feeding of rumen protected methionine and choline during transition period in Surti buffaloes and to study heat ameliorative effects of rumen protected niacin supplementation in lactating Surti buffaloes. The beneficial effects in these studies were reaped without affecting liver health or improving hepatic function as indicated by lowered as well as optimized hepatic enzymes.

REFERENCES

Allen, M.S., 2020. Control of feed intake by hepatic oxidation in ruminant animals: integration of homeostasis and homeorhesis. *Animal, 14*(S1), pp.s55-s64.

Allen, M.S., Bradford, B.J. and Oba, M., 2009. Board-invited review: The hepatic oxidation theory of the control of feed intake and its application to ruminants. *Journal of animal science, 87*(10), pp.3317-3334.

Allen, M.S. and Piantoni, P., 2013. Metabolic control of feed intake: Implications for metabolic disease of fresh cows. *Veterinary Clinics: Food Animal Practice, 29*(2), pp.279-297.

Arner, P., 1997. Obesity and the adipocyte. Regional adipocity in man. *J Endocrinol, 155*, pp.191-192.

Basic Animal Husbandry Statistics-2022 on https://dahd.nic.in/schemes/programmes/animal-husbandry-statistics

Balogh, O., Szepes, O., Kovacs, K., Kulcsar, M., Reiczigel, J., Alcazar, J.A., Keresztes, M., Febel, H., Bartyik, J., Fekete, S.G. and Fesus, L., 2008. Interrelationships of growth hormone AluI polymorphism, insulin resistance, milk production and reproductive performance in Holstein-Friesian cows. *Veterinarni Medicina, 53*(11), pp.604-616.

Bauman, D.E. and Currie, W.B., 1980. Partitioning of nutrients during pregnancy and lactation: a review of mechanisms involving homeostasis and homeorhesis. *Journal of dairy science, 63*(9), pp.1514-1529.

Baumgard, L.H., Collier, R.J. and Bauman, D.E., 2017. A 100-Year Review: Regulation of nutrient partitioning to support lactation. *Journal of Dairy Science, 100*(12), pp.10353-10366.

Bell, A.W., 1995. Regulation of organic nutrient metabolism during transition from late pregnancy to early lactation. *Journal of animal science, 73*(9), pp.2804-2819.

Bobe, G., Young, J.W. and Beitz, D.C., 2004. Invited review: pathology, etiology, prevention, and treatment of fatty liver in dairy cows. *Journal of dairy science, 87*(10), pp.3105-3124.

Bradford, B., 2011, March. Connecting transition cow physiology, behavior, and nutrition. In *Proceedings of the 10th Western Dairy Management Conference* (pp. 207-220).

Bradford, B.J. and Allen, M.S., 2007. Phlorizin administration does not attenuate hypophagia induced by intraruminal propionate infusion in lactating dairy cattle. *The Journal of nutrition, 137*(2), pp.326-330.

Bradford, B.J., Yuan, K., Farney, J.K., Mamedova, L.K. and Carpenter, A.J., 2015. Invited review: Inflammation during the transition to lactation: New adventures with an old flame. *Journal of dairy science, 98*(10), pp.6631-6650.

Butler, S.T., Marr, A.L., Pelton, S.H., Radcliff, R.P., Lucy, M.C. and Butler, W.R., 2003. Insulin restores GH responsiveness during lactation-induced negative energy balance in dairy cattle: effects on expression of IGF-I and GH receptor 1A.

Cadórniga-Valiño, C., Grummer, R.R., Armentano, L.E., Donkin, S.S. and Bertics, S.J., 1997. Effects of fatty acids and hormones on fatty acid metabolism and gluconeogenesis in bovine hepatocytes. *Journal of Dairy Science, 80*(4), pp.646-656.

Contreras, L.L., Ryan, C.M. and Overton, T.R., 2004. Effects of dry cow grouping strategy and prepartum body condition score on performance and health of transition dairy cows. *Journal of dairy science, 87*(2), pp.517-523.

De Koster, J., Urh, C., Hostens, M., Van Den Broeck, W., Sauerwein, H. and Opsomer, G., 2017. Relationship between serum adiponectin concentration, body condition score, and peripheral tissue insulin response of dairy cows during the dry period. *Domestic animal endocrinology, 59*, pp.100-104.

De Koster, J.D. and Opsomer, G., 2013. Insulin resistance in dairy cows. *Veterinary Clinics: Food Animal Practice, 29*(2), pp.299-322.

Doepel, L., Lapierre, H. and Kennelly, J.J., 2002. Peripartum performance and metabolism of dairy cows in response to prepartum energy and protein intake. *Journal of dairy science, 85*(9), pp.2315-2334.

DuriCic, D., Vince, S., Lojkic, M., Jelusic, S., Turk, R., Valpotic, H., Gracner, D., Macesic, N., Folnozic, I., Sostar, Z. and Samardzija, M., 2020. Effects of dietary clinoptilolite on reproductive performance, serum progesterone and insulin-like growth factor-1 concentrations in dairy cows during pregnancy and lactation. *Polish Journal of Veterinary Sciences, 23*(1).

Folno i , I., Samard ija, M., uri i , D., Vince, S., Perkov, S., Jeluši , S., Valpoti , H., Ljubi , B.B., Lojki , M., Gra ner, D. and aja, I. ., 2019. Effects of in-feed clinoptilolite treatment on serum metabolic and antioxidative biomarkers and acute phase response in dairy cows during pregnancy and early lactation. *Research in veterinary science, 127*, pp.57-64.

García, A., Cardoso, F.C., Campos, R., Thedy, D.X. and González, F.H., 2011. Metabolic evaluation of dairy cows submitted to three different strategies to decrease the effects of negative energy balance in early postpartum. *Pesquisa Veterinária Brasileira, 31*, pp.11-17.

Gong, J.G., 2002. Influence of metabolic hormones and nutrition on ovarian follicle development in cattle: practical implications. *Domestic Animal Endocrinology, 23*(1-2), pp.229-241.

Grabacka, M., Pierzchalska, M., Dean, M. and Reiss, K., 2016. Regulation of ketone body metabolism and the role of PPARα. *International journal of molecular sciences, 17*(12), p.2093.

Green, A.L.L.A.N. and Newsholme, E.A., 1979. Sensitivity of glucose uptake and lipolysis of white adipocytes of the rat to insulin and effects of some metabolites. *Biochemical Journal, 180*(2), pp.365-370.

Ghavipanje, Navid, Mohammad Hasan Fathi Nasri, Seyyed Homayoun Farhangfar, Seyyed Ehsan Ghiasi, and Einar Vargas-Bello-Pérez. "The impact of dietary berberine supplementation during the transition period on blood parameters, antioxidant indicators and fatty acids profile in colostrum and milk of dairy goats." *Veterinary Sciences* 9, no. 2 (2022): 76.

Ghavipanje, N., Fathi Nasri, M.H., Farhangfar, S.H., Ghiasi, S.E. and Vargas-Bello-Pérez, E., 2021. Regulation of nutritional metabolism in transition dairy goats: energy balance, liver activity, and insulin resistance in response to berberine supplementation. *Animals, 11*(8), p.2236.

Hertelendy, F., Takahashi, K., Machlin, L.J. and Kipnis, D.M., 1970. Growth hormone and insulin secretory responses to arginine in the sheep, pig, and cow. *General and comparative endocrinology, 14*(1), pp.72-77.

Hosseini, A., Tariq, M.R., Trindade da Rosa, F., Kesser, J., Iqbal, Z., Mora, O., Sauerwein, H., Drackley, J.K., Trevisi, E. and Loor, J.J., 2015. Insulin sensitivity in adipose and skeletal muscle tissue of dairy cows in response to dietary energy level and 2, 4-thiazolidinedione (TZD). *PLoS One*, *10*(11), p.e0142633.

Hove, K., 1978. Insulin secretion in lactating cows: responses to glucose infused intravenously in normal, ketonemic, and starved animals. *Journal of Dairy Science*, *61*(10), pp.1407-1413.

Janovick, N.A., Boisclair, Y.R. and Drackley, J.K., 2011. Prepartum dietary energy intake affects metabolism and health during the periparturient period in primiparous and multiparous Holstein cows. *Journal of dairy science*, *94*(3), pp.1385-1400.

Kahn, C.R., 1978. Insulin resistance, insulin insensitivity, and insulin unresponsiveness: a necessary distinction. *Metabolism*, *27*(12), pp.1893-1902.

Katz, A., Nambi, S.S., Mather, K., Baron, A.D., Follmann, D.A., Sullivan, G. and Quon, M.J., 2000. Quantitative insulin sensitivity check index: a simple, accurate method for assessing insulin sensitivity in humans. *The Journal of Clinical Endocrinology & Metabolism*, *85*(7), pp.2402-2410.

Kobayashi, Y., Boyd, C.K., Bracken, C.J., Lamberson, W.R., Keisler, D.H. and Lucy, M.C., 1999. Reduced growth hormone receptor (GHR) messenger ribonucleic acid in liver of periparturient cattle is caused by a specific down-regulation of GHR 1A that is associated with decreased insulin-like growth factor I. *Endocrinology*, *140*(9), pp.3947-3954.

Koprowski, J.A. and Allen Tucker, H., 1973. Bovine serum growth hormone, corticoids and insulin during lactation. *Endocrinology*, *93*(3), pp.645-651.

Kruszynska, Y.T., Worrall, D.S., Ofrecio, J., Frias, J.P., Macaraeg, G. and Olefsky, J.M., 2002. Fatty acid-induced insulin resistance: decreased muscle PI3K activation but unchanged Akt phosphorylation. *The Journal of Clinical Endocrinology & Metabolism*, *87*(1), pp.226-234.

Kushibiki, S., Hodate, K., Shingu, H., Ueda, Y., Mori, Y., Itoh, T. and Yokomizo, Y., 2001. Effects of long-term administration of recombinant bovine tumor necrosis factor-α on glucose metabolism and growth hormone secretion in steers. *American journal of veterinary research*, *62*(5), pp.794-798.

Li, X., Li, X., Bai, G., Chen, H., Deng, Q., Liu, Z., Zhang, L., Liu, G. and Wang, Z., 2012. Effects of non-esterified fatty acids on the gluconeogenesis in bovine hepatocytes. *Molecular and cellular biochemistry*, *359*, pp.385-388.

Lucy, M.C., Verkerk, G.A., Whyte, B.E., Macdonald, K.A., Burton, L., Cursons, R.T., Roche, J.R. and Holmes, C.W., 2009. Somatotropic axis components and nutrient partitioning in genetically diverse dairy cows managed under different feed allowances in a pasture system. *Journal of Dairy Science*, *92*(2), pp.526-539.

Maeda, N., Takahashi, M., Funahashi, T., Kihara, S., Nishizawa, H., Kishida, K., Nagaretani, H., Matsuda, M., Komuro, R., Ouchi, N. and Kuriyama, H., 2001. PPARγ ligands increase expression and plasma concentrations of adiponectin, an adipose-derived protein. *Diabetes, 50*(9), pp.2094-2099.

Manns, J.G. and Boda, J.M., 1967. Insulin release by acetate, propionate, butyrate, and glucose in lambs and adult sheep. *American Journal of Physiology-Legacy Content, 212*(4), pp.747-755.

Manns, J.G., Boda, J.M. and Willes, R.F., 1967. Probable role of propionate and butyrate in control of insulin secretion in sheep. *American Journal of Physiology-Legacy Content, 212*(4), pp.756-764.

Mann, S., Nydam, D.V., Abuelo, A., Yepes, F.L., Overton, T.R. and Wakshlag, J.J., 2016. Insulin signaling, inflammation, and lipolysis in subcutaneous adipose tissue of transition dairy cows either overfed energy during the prepartum period or fed a controlled-energy diet. *Journal of Dairy Science, 99*(8), pp.6737-6752.

Mekuriaw, Y., 2023. Negative energy balance and its implication on productive and reproductive performance of early lactating dairy cows. *Journal of Applied Animal Research, 51*(1), pp.220-229.

Mitrakou, A., Vuorinen-Markkola, H., Raptis, G., Toft, I., Mokan, M., Strumph, P., Pimenta, W., Veneman, T., Jenssen, T. and Bolli, G., 1992. Simultaneous assessment of insulin secretion and insulin sensitivity using a hyperglycemia clamp. *The Journal of Clinical Endocrinology & Metabolism, 75*(2), pp.379-382.

Muller, G., Ertl, J., Gerl, M. and Preibisch, G., 1997. Leptin impairs metabolic actions of insulin in isolated rat adipocytes. *Journal of Biological Chemistry, 272*(16), pp.10585-10593.

Muniyappa, R., Lee, S., Chen, H. and Quon, M.J., 2008. Current approaches for assessing insulin sensitivity and resistance in vivo: advantages, limitations, and appropriate usage. *American Journal of Physiology-Endocrinology and Metabolism, 294*(1), pp.E15-E26.

Ospina, P.A., Nydam, D.V., Stokol, T. and Overton, T.R., 2010. Associations of elevated nonesterified fatty acids and -hydroxybutyrate concentrations with early lactation reproductive performance and milk production in transition dairy cattle in the northeastern United States. *Journal of dairy science, 93*(4), pp.1596-1603.

Overton, T.R. and Waldron, M.R., 2004. Nutritional management of transition dairy cows: strategies to optimize metabolic health. *Journal of dairy science, 87*, pp.E105-E119.

Patton, R.S., Sorenson, C.E. and Hippen, A.R., 2004. Effects of dietary glucogenic precursors and fat on feed intake and carbohydrate status of transition dairy cows. *Journal of Dairy Science, 87*(7), pp.2122-2129.

Perseghin, G., Caumo, A., Caloni, M., Testolin, G. and Luzi, L., 2001. Incorporation of the fasting plasma FFA concentration into QUICKI improves its association with insulin sensitivity in nonobese individuals. *The Journal of Clinical Endocrinology & Metabolism, 86*(10), pp.4776-4781.

Piantoni, P. and VandeHaar, M.J., 2022. Symposium review: The impact of absorbed nutrients on energy partitioning throughout lactation. *Journal of Dairy Science.*

Piantoni, P., Ylioja, C.M. and Allen, M.S., 2015. Feed intake is related to changes in plasma nonesterified fatty acid concentration and hepatic acetyl CoA content following feeding in lactating dairy cows. *Journal of Dairy Science, 98*(10), pp.6839-6847.

Pires, J.A.A., Pescara, J.B. and Grummer, R.R., 2007. Reduction of plasma NEFA concentration by nicotinic acid enhances the response to insulin in feed-restricted Holstein cows. *Journal of Dairy Science, 90*(10), pp.4635-4642.

Rulquin, H. and Delaby, L., 1997. Effects of the energy balance of dairy cows on lactational responses to rumen-protected methionine. *Journal of dairy science, 80*(10), pp.2513-2522.

Scalia, D., Lacetera, N., Bernabucci, U., Demeyere, K., Duchateau, L. and Burvenich, C., 2006. In vitro effects of nonesterified fatty acids on bovine neutrophils oxidative burst and viability. *Journal of Dairy Science, 89*(1), pp.147-154.

Schoenberg, K.M., Perfield, K.L., Farney, J.K., Bradford, B.J., Boisclair, Y.R. and Overton, T.R., 2011. Effects of prepartum 2, 4-thiazolidinedione on insulin sensitivity, plasma concentrations of tumor necrosis factor-α and leptin, and adipose tissue gene expression. *Journal of Dairy Science, 94*(11), pp.5523-5532.

Sharma, B.K., Vandehaar, M.J. and Ames, N.K., 1994. Expression of insulin-like growth factor-I in cows at different stages of lactation and in late lactation cows treated with somatotropin. *Journal of dairy science, 77*(8), pp.2232-2241.

Shelke, S.K., Thakur, S.S. and Shete, S.M., 2012. Protected nutrients technology and the impact of feeding protected nutrients to dairy animals: a review. *Int J Dairy Sci, 7*, pp.51-62.

Simmons, C.R., Bergen, W.G., Vandehaar, M.J., Sprecher, D.J., Sniffen, C.J., Stanisiewski, E.P. and Tucker, H.A., 1994. Protein and fat metabolism in cows given somavubove before parturition. *Journal of dairy science, 77*(7), pp.1835-1847.

Sordillo, L.M. and Raphael, W., 2013. Significance of metabolic stress, lipid mobilization, and inflammation on transition cow disorders. *Veterinary Clinics: Food Animal Practice, 29*(2), pp.267-278.

Sretenovi , L., Petrovi , M.P., Aleksi , S., Panteli , V., Kati , V., Bogdanovi , V. and Beskorovajni, R., 2008. Influence of yeast, probiotics and enzymes in rations on dairy cows performances during transition. *Biotechnology in Animal Husbandry, 24*(5-6), pp.33-43.

Tedesco, D., Tava, A., Galletti, S., Tameni, M., Varisco, G., Costa, A. and Steidler, S., 2004. Effects of silymarin, a natural hepatoprotector, in periparturient dairy cows. *Journal of dairy science, 87*(7), pp.2239-2247.

Tucker, H.A., 2000. Hormones, mammary growth, and lactation: a 41-year perspective. *Journal of dairy science, 83*(4), pp.874-884.

Vandehaar, M.J., Yousif, G., Sharma, B.K., Herdt, T.H., Emery, R.S., Allen, M.S. and Liesman, J.S., 1999. Effect of energy and protein density of prepartum diets on fat and protein metabolism of dairy cattle in the periparturient period. *Journal of Dairy Science, 82*(6), pp.1282-1295.

Vernon, R.G., Faulkner, A., Hay Jr, W.W., Calvert, D.T. and Flint, D.J., 1990. Insulin resistance of hind-limb tissues in vivo in lactating sheep. *Biochemical journal, 270*(3), pp.783-786.

Weiss, W.P. and Gonzalo, F., 2006. Are your cows getting the vitamin they need. *J. WCDS advances in Dairy Technology, 18*, pp.249-259.

Yamauchi, T., Kamon, J., Waki, H., Terauchi, Y., Kubota, N., Hara, K., Mori, Y., Ide, T., Murakami, K., Tsuboyama-Kasaoka, N. and Ezaki, O., 2001. The fat-derived hormone adiponectin reverses insulin resistance associated with both lipoatrophy and obesity. *Nature medicine, 7*(8), pp.941-946.

Zachut, M., Honig, H., Striem, S., Zick, Y., Boura-Halfon, S. and Moallem, U., 2013. Periparturient dairy cows do not exhibit hepatic insulin resistance, yet adipose-specific insulin resistance occurs in cows prone to high weight loss. *Journal of Dairy Science, 96*(9), pp.5656-5669.

Zebeli, Q., Mansmann, D., Steingass, H. and Ametaj, B.N., 2010. Balancing diets for physically effective fibre and ruminally degradable starch: A key to lower the risk of sub-acute rumen acidosis and improve productivity of dairy cattle. *Livestock Science, 127*(1), pp.1-10.

Zenobi, M.G., Scheffler, T.L., Zuniga, J.E., Poindexter, M.B., Campagna, S.R., Gonzalez, H.C., Farmer, A.T., Barton, B.A., Santos, J.E.P. and Staples, C.R., 2018. Feeding increasing amounts of ruminally protected choline decreased fatty liver in nonlactating, pregnant Holstein cows in negative energy status. *Journal of dairy science, 101*(7), pp.5902-5923.

Zhang, F., Nan, X., Wang, H., Zhao, Y., Guo, Y. and Xiong, B., 2020. Effects of propylene glycol on negative energy balance of postpartum dairy cows. *Animals, 10*(9), p.1526.

Zinicola, M. and Bicalho, R.C., 2019. Association of peripartum plasma insulin concentration with milk production, colostrum insulin levels, and plasma metabolites of Holstein cows. *Journal of dairy science, 102*(2), pp.1473-1482.

Chapter 18

Emerging Tissue Engineering Strategies in Neurodegenerative Disease Therapy

Uroos Ali*, Sumeira Shafi*, Nowsheen Amin*, Aasif A. Sheikh, Z. A. Pampori, D. Hasin, Fozia Shah, O. Aarif and M. R. Dar

Division of Veterinary Physiology, FVSc & AH, Shuhama, SKUAST-Kashmir, J&K

INTRODUCTION

Neural stem cell (NSC), a landmark discovery has extended the treatment strategies beyond symptomatic relief and opened the possibility of neural regeneration driven by neuronal circuits. NSCs are self-renewing multipotent cells capable of differentiating into any of the three elementary neuroectodermal specifications, including neurons, astrocytes and oligodendrocytes. Tissue engineering combines principles and techniques of cell biology, material science, and engineering to fabricate tissue substitutes that mimic the structural and physiological nature of native tissue with the fundamental aim to regenerate the functional properties of an injured or diseased tissue (Boni et al., 2018). The aim of tissue engineering is served by using scaffolds, cells, and bioactive molecules. Using scaffolds should mimic extracellular matrix (ECM) in morphological, biochemical and mechanical aspects to improve cell adhesion, proliferation, and differentiation (Tonda-Turo et al., 2016 & Amani et al., 2018). The main challenge of the tissue engineering is designing of appropriate biomaterials for effective mimicking of the native extracellular matrix (ECM). Among different materials, polymers due to their biocompatibility, biodegradability and easy processing are widely used for making scaffolds. The absence of bio-active sites in the synthetic polymers has limited their application in inducing tissue-specific regeneration. In recent years, incorporation of the ECM components or decellularized ECM matrix into synthetic scaffolds has overcome this limitation (Mao et al., 2017). Scaffolds, cells, and bioactive factors (Triad) are used in isolation or in combination (Figure 1) to recapitulate the desired tissue (Doblado et al., 2021).

The regeneration and repair of both the central nervous system (CNS) and peripheral nervous system (PNS) remain crucial challenges in tissue engineering, reason being their limited self-regeneration capacity (Lombardi V, 2012). The CNS can be impaired due trauma, car accidents, assaults, etc which are the leading causes of long-term disability in both urban and rural population worldwide. Neurodegenerative diseases, such as Alzheimer's disease, Parkinson's disease, Huntington disease and Amyotrophic Lateral Sclerosis are serious health problems resulting in discrete cell loss in specific brain regions and their incidence is more in aging population (Checkoway et al., 2011). Stroke is also a leading cause of adult disability because of the brain's limited capacity for repair, with most surviving the stroke, but living with a lasting impairment (Benjamin et al., 2018). Most of the current research is focused towards preventing further damage to the affected area. In addition, the PNS is also vulnerable to different kinds of traumatic injuries due to the extensive presence of nerves throughout the body. The most common types of traumatic peripheral nerve injuries are penetrating injury, crush injury, traction injury, ischemia, laceration, compression, and thermal injury (Adiguzel et al., 2016). Nerve injuries have devastating consequences due to sensory and motor function defects leading to paralysis and excruciating neuropathic pain (Boni et al., 2018).

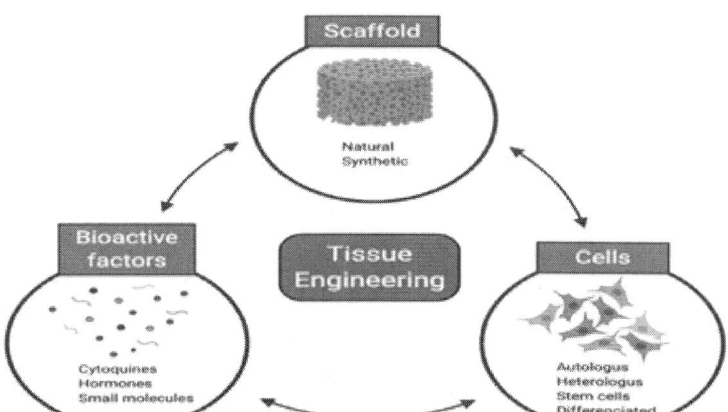

Figure 1: Tissue Engineering Triad

CELLS FOR NEURAL TISSUE ENGINEERING

There are three types of cell sources that can be used for tissue engineering: namely, autologous, allogenic and xenogeneic. Autologous cells are harvested from the patient, cultured *ex vivo* and then re-implanted at the site of injury in the patient. It is an ideal choice from an immunological perspective, as the cells used from one's own body don't elicit any immune reaction. The second cell source is allogeneic, which requires immune suppression or other strategies to reduce the immunogenicity of the allogenic cells. This has found limited success. One of the mostly widely used allogenic cell-based grafts is Apligraf, a bilayered tissue composed of a bovine type I collagen matrix populated with human male neonatal fibroblasts and an epidermal sheet derived from male neonatal epidermal keratinocytes. The third usable cell source is referred to as xenogeneic, where cross-species transplantation takes place. The immune response poses a major hurdle, along with cross-species pathogen infectivity. The cells used specifically in neural tissue regeneration (Figure 2) include Schwann cells, bone marrow derived mesenchymal stem cells (MSC) and other stem cell sources like embryonic Stem cells (ESC), nerve stem cells (NSC), and induced pluripotent stem cells (iPSC) (Sensharma et al., 2017).

Schwann Cells

Schwann cells produce neurotrophic factors and cause neurite outgrowth in the cells which helps in the repair of peripheral nerve injuries. Schwann cells play an important role in the process of axonal outgrowth. Schwann cells get activated when an injury takes place and secretes N-cadherin, neurotrophins, gamma integrins, neural cell adhesion molecules (N-CAM) as well as collagen and lamin in for ECM production (Sensharma et al., 2017). Conduits seeded with Schwann cells have been used successfully to repair defects in rat sciatic nerve, with functional recovery equivalent to nerve autograft at 6 months post-surgery (Zhang et al., 2014).

Bone Marrow Derived Mesenchymal Stem Cells (BM-MSC)

These are stromal cells which have the potential to differentiate into different cell lineages and can thus be investigated as a plausible alternative to the use of SCs. This cell type overcomes most of the drawbacks that the use of SCs present: multi-directional differentiation potential, and have many clinical advantages, such as the ease of accessibility, rapid proliferation in culture and successful integration into the host tissue without producing an eminent immune response.

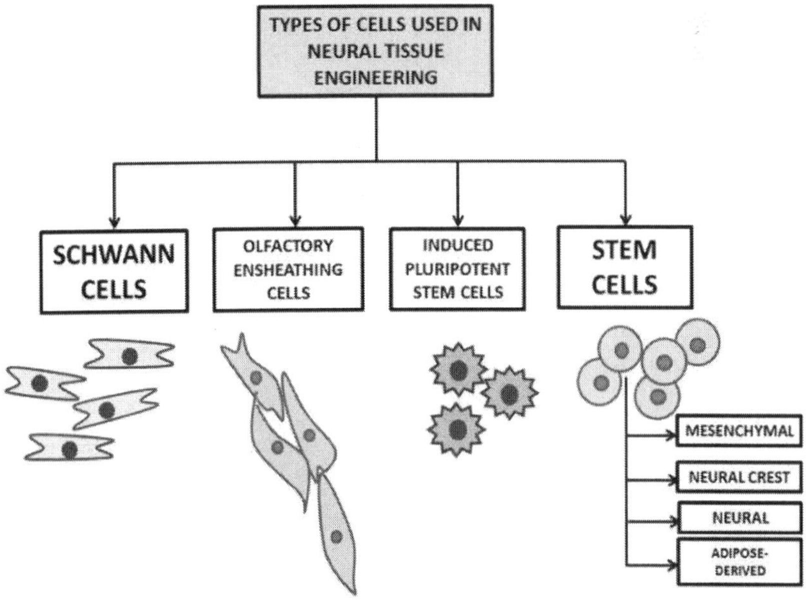

Figure 2: Types of cells used in Neural Tissue Engineering

Other Sources

1. Embryonic Stem Cells originate from embryos. Embryonic stem cells are pluripotent stem cells harvested from the human blastocyst with immense proliferation capacity. The advantage of using these cells is that they are bereft of the impact of age and disease and cause no discomfort upon extraction (Sensharma et al., 2017).
2. Adult Stem Cells are found inside the body among regular cells. They can multiply by cell division to replenish dying cells and tissue.
3. Neural stem cells are multipotent stem cells that give rise to different cell types within the neuronal lineage like astrocytes, oligodendrocytes, etc. Studies have reported that they play a regenerative role in response to events like ischemic stroke, multiple sclerosis and other neurodegenerative occurrences. Thus, the plasticity of the neural stem cells can be manipulated to give regenerative functions.
4. Autologous neural stem cells, mesenchymal stems cells (MSCs), and induced pluripotent stem cells (iPSC) provide alternative sources of trophic cells to autologous Schwann cells for neural tissue engineering. These cells can differentiate into any neural cell type.

NEURAL TISSUE ENGINEERING

Last two decades have witnessed an enormous progress with regards to understanding biological mechanisms regulating CNS and PNS. Polymers have been used in neural tissue engineering due to their range of versatility that is unmatched by other biomaterials like metals and ceramics.

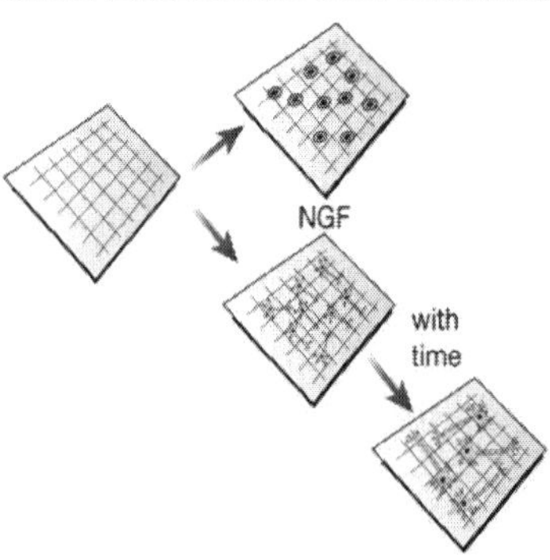

Figure 3: Polymeric structure for neural regeneration

The different polymers vary depending on the application they are being used for, such as 3D cell culture for PC12 cells, drug delivery vehicles, hydrogels, nerve conduits and scaffolds. Polymeric structures not only offer mechanical support for growing neurites but they also regulate biological cues to guide axonal growth, promote regeneration and stimulate integration into the existing healthy tissue (Figure 3). Polymer nanoparticles are considered an optimal and versatile drug delivery system for regions like the brain. Polymer nanoparticles are able to cross blood-brain barrier (BBB) and efficiently deliver drugs into damaged areas. Polymeric neural probes and electrodes have been successfully used to treat neurodegenerative diseases, dystonia, chronic pain, and deep brain stimulation, becoming an invaluable clinical and diagnostic tool (Boni et al., 2018). Polymeric structures seeded with nerve growth factor (NGF) offer mechanical support for growing neurites that differentiate into fully matured neurons. They regulate biological cues to guide axonal growth and sprouting to promote the regeneration of the nerves.

NATURAL POLYMERS FOR NEURAL TISSUE ENGINEERING

In neural tissue engineering, the use of natural polymers is highly beneficial due to their high biocompatibility and natural biodegradation kinetics combined with chemically tunable properties. Often, natural polymers are analogues to substances already present in the human body, minimizing the risks of cytotoxicity and immunogenic reaction upon implantation in the body e.g., Collagen. Natural polymers applied in neural tissue engineering have different origins, such as extracellular matrix components (ECM), like collagen, alginate, chitosan and silk. Natural polymers are the most researched type of polymer in neural tissue engineering. Collagen is the only biopolymer currently approved for clinical studies aimed at peripheral nerve regeneration (Boni et al., 2018).

Collagen

The most common, type I, a fibrillary type of collagen, provides structure and support. Collagen-based nerve guide conduits have been used to repair small nerve injuries. However, they have also given good results in the regeneration of larger injuries as in 15-mm gap in rat sciatic nerve or in combination with NGF, partially reconstructing a 35-mm gap in dog sciatic nerve model (Doblado et al., 2021). Collagen is also used in combination with other polymers and proteins in neural tissue engineering.

Gelatin

Gelatin is a denatured protein obtained by hydrolysis of animal collagen. Gelatin electrospun, in combination with other polymers supports the neurite outgrowth and SC proliferation e.g., gelatin/polycaprolactone (PCL). Gelatin nanoparticles too have been developed for neural tissue engineering (Doblado et al., 2021).

Elastin

Elastin-like polypeptides (ELPs) have found specialized applications in neural tissue engineering. ELPs enhance the biocompatibility and stability of polymeric structures and act as robust drug delivery systems targeting the brain. For example, ELPs can be tailored to be thermally responsive and target specific areas of the CNS for treatment of neurodegenerative disorders. ELPs fused with neurotrophin serve as a drug depot, limiting neurotrophin loss due to diffusion. Moreover, the controlled characteristics of ELPs allowed intranasal administration aimed at therapeutic drug delivery to the CNS (Boni et al., 2018).

Hyaluronic Acid

Hyaluronic acid (HA) is an un-branched glycosaminoglycan present naturally as ECM in all vertebrates including humans. It has gained significant interest in the area of neural tissue engineering, supporting neurite outgrowth. HA hydrogels enhance the survival rates and proliferation of neural precursors in the PNS and the CNS. HA can be used in combination with other natural polymers like collagen, chitosan, etc to promote regeneration (Boni et al., 2018).

Alginate

Alginate gels, polysaccharides obtained from brown algae and bacteria promote peripheral nerve regeneration across a 50-mm-long gap in cat sciatic nerve and a 10-mm nerve gap in rats, increasing the regenerating axon diameter. Alginate can be used in combination with other polymers to develop scaffolds, showing great potential for peripheral nerve regeneration and SCI treatment (Doblado et al., 2021).

Chitosan

Chitosan, derived by the chemical deacetylation of chitin, structural polysaccharide naturally is found in crustaceans and shellfish. Chitosan hydrogels promote cell adhesion, cell interaction, cell survival, and neurite outgrowth. Chitosan scaffolds with NGF show regeneration in PNS and CNS (Doblado et al., 2021).

SYNTHETIC BIOMATERIALS

Another approach for neural tissue engineering is the use of biomaterials of synthetic origin. For example, polycaprolactone (PCL), poly-L-lactic acid (PLLA), poly-D, L-lactic-co- glycolic acid (PLGA). A wide variety of formats can be obtained, such as aligned scaffolds, fibers or filaments, and tubular structures. However, they also have certain limitations, such as reduced bioactivity that increases the risk of rejection after implantation. Therefore, the choice of the origin of the biomaterials to be used is especially important.

Polycaprolactone (PCL)

Polycaprolactone (PCL) fibers have most commonly been generated by the method of electrospinning. PCL can be combined with natural polymers or coated with cells to improve its biocompatibility, cell adhesion properties, and promote regeneration of nerve fibers or assist the directional growth of regenerating axons in peripheral nerves.

Poly-L-Lactic Acid (PLLA)

Poly-L-lactic acid (PLLA) has been employed in the development of single or multilayer guidance conduits, nanofibrous conduit scaffolds with single or multiple microchannels, or like fibers allocated in the lumen of tubular conduits providing a support for cell adhesion, migration and elongation in a guided manner.

Poly-D, L-Lactic-co-Glycolic Acid (PLGA)

Poly-D, L-lactic-co-glycolic acid (PLGA) is a copolymer of polylactic acid (PLA) and polyglycolic acid (PGA). PLGA has been successful in drug delivery microparticles and conduits for nerve regeneration. PLGA seems to be extremely useful in transporting therapeutic agents across the BBB.

HYDROGELS

Hydrogels are 3D cross-linked hydrophilic polymer networks capable of swelling and de-swelling reversibly in water and can retain large volume of liquid in a swollen state. In neural tissue engineering, the two most common polymers used to create synthetic hydrogels are polyethylene glycol (PEG) and poly (2-hydroxyethyl methacrylate)/(pHEMA).

PEG is a biodegradable synthetic polymer of ethylene oxide (EO) units. PEG is highly biocompatible and well suited for use in hydrogels due to its hydrophilic properties, crucial for nutrient and waste transport, and is also biochemically inert. In addition, PEG is non-immunogenic and resistant to protein absorption. However, unlike natural polymers used in hydrogels, PEG is not bioactive; hence it is used in combination with other polymers. PEG hydrogels have been extensively used for neural tissue engineering. Neuronal cell growth on PEG platforms improves neural cell survival, proliferation, and differentiation, showing great potential for the treatment of CNS injuries. Lampe et al (2010) showed that in PEG 2D cultures hydrogel properties did not affect metabolic or apoptotic activity but affects cell proliferation and glial cell reactivity. Conversely, in PEG 3D cultures that closely matched the stiffness of the native brain, cells had increased metabolic activity and proliferation and lower rates of apoptosis.

The versatile and non-toxic nature of PEG meant it could be trialed preclinically and administered intravenously following head injury. Liu et al (2015) showed enhanced cell growth and migration along with improved functional recovery in rats after transection of the spinal cord using an electrospun PLGA/PEG scaffold.

pHEMA is a polymer that forms hydrogels in water due to its extremely hydrophilic nature, is biocompatible, and it can polymerize at low temperatures, (-20 C to +10 C), which allows immobilisation of proteins into hydrogels. Dalton et al (2002) development multiple pHEMA hydrogels capable of guiding neurite outgrowth. By controlling the formulation and surface chemistry, pHEMA hydrogels can be tailor made to suit a particular application in either the CNS or the PNS. Some pHEMA hydrogels were more suitable for peripheral nerve regeneration, and others have been developed with a photochemically bound nerve growth factor that promoted neurite outgrowth on 3D surfaces *in vitro*.

One of the main advantages of the use of hydrogels (PEG and pHEMA), in neural tissue engineering is the variety of characteristics that can be achieved. They can be applied as nerve guidance conduits, intravenous inhibitors of cell death, and as 3D structures that support the formation of nervous tissue. Figure 4 represents a simple schematic of an implanted hydrogel establishing new functional reconnections between seeded cells and the host's neurons.

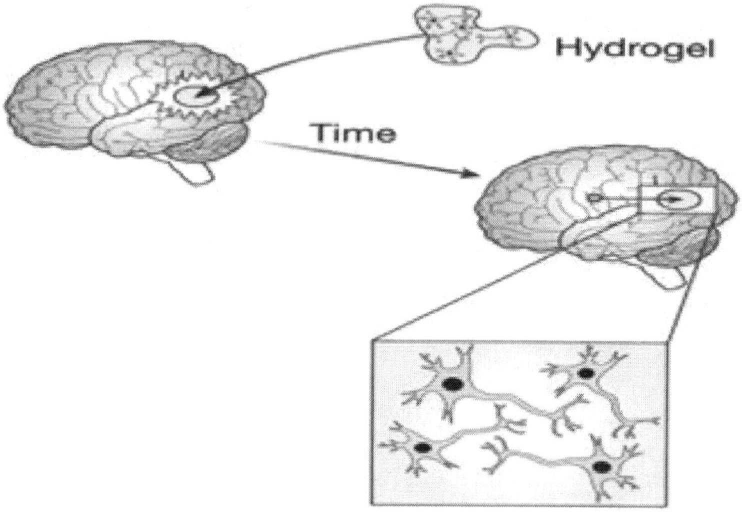

Figure 4: Polymer hydrogel supports the regeneration of the brain tissue

Conductive polymers are those with electrons present in their backbone, which enable them to conduct electricity. Nerve cells respond to electrical stimulation. Some common conductive polymers used are polypyrrole (PPY) and carbon nanotubes. Carbon-based nanomaterials present exclusive electrical, mechanical, and biological characteristics, which make them particularly useful for tissue engineering. In particular, neural tissue engineering mainly utilizes graphene and carbon nanotubes because of their inherent properties of conductivity, flexibility, and biocompatibility.

Wang et al (2011) derived Neural Crest-Derived Stem Cells (NCSCs) from ESCs or iPSCs as described in Figure 5. ESCs lost the expression of pluripotency markers Oct3/4 and Nanog upon differentiation. In contrast, the expression of various neural crest markers including AP2, Sox10, Slug and Brn3a increase during the differentiation process. ESC-NCSCs and iPSC-NCSCs formed neural sphere like aggregates when cultured on ultra-low-attachment plates in the presence of basic fibroblast growth factor (bFGF) and epidermal growth factor (EGF), and the cells within the spheres retained the expression of NCSC markers nestin, vimentin, p75 and HNK1.

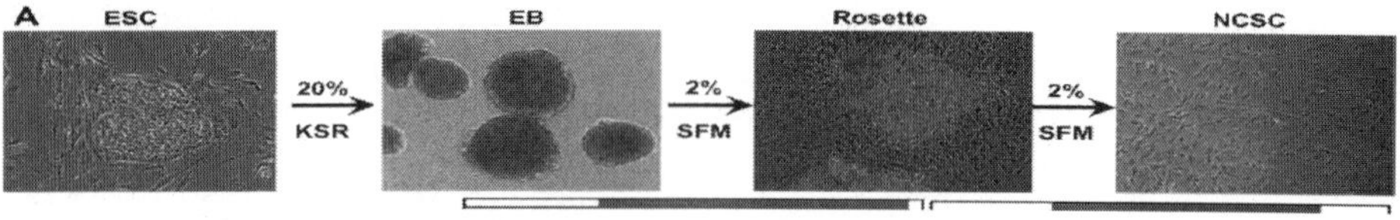

Figure 5: NCSC derived from iPSCs and ESCs

Besides the peripheral neural lineages, NCSCs could also differentiate into various mesenchymal lineages. Under specific conditions ESC-NCSCs and iPSC-NCSCs differentiated into chondrocytes, osteoblasts, adipocytes and smooth muscle precursors. The tissue engineering approach is schematically outlined in Figure 6.

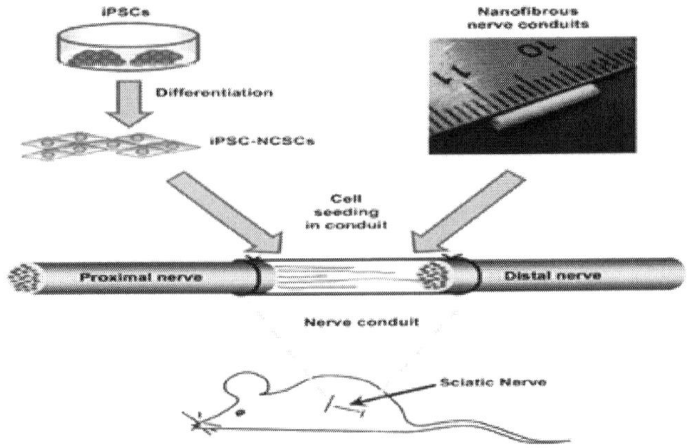

Figure 6: Tissue engineered nanofibrous nerve conduits for peripheral nerve regeneration

REGENERATIVE THERAPIES FOR NEURODEGENERATIVE DISEASES BY SCAFFOLDS

Amongst all the organs, the brain possibly represents the biggest challenge in terms of the modeling and development of therapeutic strategies. Its structural complexity and the inability to retrieve samples without highly invasive, and often unfeasible, approaches represent the major limitation in the study of physiological and pathological brain activity.

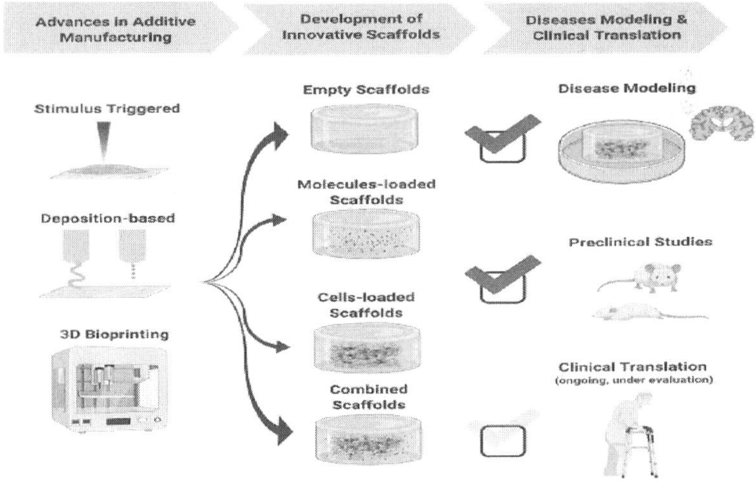

Figure 7: Use of additive manufacturing techniques in neurodegenerative diseases

The use of scaffolds becomes of great relevance in this field, as they can be used to mimic the brain's morphology and function, to improve cellular growth for transplantation means, to improve drug delivery, and even to be directly transplanted at the lesion site. Although the lack of successful replacement therapy for damaged brain tissue is worth looking at recent advances made in specific diseases, some common patterns can be highlighted. It is possible to discriminate between the transplantation of empty scaffolds, scaffolds carrying specific therapeutic agents, cell-loaded scaffolds, or scaffolds combining cells and molecules. The use of scaffolds improves the therapeutic efficacy as the contained agents are "protected" by the hydrogel and thus present a decreased degradation rate. Similarly, cell-loaded scaffolds can bridge stem cell therapy with tissue engineering, improving the delivery of stem cells to the lesioned site. Of late, the combined approach is being tried to deliver both drugs and cells or even different drugs contained in the same scaffold but released at different times after scaffold delivery (Figure 7).

Alzheimer's Disease (AD)

AD is the most common form of dementia and is characterized by progressive memory loss and declining cognitive functions, which eventually lead to patient's death. The two cellular hallmarks of the disease are the presence of extracellular amyloid plaques and intracellular neurofibrillary tangles (Karch et al., 2014). To date, there is no known therapy for the disease and the root cause of the disease is also unknown. Thus, there is a need to evolve from current pharmacological strategies, which, for now, are only symptomatic remedies. A therapeutic advancement involves the use of scaffolds, advantageous for both drug delivery and for promoting stem cell delivery and survival in the hostile AD microenvironment. In this context, hydrogels are of key importance for the delivery of therapeutic agents, to increase their bioavailability. Examples include biodegradable microspheres loaded with huperzine A, microemulsion loaded with tacrine, microspheres optimized to deliver NGF, PLGA nanoparticles loaded with estradiol or tempol, and thiolated chitosan hydrogels loaded with donepezil. Recently, a combinatory approach has also been tested, combining liposomes with hydrogels and delivering an active pharmaceutical ingredient, to improve bioavailability. (Bordoni et al., 2018; Rey et al., 2020).

Parkinson's Disease (PD)

Parkinson's disease (PD) is the second most common neurodegenerative disorder, with a prevalence of 1% in individuals over age 60 and 4% in individuals over age 85, characterized by the loss of dopaminergic neurons in the substantia nigra pars compacta (SNpc) and the presence of alpha-synuclein, which aggregates in toxic components termed Lewy bodies. The first line of therapy for the treatment of PD is dopaminergic agonists (such as L-DOPA, combined with other tested drugs). Several works have investigated the potentiality of hydrogels in the delivery of therapeutic agents (both pharmacological and biological) *in vivo* models of PD. The scaffolds "protect" the delivered neurotrophic agents (e.g., Glial cell-derived neurotrophic factor GDNF, NGF) and promote a controlled and localized release. A hydrogel-based system developed aims at improving transdermal dopamine delivery and a biodegradable polymer matrix releasing dopamine in the striatum of a hemi parkinsonian animal model.

Hydrogels have also been used for the delivery of less canonical therapeutic agents, such as Tat-fused protein, Heat Shock Protein 70 (Hsp70), activin-B, or even the secretome of mesenchymal stem cells. Hydrogels can also be used to ameliorate the differentiation of iPSCs to a dopaminergic phenotype, which could prove useful in drug screening and disease modeling. Another novel 3-D nanofiber scaffold has been developed using electrospun PAN, a pure carbon-based polymer, and Jeffamine polymer-infused PAN. Both scaffolds are capable of promoting the survival and proliferation of SH-SY5Y and U-87MG cells.

Amyotrophic Lateral Sclerosis (ALS)

Amyotrophic lateral sclerosis (ALS) is the most prevalent motor neuron disease and is characterized by the progressive loss of upper and lower motor neurons (MNs), leading to muscle atrophy, paralysis, and death 2–5 years after the first diagnosis. MNs derived from iPSCs are the most common neural cell type used in ALS. An increase in oxidative stress and DNA damage was found in iPSC derived C9ORF72 MNs, confirming that the reduction of oxidative stress could help to delay patient's death (Bordoni et al., 2018). Gingras and colleagues developed a 3-D tissue-engineered model to study motor neuronal axonal migration and myelination. The gold standard model that recapitulates all of the disease aspects observed in ALS would have to be a whole spinal cord organoid obtained from ALS patient-derived iPSCs. IPSCs MNs also proved to be a useful model for drug screening. Small molecule compounds that regulate IGF-II expression were found to increase MN resilience. Furthermore, Egawa and colleagues, which first generated and characterized MNs from iPSCs of TDP43 mutated patients, found some pathological hallmarks, such as short neurites and abnormal insoluble TDP43. They then tested trichostatin A, spliceostatin A, garcinol, and anacardic acid and wherein the last one, an inhibitor of histone deacetylase, rescued the pathogenic abnormalities. The devices, such as the "syringe-injectable nano-scale electronic scaffolds", which can be used to monitor neural activity, stimulate tissues, and promote neuronal regeneration, could be of great relevance in the treatment of the disease (Rey et al., 2020).

Acute Ischemic Stroke (AIS)

Acute ischemic stroke (AIS) is caused by a transient or permanent reduction in cerebral blood flow, generally caused by the occlusion of a cerebral artery, an embolus, or local thrombosis. The consequences of AIS are hypoxia, an increase in radical oxygen species, and an excessive inflammatory response, which can lead to long-term consequences. The first evidence that supported the use of scaffold in AIS was determined after the transplantation of NSCs on polymeric scaffolds. Hydrogels improved the interaction between NSCs and the host tissue, through neuronal differentiation, re-formation of cortical tissue, increased connectivity, reduced inflammation, and reduced scarring. Other types of cells, such as iPSCs and bone marrow mesenchymal stem cells, can be transplanted together with other kinds of scaffolds (e.g., gel-like scaffold from plasma). Hydrogels can be used for the delivery of pharmacological agents, which proved beneficial for stroke, such as erythropoietin (EPO), a cytokine found to promote neurogenesis after AIS; or vascular endothelial growth factor (VEGF), capable of inducing structural protection after AIS; and brain-derived neurotrophic factor (BDNF). Hydrogels have also been developed for sustained delivery of cyclosporine A, stimulating neurogenesis in the damaged tissue of the rodent brain.

Spinal Cord Injury (SCI)

SCI is a devastating disease caused by high-energy trauma, which leads to severe neurological dysfunctions. To this day, there is no curative therapy, and treatments are aimed at reducing secondary degeneration with high-dose corticosteroids, surgical stabilization, and decompression. It is especially during surgical stabilization that scaffolds could prove to be efficient and may be improving current lines of therapy. Synthetic scaffolds (e.g., physical chitosan micro hydrogels) implanted with drugs, growth factors and even stem cells are used to bridge the extremities of damaged spinal cords to promote regeneration and connectivity. Bhat et al (2019) showed that allogenic canine BMSCs can serve as potent therapeutic candidate for SCI. Biodegradable synthetic polymer scaffolds (PCL, PLA, PLGA, PEG), non-biodegradable synthetic polymer scaffolds (PHEMA, PHPMA, PAN/ PVC, conductive polymers), and natural polymer scaffolds (collagen, chitosan, alginate, fibrin) have a potential for SCI therapy. An interesting and promising technology is represented by graphene oxide (GO) 3-D nano-structured scaffolds, capable of stimulating neuronal differentiation through unique electro-physico-chemical properties. The MSC present inside the adipose tissue promoted regeneration and recovery of function, and reduced the inflammatory response (Li et al., 2019). Bio-scaffolds can also be used to deliver stem cells which are widely used in the treatment of the disease, but scaffolds complexed with NPCs have also been developed.

CONCLUSION

The repair of the nervous system is one of the great challenges of modern medicine. The cell-based therapies are not sufficient for the repair of neural tissue after damage. Tissue engineering advocates the combination of biomaterials together with cells and bioactive molecules to regenerate and support the repair of new tissue. More multidisciplinary approaches are needed in the future to apply these therapeutic strategies in clinics.

REFERENCES

Adiguzel E, Ya ar E, Tecer D, Güzelküçük Ü, Ta kaynatan MA, Kesikburun S, Özgül A. 2016. Peripheral nerve injuries: Long term follow-up results of rehabilitation. *Journal of Back and Musculoskeletal Rehabilitation*. 29(2):367-371.

Amani H, Mostafavi E, Arzaghi H, Davaran S, Akbarzadeh A, Akhavan O, Pazoki-Toroudi H, Webster TJ. 2018. Three-dimensional graphene foams: synthesis, properties, biocompatibility, biodegradability, and applications in tissue engineering. ACS *Biomaterials Science & Engineering*. 5(1):193-214.

Benjamin EJ, Virani SS, Callaway CW, Chamberlain AM, Chang AR, Cheng S, Chiuve SE, Cushman M, Delling FN, Deo R, de Ferranti SD. 2018. Heart disease and stroke statistics—2018 update: a report from the American Heart Association. *Circulation*. 137(12):e67-492.

Bhat IA, TB S, Somal A, Pandey S, Bharti MK, Panda BS, Verma M, Sonwane A, Kumar GS, Chandra V, Sharma GT. 2019. An allogenic therapeutic strategy for canine spinal cord injury using mesenchymal stem cells. *Journal of Cellular Physiology*. 234(3):2705-18.

Boni R, Ali A, Shavandi A, Clarkson AN. 2018. Current and novel polymeric biomaterials for neural tissue engineering. *Journal Of Biomedical Science*. 25:1-21.

Bordoni M, Rey F, Fantini V, Pansarasa O, Di Giulio AM, Carelli S, Cereda C. 2018. From neuronal differentiation of iPSCs to 3D neuro-organoids: Modelling and therapy of neurodegenerative diseases. *International Journal of Molecular Sciences*. 19(12):3972.

Checkoway H, Lundin JI, Kelada SN. 2011. Neurodegenerative diseases. IARC *Scientific Publications*. 163:407-419.

Dalton PD, Flynn L, Shoichet MS. 2002. Manufacture of poly (2-hydroxyethyl methacrylate-co-methyl methacrylate) hydrogel tubes for use as nerve guidance channels. *Biomaterials*. 23(18):3843-3851.

Doblado LR, Martínez-Ramos C, Pradas MM. 2021. Biomaterials for neural tissue engineering. *Frontiers in Nanotechnology*. 3:643507.

Karch CM, Cruchaga C, Goate AM. 2014. Alzheimer's disease genetics: from the bench to the clinic. *Neuron*. 83(1):11-26.

Lampe KJ, Mooney RG, Bjugstad KB, Mahoney MJ. 2010. Effect of macromer weight percent on neural cell growth in 2D and 3D nondegradable PEG hydrogel culture. *Journal of Biomedical Materials Research* (Part A). 94(4):1162-1171.

Li X, Liu D, Xiao Z, Zhao Y, Han S, Chen B, Dai J. 2019. Scaffold-facilitated locomotor improvement post complete spinal cord injury: Motor axon regeneration versus endogenous neuronal relay formation. *Biomaterials*. 197:20-31.

Liu C, Huang Y, Pang M, Yang Y, Li S, Liu L, Shu T, Zhou W, Wang X, Rong L, Liu B. 2015. Tissue-engineered regeneration of completely transected spinal cord using induced neural stem cells and gelatin-electrospun poly (lactide-co-glycolide)/polyethylene glycol scaffolds. *PloS One*. 10(3):e0117709.

Lombardi V. 2012. New challenges in CNS repair: the immune and nervous connection. *Current Immunology Reviews*. 8(1):87-93.

Mao Y, Hoffman T, Wu A, Goyal R, Kohn J. 2017. Cell type–specific extracellular matrix guided the differentiation of human mesenchymal stem cells in 3D polymeric scaffolds. *Journal of Materials Science: Materials in Medicine*. 28:1-8.

Rey F, Barzaghini B, Nardini A, Bordoni M, Zuccotti GV, Cereda C, Raimondi MT, Carelli S. 2020. Advances in tissue engineering and innovative fabrication techniques for 3-D-structures: translational applications in neurodegenerative diseases. *Cells*. 9(7):1636.

Sensharma P, Madhumathi G, Jayant RD, Jaiswal AK. 2017. Biomaterials and cells for neural tissue engineering: Current choices. *Materials Science and Engineering*. 77:1302-15.

Tonda-Turo C, Boffito M, Cassino C, Gentile P, Ciardelli G. 2016. Biomimetic polyurethane–Based fibrous scaffolds. Materials *Letters*. 167:9-12.

Wang A, Tang Z, Park IH, Zhu Y, Patel S, Daley GQ, Li S. 2011. Induced pluripotent stem cells for neural tissue engineering. *Biomaterials*. 32(22):5023-5032.

Zhang BG, Quigley AF, Myers DE, Wallace GG, Kapsa RM, Choong PF. 2014. Recent advances in nerve tissue engineering. *The International Journal of Artificial Organs*. 37(4):277-291.

Chapter 19

Heat Stress Effects on Mammogenesis and Amelioration Measures in Transition Cattle

Dr. Mahendra Singh[1], Mohammad Rayees Dar[2]

[1]Division of Animal Physiology, ICAR-National Dairy Research Institute, Karnal-132001,

** Email; chhokar.ms@gmail.com*

[2]Division of Veterinary Physiology, FVSc & AH, SKUAST-Kashmir – 190006

Milk has been recognized as a valuable food of pastoralist diets due to high proportion of the nutrients in the entire world. Different factors, such as race of animals, genetic variants, stage of lactation and environmental factors can significantly affect milk component and properties of milk. At present about 7.08 billion people inhabit on the earth and the estimated milk requirement is around 910.10 million tons, against a global production of 720.98 mt. milk. This demand can be met by intensive care of lactating animals for milking, feeding and reproductive management. However, climate has posed a formidable challenge to augment the milk production potential of elite animals. This situation is also being faced by the livestock sector in India to meet the increased demand of milk and milk products. The predicted anticipated rise in the global temperature (2.3-4.8 °C) together with high precipitation is likely to aggravate the heat stress in crossbred cows as compared to Indigenous ones. The net adverse effect of climate change on livestock is low productive, poor reproductive performance, reduced growth, immunity and increased incidence of disease in dairy farms. To assess the heat stress, many indices and index are being used in cows and buffaloes. The Temperature- Humidity Index (THI) is often used to relate animal stress with milk production in buffaloes, crossbred and indigenous cows, however comfort range of THI varies between breeds. The range of THI comfort in indigenous cows (Sahiwal,SW: Tharparkar,TP) ranges from 66-75, cold stress THI 55-65 and the heat stress THI is >76. It has been found that TP cows exhibit less magnitude of change in RT in TP cows than SW and Gir (GR) cows and have higher aldosterone level to regulate electrolyte balance of body. However, microclimatic alterations using mist and fan in the buffaloes shed augmented feed intake and more milk yield. Crossbred cows exhibit heat stress when THI>72 while thermal comfort (thermoneutral) zone temperature range between 16-25 °C which is beneficial to physiological functions i.e. lactation, growth and reproduction.

Ambient temperature >25 °C in temperate climate (crossbred/purebreds) and >30 °C in tropical climate (India) influence the production potential of animals. The Indigenous cows like Sahiwal, Tharparkar, Red Sindhi, Gir and Rathi are comfortable in hot-dry season between 33-35 °C. A rise in ambient temperature above this impairs the heat loss and heat gain balance. When the heat gain exceeds beyond heat loss from the body in hot dry and hot humid season, it results in heat stress in animals. The lactating animals are more vulnerable to heat stress due to being more active metabolically then the dry cows. The quality and quantity of the feed in summer season is also impaired which results in poor health, welfare, productivity (growth, reproduction, health and immunity. The climate change & warming effect is likely to continue and health and production, despite all mitigation measures taken in an animal farm, but we can minimize such adverse effects by adopting suitable management tools viz., shelter, feeding and milking management.

Lecture delivered in SAPICON 2023 organized by FVSc& AH, SKAUST, Srinagar, from 3rd-5th May, 2023

The physiological and behavioral responses are the integral part of thermoregulation to maintain body temperature within a safe range. Heat stress induces the following physiological indices at high temperature;

- Increased rectal temperature (body temperature)
- Increased respiration rate
- Increased pulse rate
- Increased heart rate
- Skin temperature changes
- Panting/ sweating

The impact of heat stress on the animal is further determined by;

1. Greater intensity of ambient temperature
2. Duration of heat exposure

Both the above factors can exceed to thermoregulatory capacity and evokes different animal responses as above. The observations on visible response of individual animal to heat stress in a dairy farm is labour intensive and time consuming and subjective.

Various sensor-based approaches to shift the focus of heat stress management to the individual animal level are now in use with following advantages.

- Strategies for heat-susceptible cattle and stress amelioration
- Save time and heat management costs
- Focus animal welfare and productivity.

◈ Real-time solutions to animal responses

RELEVANCE OF TRANSITION PERIOD

Mammary gland involution is a complex physiological process that transforms the lactating mammary gland to a non-secretary state. Transition phase is characterized by a high degree of programmed epithelial cell death, redevelopment of the mammary non-parenchyma tissue (adipose tissue) and its remodeling. Therefore transition phase is crucial to determine the milk production potential of animal in ensuing lactation. If cows are stressed in transition period the growth of fast growing fetus and mammary gland remodeling is impaired due to decrease in feed intake and low immunity.

EFFECT OF TEMPERATURE-PHOTOPERIOD

Photoperiod and temperature effects can be manipulated during the dry period in way that influence a cow's performance in the subsequent lactation. Dry cows exposed to short-day photoperiod (SDPP) produce more milk in the next lactation with improved immune function compared to cows managed with long day photoperiods (LDPP) due to altered PRL signaling (decrease PRL levels) and increase of PRL-Receptor (PRL-R) gene expression in mammary gland and other tissues of the body. This result in increased remodeling viz., increased cell proliferation, decreased cell apoptosis and increased mammogenesis. However, a narrow window of dry period during 3–6 wk prepartum is highly crucial to allow this.

Heat Stress and Cooling Effects on Mammogenesis

It has been found that heat stress in dry cows has tremendous adverse effects on next lactation production performance. HS decrease milk production by 10-15% and 15-20% in GD and HH season and negatively impact liver metabolism in early lactation. However lactating cows provided with mist and fan cooling have beneficial effects on feed intake and milk production by decrease in heat load. Dry cows provided with mist/ cooling facilities had greater mammary epithelial cell proliferation and increased expression of the hormone-sensitive lipase gene in the mammary gland in close-up period then non-cooled cows. Further gene expression profile of a lipid synthetic pathway is more associated with cell secretory state rather than mammary gland growth.

Heat Stress Influence Involution of Mammary Gland

The mammary gland undergoes following 3 stages of involution when dried off.

1. Active phase of involution
2. Steady phase of development
3. Regenerative and colostrogenesis phase

During initial active phase of involution (30 days), the migration of leucocytes and phagocytes in mammary gland results in phagocytosis of epithelial cells due to cessation of milking (drying off). Increased intramammary pressure causes release of cytosomal enzymes, growth factors which leads to necrosis and apoptosis of epithelial cells and growth of non-parenchyma tissue. Heat stress attenuates mammary involution through the altered endocrine profile. High temperature reduces placental estrone sulfate, placental lactogen (PL) levels and increase prolactin concentration which impair autophagy and apoptosis process taking place in epithelial cells during involution (drying off). The altered synchrony of hormones results in less mammary growth (new epithelial cells). These changes are also associated with prepartum reduction in DMI resulting in low milk production in the ensuring lactation.

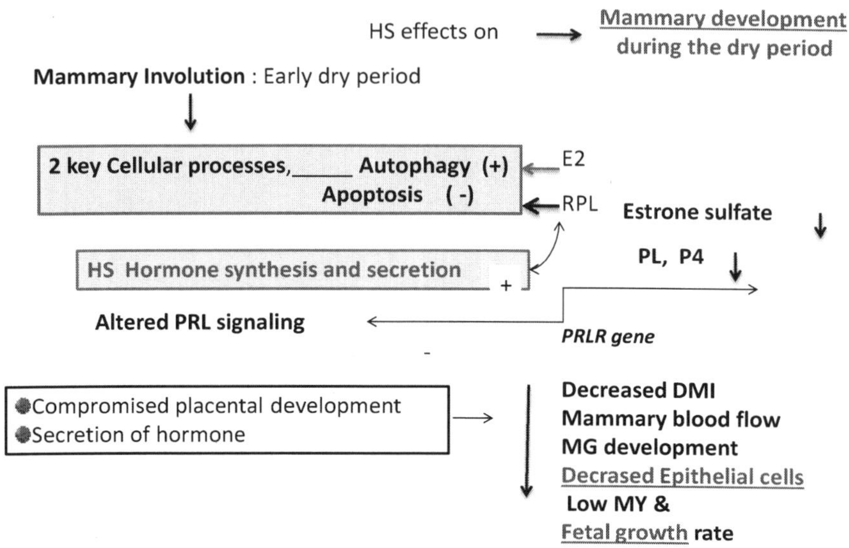

Heat stress disturb the positive relationship between the mediators of blood hormone: estrogen, progesterone, and PRL signaling in mammary and results in above shown effects in dry cows.

Thus removal of senescent cells within the mammary gland and their replenishment (cell proliferation) with new mammary cells takes place after drying off the animals.

Heat Stress Effects on Mammogenesis

- Decreased mammogenesis in late dry period
- Decreased mammary blood flow
- Increased expression of HSP (cytoprotective role) in MG
- Increased Anti-apoptotic cell properties
- Number of epithelial cells/ alveolus decrease
- No effect on postpartum synthetic capacity of cells
- Altered post-absorptive metabolism limits nutrient availability in mammary gland thereby influence mammary function and growth.
- Dry cows maintains positive EBAL, despite 10 to 15% decrease in DMI,

- No effect on blood glucose, insulin and plasma NEFA levels
- MEC apoptotic rates higher than cellular proliferation in dry period.

Effects on Colostrum and Milk Yield

- Cows produce less milk yield and protein.
- Colostrums yield (0.12kg), protein (0.08 kg) and fat (0.9%) decrease.
- Milk fat: protein ratio increases in dry-heat stressed cows
- Milk lactose remain unaffected
- Heat-stress in late-gestation –severe reduction in milk yield (3-7.5 kg/d) vis a vis cooled cows (fan, shade or foggers).

Amelioration of Heat Stress by Cooling Practices

Adoption of cooling measures which are frequently used by the organized dairy farms and progressive dairy farmers helps to alleviate heat stress. Cooling measure includes; use of fan, foggers, mist, water showers and ceiling fan usage in cows and buffaloes are being used frequently, however wallowing (buffalo) have more efficacious in amelioration of summer stress. Cows subjected to cooling practices (mist, foggers, fan) in transition period improves mammary growth and postpartum milk yield due to the comfort. Such animals have low stress indices like respiration rate, pulse rate, heart rate and skin temperature compared to non-cooled transition cows.

Postpartum Advantages of Cooling Practices

1. Higher milk yield due to increase in DMI (1 to 1.5 kg/d).
2. Cows cooled during dry period produce 4 to 5 kg/d more milk and have least adverse effects on alveolar morphogenesis and lactogenesis enzymes and hormones.
3. Non-cooled cows have low alveolar morphogenesis prepartum and low milk production postpartum due to less number of epithelial cells.
4. Heat stress also limits availability of milk precursors thus influence mammary seceretory functions and growth.
5. Heat stress does not influence adipose tissue mobilization but causes mobilization of protein in comparison to cooled cows.
6. Mammary gland of non-cooled cows had higher gene expression of Acetyl CoA carboxylase enzyme and fatty acid synthetase enzyme relative to cooled cows.
7. Heat stressed mammary gland of cow's partitions more energy for fatty acid synthesis and not for mammary cell proliferation.

During late dry period, the adverse effects of environmental factors like light (photoperiod) and temperature are more intense due to increased rate of fetus growth and onset of lactogenesis phase-I. Fetus achieves fastest growth in body weight i.e. 60% of calf birth weight is achieved in late dry period. Heat stress also causes immune dysfunctions, increased NEBAL and higher incidence of health and metabolic disorders during peri-parturient period.

Mammary Histological Changes

- Heat stress impairs mammary cell proliferation in dry period by down regulating the expression of genes associated with epithelial growth, branching of ducts and mammary immunity. However, expression of genes relating to apoptosis, phagocytic activity and cell survival are up-regulated.
- In HS in cows, the apoptotic rates exceed then rates of cellular proliferation.
- Proliferating epithelial cell decrease and adipose tissue cell increases.
- Reduction in alveoli numbers, alveolar area and an increase in non-parenchyma tissue.

Management Measures to Ameliorate Heat Stress

- Trees are very effective and serve as natural shade to cool the animals. The moisture evaporating from the plant leaves lowers the temperature between 4-°C.
- Artificial shades are also used to protect livestock's from adverse effects of solar radiation in absence of natural shade.
- Various types of roofing materials from metal to synthetic materials can be used for shade structures depending on the agro-climatic zones.
- Galvanized or aluminum roof reflect solar radiations and are considered best for animal shed.
- Cooling practices like use of Fan, Mist, Foggers, Showers etc. can be practiced to augment milk. It has been found that these practices increases milk yield between 10-15% in hot-dry and 15-20% in hot-humid season concomitant to higher DMI in crossbred, Indigenous cows (fan only) and buffaloes.
- Provision of sand bedding and use of ceiling fan in sheds in hot-humid season sustain the milk yield and dry matter intake.
- Use of mist or foggers in conjunction with fan is effective to alleviate heat stress in hot-dry season.

Feeding Interventions in Summer

Feeding interventions are essential to address the decline in DMI during the summer season in transition cattle and buffaloes. The adverse effects of heat waves further attenuate the deleterious effects due to low quality and less availability of nutrients. This situation becomes worst due to the reduced periparturient DMI (upto 20%). Transition phase is crucial period for the normal growth of fetus and mammogenesis. Therefore it is essential to reduce the decline in feed intake in periparturient cows in summer. The decreased DMI in conjunction with heat stress in transition period results in following effects.

- ◈ Reduced Body weight and Body condition score
- ◈ Diminished plasma concentrations of fat soluble vitamins
- ◈ Immuno-suppression
- ◈ Increased susceptibility to mastitis and metritis
- ◈ Enhanced vulnerability to metabolic diseases
- ◈ Poor growth of fetus
- ◈ Poor mammary gland fat pad &
- ◈ Poor growth of MG

Few important salient points to correct this problem are listed below.

a. Feed high quality forages,
b. Maintain a balanced ration (pregnancy +maintenance allowance)
c. Maintain dietary crude fiber level >18-19 %
d. Dietary ADF and NDF should be 25-28 %
e. Use by pass fat/ protein in ensuing lactation

ROLE OF PA-PG-PL SYSTEM ON MILK SECRETION DURING STRESS

Fast modulation of milk secretion in response to external factors, such as emotional stress, and severe physical conditions such as heat stress and water scarcity depends on such negative-feedback regulatory system (Figure 1), which enhances the potential to survive in stress conditions. Hence, the milk secretion and mammary functions are regulated acutely by local autocrine feedback mechanisms that involve milk-borne factors, sensitive to the frequency and efficiency of milking. The factors like negative energy balance and stress lead to an alteration in the milk and plasma plasminogen.

The principal enzyme in milk is plasmin which originates from blood and enters milk either in soluble form or associates with casein micelles. Adipose tissue mobilization has correlated with the highest expression of plasminogen activator receptor. The plasminogen activator along with plasmin and plasminogen constitute PA-PG-PL system, a milk-borne factor which down-regulates milk secretion during stress conditions. Factors like stages of lactation, seasonal, stress, type of diet and mastitis effects PA-PG-PL system. Hypothalamus-pituitary-adrenocortical axis activation by external stress liberates cortisol into blood plasma, which in turn induces the liberation of Plasminogen Activator (PA) from the mammary epithelial cells, where it stimulates the Plasminogen-Plasmin (PG-PL) system. This is the negative feedback system specifically forms β-casein (CN) fragment (f) (1-28) from β-CN, which acts as the negative control signal to down-regulate milk secretion by closing the potassium channels on the apical membrane of the epithelial cells of the mammary gland. Down-regulation of these channels persuades cellular signals that inhibit milk secretion.

The PA-PG-PL system is expressed in the milk of humans, ruminants and rodents and is related with regulation of milk secretion in both cows and goats and initiation of involution in goats, cows and rodents. Plasminogen/plasmin, a serine-proteinase system, is principal hydrolytic system in milk of many species. This system is associated to casein micelles which signify its substrate. In bovine milk most of the enzyme is in the form of the inactive zymogen PG, which is converted to active PL by the action of enzymes called PA. The action of PL and PA in milk is controlled by a heterogeneous system of inhibitors.

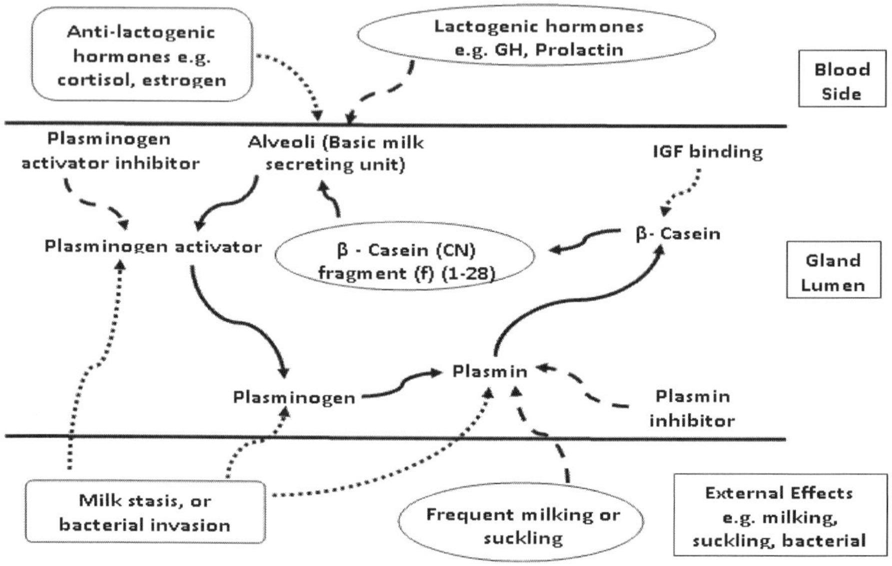

Figure 1: Overview of the PA-plasminogen-plasmin negative feedback mechanism that down-regulate milk secretion. (Bold arrows indicate flow signal along the feedback loop, dotted arrows positive effects and dashed arrows suppressive effects).

Summary: The fetal temperature is determined primarily by maternal environment of a heat stressed cows. The prenatal exposure of developing calf to hyperthermia in late gestation probably establishes a different intrauterine environment that may limit nutrient availability to growing fetus. Thus maternal insults (thermal stress) during dry period have significant impact on remodeling of mammary gland tissue and cell secretory functions thereby reducing postpartum milk production performance. Availability of cooling facilities ameliorates the adverse effect of heat stress and has beneficial effects on mammogenesis and milk production in ensuing lactation. Negative feedback system specifically forms β-casein (CN) fragment (f) (1-28) from β-CN, which acts as the negative control signal to down-regulate milk secretion by closing the potassium channels on the apical membrane of the epithelial cells of the mammary gland. Down-regulation of these channels persuades cellular signals that inhibit milk secretion during the stress conditions.

REFERENCES

Aggarwal, A. and Mahendra Singh. 2008. Changes in skin and rectal temperature in lactating buffaloes provided with showers and wallowing during hot-dry season, 40(3):223-8. doi: 10.1007/s11250-007-9084-3.

Aggarwal, A. and Mahendra Singh.2010. Hormonal changes in heat-stressed Murrah buffaloes under two different cooling systems. Buffalo Bulletin 291(1):1-6.

Aggarwal, A. and Mahendra Singh. 2007. Economics of using mist and fan system during summer and in-house shelter during winter for alleviating environmental stress in dairy animals. Ind. J. Agri. Econ. 62 (2): 272-79.

Amaral, do.B.C.; Connor, E.E.; Tao, S.; Hayen, J.; Bubolz, J.; Dahl, G.E. 2009.Heat-Stress Abatement during the Dry Period: Does Cooling Improve Transition into Lactation? *J. Dairy Sci. 92*, 5988–5999.

Bethany, D.S., Amy, L.S, Dahl, G. E., Sebastian, I.A.A, Laporta, J. 2021. Dry period heat stress impacts mammary protein metabolism in the subsequent lactation. *Animals, 11*(9), 2676

Daly SE, Owens RA, Hartmann PE. The short term synthesis and infant regulated removal of milk in lactating women. Experimental physiology. 1993; 78: 209-220.

Fantuz F, Pedron O, Polidori F, Tedesco D, Baldi A. Milchwissenschaft (Dairy Science) 2001; 3: 150-153.

Gerbens-Leenes, W. 2017. Dietary transition: Long term trends, animal versus plant energy intake, and sustainability issues. Vegetarian and plant-based diets in health and disease prevention, in book: Vegetarian and Plant-Based Diets in Health and Disease Prevention (pp.117-134), DOI: 10.1016/B978-0-12-803968-7.00008-3

Haque N, Singh M, Hossain SA. PA-PG-PL system in dairy animals and its significance: a review. International Journal of Dairy Science. 2015; 10(3): 95–106.

Haque, N., Hossain,S.A. and Singh,M. 2017. Effect of Management Practices on Milk Yield and Composition of Lactating Murrah Buffaloes during Different Seasons. Bull. Env. Pharmacol. Life Sci., Vol 6 Special issue [3]: 447-450

Heegaard CW, Rasmussen LK, Andreasen PA. The plasminogen activation system in bovine milk. Differential localization of tissue-type plasminogen activator and urokinase in milk fractions is caused by binding to casein and urokinase receptor. Biochimica et Biophysica Acta. 1994; 1222: 45–55.

Kelly AL and McSweeney PLH. Indigenous Proteinases in Milk. In: Advanced Dairy Chemistry, Fox, P.F. and P.L.H. McSweeney (Eds.). Kluwer Academic/ Plenum Publishers, New York, USA. 2003; 1: 495-521.

Maurya, S., Mahendra Singh, Aggarwal, A. and Sharma, R. 2020.Effect of seasons on physiological responses, milk production and composition in Indigenous cows. J. Anim. Sci. Vet. Med. Volume 5(1):11-20.

Ouellet, V.; Laporta, J.; Dahl, G.E.2020. Late Gestation Heat Stress in Dairy Cows: Effects on Dam and Daughter. Theriogenology, 150: 471–479 (PLoS One. 2019; 14(9):e0222120)

Politis I. Plasminogen activator system: implications for mammary cell growth and involution. Journal of Dairy Science. 1996; 79: 1097–1107.

Shamay A, Shapiro F, Mabjeesh SJ, Silanikove N. Casein-derived phosphopeptides disrupt tight junction integrity and precipitously dry up milk secretion in goats. Life Science. 2002; 70: 2707-2719.

Shangguan Tao, J.W. Bubolz , B.C. do Amaral, I.M. Thompson. 2011. J. Dairy Sci., 94(12):5976-86

Silanikove N, Iscovich J, Leitner G. Therapeutic treatment with casein hydrolyzate eradicate effectively bacterial infection in treated mammary quarters in cows. In: Hogeveen, H. (Ed.), Mastitis in Dairy Production: Current Knowledge and Future Solutions. Wageningen Academic Publishers, Wageningen. The Netherlands, 2005b; 327–332.

Silanikove N, Merine U, Leitner G. Physiological role of indigenous milk enzymes: an overview of an evolving picture. International Dairy Journal. 2006; 16, 533–545.

Silanikove N, Shamay A, Shinder D, Moran A. Stress down regulates milk yield in cows by plasmin induced β-casein product that blocks K+ channels on the apical membranes. Life Sciences. 2000; 67: 2201–2212.

Silanikove N, Shapiro F, Shinder D. Acute heat stress brings down milk secretion in dairy cows by up-regulating the activity of the milk-borne negative feedback regulatory system. BMC Physiology. 2009; 9: 13.

Skibiel, A.L., Jin Koh, Ning Zhu, Fanchao Zhu, Mi-Jeong Yoo and Jimena Laport. 2022. Carry-over effects of dry period heat stress on the mammary gland proteome and phosphoproteome in the subsequent lactation of dairy cows. *Scientific Reports*, 12: 6637

Sreenivasaiah, K. et al. 2016.Climate Change and Its Impact on Milk Production in India, book on ; Climate Change Challenge (3C) and Social-Economic-Ecological Interface-Building pp.531-547; DOI:10.1007/978-3-319-31014-5_32.

Tao, S., R.M., Orellana, X.Weng, T.N., Marins, G., E.Dahl, J.K. Bernard. 2018. Symposium review:The influences of heat stress on bovine mammary gland function. J. dairy sci., 101:60:5642-5654

Tao, S.; Bubolz, J.W.; do Amaral, B.C.; Thompson, I.M.; Hayen, M.J.; Johnson, S.E.; Dahl, G.E. 2011.Effect of Heat Stress during the Dry Period on Mammary Gland Development. *J. Dairy Sci.* 2011, 94, 5976–5986

Tonner E, Allan GJ, Flint DJ. Hormonal control of plasmin and tissue-type plasminogen activator activity in rat milk during involution of the mammary gland. Journal of Endocrinology. 2000; 167: 265–273.

Chapter 20

Extreme Weather Events: Impacts on Livestock and Ameliorating Strategies

Sohan Vir Singh
Animal Physiology Division
ICAR-National Dairy Research Institute
Karnal, India

India has vast livestock resources which are also an important source of income for landless and marginal farmers and plays an important role in national economy. It is an important part of Indian agriculture, supporting livelihood of about 55% of the rural population. Which are economically valuable. Growth in demand for livestock products is primarily expected to escalate due to increase in human population, increasing urbanization and rising income, as the demand for livestock products is income elastic. These developments present enormous opportunities to boost farmer's income, especially in less developed region (Saxena et al. 2017) and accelerate the pace of poverty reduction. The gross value added (GVA) from livestock sector contributed 4.1 percent to the total GVA and 27.5 percent to the agricultural GVA in 2017-18. This sector is also being considered to play promising role in the ambitious goal of the government to double the farmer's income (Chand, 2017; Das and Kumar, 2017). Animal rearing has multidimensional potential so the Indian government and state governments have made significant efforts to boost milk output and milk availability per capita. In 1970, Operation Flood has helped dairy farmers in directing their own growth, increasing milk output ("a flood of milk"), boosting rural incomes, and ensuring fair prices for milk consumers. The demand for animal food products is growing fast and so the necessity of consumers awareness about food safety (Kumar et al. 2017 and Joshiand Kumar, 2016).

Livestock in India are low-yielding and livestock producers face several risks or constraints related to animal health, nutrition and breeding in improving livestock productivity. Gradual stress induced by global warming and climate change is also influencing fertility and productivity of livestock. Birthal et al. (2008) estimated that more than26% of the milk production in India was lost due to these constraints and half of these were due to insufficient availability of feed and fodder and the rest were shared by diseases (21%), breeding problems (18%) and inappropriate management (11%).

Climate change also has complicated impact on livestock performance. Increasing climate variability is expected to surge livestock production risks in addition to reduced capacity of farmers to cope up with the serisks. It has been seen that extreme events such as floods and prolonged summer droughts/dry spells and heat and cold waves were on increasing trend from the last two-and-half-a-decades in a projected climate change scenario. The 20-years data of extreme weather events were compared between 1980-1999 and 2000-2019 and that an increase of 138% in heat waves, 193% in lightning strikes, 25% in cold waves, 28% in floods, and a decrease of 19% in tropical cyclones. These extreme weather events can affect the animal productivity and reproduction both directly such as heat stress due to heat wave and indirectly through water scarcity, tides or floods, soil infertility, poor grain yield and quality because of draught and distribution of pathogens. It has been estimated that up to 2050 the world population will increase by 60% and the consumption will increase to double (Cohen, 2001). Thus, it becomes important to pay attention on sustainable livestock production to meet up the future demand. Extreme climate is a major hurdle to meet up the goal. So, it is important first to know about various extreme weather conditions and how it is affecting the livestock production and reproduction.

Recent 6thsynthesis report of IPCC (2023) predicted that with every increment of global warming, climatic extremes will become more widespread and pronounced. The CO2 absorption capacity of land and ocean sinks is likely to decrease, ocean acidification is likely to increase, and compound heat waves and droughts are projected to become more frequent.

Climate strongly influences the growth, production (Choudhary and Sirohi, 2019; Choudhary, 2017; Kanwal, 2018), reproduction (Nardone et al. 2010), health and well-being ofthe livestock through affecting animal physiology, incidence of disease (Nardone et al. 2010;Thorntonetal. 2009) feed, fodder and water availability etc. Increased climatic variability particularly in terms of rainfall and temperature is likely to negatively influence the live stock productivity. Animal health can be directly or indirectly affected by climate change, particularly rising temperatures (Nardoneetal.2010). These direct and indirect effects may be due to the consequence of individual or combined changes of air temperature, humidity and magnitude of extreme weather events.

The direct effects are related to the increased temperature, which increases the potential for morbidity and death. The indirect effects are related to the impacts of climate change on microbial communities (pathogens or parasites), spreading of vector-bornediseases, food-bornediseases, hostresistance and feed and waters car city (Nardone et al. 2010; Thornton et al. 2009).

CLIMATE CHANGE AND PRODUCTION

In general, India's climate is dominated by the summer monsoon (June to September). Whole year is divided into four seasons:

i. Winter (January and February)

ii. Pre-monsoon or Hot Weather season (March–May)

iii. Southwest or Summer Monsoon season (June–September)

iv. Post monsoon season (October–December).

The IPCC's (IPCC, 2007) anticipated average increase by 0.74 ± 0.18 °C (1.33 ± 0.32 °F) surface temperatures is mostly due to an increase in global atmospheric temperature and greenhouse gases, particularly carbon dioxide concentration, precipitation variation and a combination of these variables.

Zebu cattle, which are more acclimated to India's tropical environment, show a change in milk production during different climatic conditions. As the temperature increases, reduction in total dry matter intake and milk yield is observed in Haryana cattle (Lal et al. 1987).The production of Sahiwal cows has similarly decreased when the temperature and relative humidity have increased (Mandal et al. 2002b).The milk yield of crossbred cows (e.g., Karan Fries, Karan Swiss, and various Holstein and Jersey crosses) is negatively associated with the temperature-humidity index (Mandal et al. 2002a).Bovines under heat stress lose a large proportion of body weight and body score because of the drop in energy intake caused by reduced feed intake, which causes a negative energy balance (Lacetera et al., 1996). Several studies are available that demonstrates the alteration of glucose, protein and lipid metabolism and alteration of liver functionality in heat stressed subjects (Moore et al., 2005). Martin et al. (1975) showed that summer calves had higher mortality rates. Others have claimed that heat stress could be responsible for the diminished protective efficacy of colostrum in cows (Nardone et al., 1997), and also for modification of passive immunoglobulin transfer in neonatal calves (Lacetera, 1998).

Buffaloes are well-suited to hot and humid areas due to their morphological and anatomical traits; however heat stress has a negative impact on buffalo reproduction (Tailor and Nagda 2005).

IMPACTS OF EXTREME WHETHER EVENTS ON LIVESTOCK

Weather refers to the physical state of the atmosphere at a specific location at a particular time. The instantaneous or short-term mean value of several atmospheric variables such as atmospheric pressure, temperature, humidity, cloudiness and sunshine, evaporation, and rainfall are used to characterise weather. Weather affects livestock husbandry operations and comfort and discomfort on a daily basis.

There are an estimated 535.78 million livestock in India; they are vital to the rural communities where they mostly live. Rural families keep an average of five to seven animals. These are usually a combination of bovine (cattle and buffaloes), sheep, goats, pigs, chickens and ducks. Their owners depend on them for their income, livelihoods and companionship.

According to the Directorate of Animal Husbandry and Veterinary Services, 4393 animals died in 13 districts in Odisha as a result of cyclone "phailin" in October 2013. It was also stated that the hurricane killed 166579 poultry birds in five areas. Ganjam, Kendrapada, Khordha, Puri, Jajpur, Gajapati, Balasore, and Bhadrak were the most impacted districts. In the ten cyclone-affected areas of the state, carcasses of 1169 large animals, 2,728 small animals, and 161,949 birds were disposed of.

The success or failure of animal husbandry is determined by a complex chain of factors including breed, nutrition management and the environment and its interactions, such as weather and climate. Any weak link in the chain finally decreases the animal production. Nowadays livestock farmers are encountering new challenges of increased weather/climate risks. The vulnerability of animals to extreme weather events is generally higher than vulnerability to changing average climatic conditions. During these events the economy of farmers are badly affected. Severe storms and hurricanes that are accompanied by excessive flooding and high winds have also proven deadly for farm animals, killing millions of birds and thousands of pigs in recent years. Floods and drought contribute for 83 percent of total crop and livestock production losses, with drought accounting for 44% of losses and floods accounting for 39% (FAO, 2015). The occurrence of whether extremes are as follows:

i. Cold wave, Fog, Snow storms and Avalanches
ii. Hailstorm, Thunderstorm and Dust storms
iii. Heat wave
iv. Tropical cyclones and Tidal waves
v. Floods, Heavy rain and Landslides
vi. Droughts

These are all related to weather, flood and drought are more frequent due to adverse changes in temperature and precipitation whereas earthquakes, volcanoes, and tsunamis are examples of geophysically generated calamities.

No. of cattle lost in India due to natural disaster from 2018-2019

Year	No. of cattle loss
2008	119218
2009	53833
2010	128452
2011	48778
2012	9126
2013	24293
2014	102998
2015	92180
2016	59057

2017	41965
2018	46488
2019	123014

(Source:- Statista, 2021)

Heat Wave

Heat waves occur during the summer season when extreme positive deviations from the normal maximum temperature occur. In the northwestern areas of the country, the rising maximum temperature during the pre-monsoon months often lasts through June and in exceptional occasions, until July. Heat waves and high temperatures throughout the summer months put all farm animals, whether housed outdoors or in building structure, at risk of heat stress and hyperthermia.

Cold Wave

Cold waves are defined as periods of extremely low temperatures associated with the arrival of dry cold winds from the north into the subcontinent. Extreme cold, wind, and snow make animals housed outside, particularly cattle, sheep, and goats, vulnerable to cold-weather-related injuries and illnesses including frostbite and hypothermia, throughout the winter. Transient disturbances in the mid-latitude westerlies, which typically have mild frontal characteristics, affect the northern areas of India, particularly the mountainous regions and bordering plains called western disturbances. The maximum number of cold waves occurs in Jammu and Kashmir followed by Rajasthan and Uttar Pradesh.

Land Slide

Landslides are mass movements of rocks and debris caused by gravity following a storm, volcano, or earthquake (Cruden and Varnes, 1996). The Himalayan and Western Ghats regions of India are the most prone to land-slides. Sliding of vast swaths of land has been a typical natural calamity in India's mountainous regions, causing bad impact on lives and property. Weak, weathered materials, physical property variations, ground uplift, erosion, earthquakes and volcanic eruptions are the main causes of landslides. Drainage correction, reforestation, and public awareness are examples of general and easy mitigation that are used. In 2014, 15 buffaloes and 12 cow were died due to the landslide in Uttrakashi.

Tropical Cyclones

The frequency of tropical storms in the north Indian ocean has increased significantly in recent decades (20% every hundred years) between November and May, when the most intense cyclones occur (Singh et al., 2000). Because to the unique nature of the coastline, weak coastal bathymetry and tide characteristics, tropical cyclones affecting the east coast of India and Bangladesh frequently create higher storm surge than elsewhere in the world. The storm in Andhra Pradesh, which struck from November 14 to 20, 1977, killed an estimated 2,30,146 cattle and 3,44,056 other livestock, compared to 8,515 people. Similarly, after the Orissa storm on June 4, 1982, 11,468 livestock were lost compared to 243 human deaths.

Cyclones also cause huge losses of animal life in India – most notably the 1999 Orissa Super Cyclone killed 3,205,689 animals (mainly cattle, small animals and poultry birds) in Orissa state. The lessons learned from this terrible disaster meant that the Orissa State government was prepared for 2013's Cyclone Phailin. They conducted India's biggest evacuation in 23 years evacuating nearly 1.2 million people and 30,000 animals.

Earthquakes

Infrastructure, such as bridges, dams, roads, and trains, can be damaged by an earthquake. Apart from a lack of feed and fodder, contamination of water caused by drainage water seepage causes severe discomfort to people and animals. Physical injuries are unlikely if animals are tied outside or housed in thatched sheds. When animals are tethered or imprisoned, their chances of escaping are restricted and they may suffer serious injuries.

Animal lives lost and human population affected due to major earthquakes in India

Date	Place	Magnitude (on Richter scale)	Population affected	Livestock losses	Damage to property US$)
25 April, 2015	India & Nepal	7.8	8,964 (78 death)	Not known	$10 billion
08 October, 2005	Kashmir	7.6	86,000–87,351	Thousands in number	2.8 million displaced
26 January, 2001	Gujarat	7.9	38 million	20,000 heads, worth 4,519 million (a)	US$1.22 million (a)
29 March, 1999	Chamoli, Northern India	6.6	372,000(b)	Very high	Not known
30 September, 1993	Latur and Osmanabad (Maharashtra)	6.4	30,000(c)	15,800 heads(c)	11 billion (c)
20 October 1991	Uttarkashi, Tehri and Chamoli (Uttar Pradesh)	6.1	307,000 (d)	3, 096 heads (d)	Not known

Sources: Sharma and Wason (2000)

Agriculture and livestock industry sectors are most affected by the earthquake (ADBWB,2005). Agriculture and livestock provide employment about 33.6% in Jammu and Kashmir where majority of the rural population engaged in agriculture. The significant loss of agricultural assets worth Rs.12.9 billion, where a reduction in production capacity might affect the food security and livelihoods.

According to Sobia et al. (2008) about 26% complained poor agriculture production as a result of the earthquake, 31% believed in food shortage, 27% reported loss of livestock and poultry, 22% reported loss of land, 24% reported about market fluctuation and inflation and 14% reported loss of jobs during earthquake 2005.

Drought

Drought is a condition in which there is a lack of rainfall for an extended period of time. Water levels in ponds, reservoirs, rivers, streams, and groundwater may be lower than usual, resulting in a hydrological imbalance. Drought causes a reduction in the amount of water available for drinking, as well as a shortage of feeds and fodders and the animals may become stressed, lowering their output. On a dry matter basis, India is already lacking in feed and fodder, with 40% dry fodder, 36% green fodder and 52% concentrate (DAHDF, 2013-14) and poor quality roughage, largely agricultural leftovers, is already one of the key restrictions. Various forms of disasters in India would expand the gap even more. In comparison to the other extremes, about 44% of the country's livestock are perpetually affected by droughts.

According to the Standardized Precipitation Index (SPI), just seven years (1988, 1992, 1994, 1995, 2011, 2012 and 2013) in Rajasthan have seen normal rainfall with no drought. Droughts of varied intensities occurred in various districts around the state in the remaining years, though the official drought years were 1987, 1999, 2000, and 2002. During these years cattle losses were substantially larger than buffaloes. According to Rathore (2004) local livestock become unproductive and weak during drought years. After the drought of 2002, the number of dry cattle (crossbred) and buffalo increased, which is reflected in a decrease in buffalo in-milk and adult female cattle ratios. Sheep and goats numbers dropped dramatically during drought years, which is a major part of the total livestock. The change in livestock population shown in the table-

Particular	Category	1983	1988	1992	1997	2003	2007	2012
Cross-bred	AFC*	15 -86-7	28 -86.7	56 -100	85 -51.8	249 -192.9	420 -68.7	929 -121.2
	IM**	10	15 -50	28 -86.7	54 -92.9	173 -220.4	316 -82.7	654 -107
Indigenous-cattle	IM-:AFC	0.64	0.54	0.5	0.64	0.69	0.75	0.7
	AFC	5099	4342 (-14.8)	4566 -5.2	4993 -9.4	4652 (-6.8)	5093 -9.5	5540 -8.8
	IM	2110	1762 (-16.5)	2100 19-.2	2411 -14.8	2208 (-8.4)	2726 -23.5	3091 -13.4
	IM:AFC	0.41	0.41	0.46	0.48	0.47	0.54	0.56

Particular	Category	1983	1988	1992	1997	2003	2007	2012
Total cattle		13504	10920 (-19.1)	11666 -6.8	12141 -4.1	10854 (-10.6)	12119 -11.7	13324 -9.9
Buffalo	AFC	3115	3467 -11.3	4133 -19.2	5221 -26.3	5658 -8.4	5824 -2.9	6733 -15.6
	IM	1590	1863 -17.2	2429 -30.4	3136 -29.1	3392 -8.2	3929 -15.8	4448 -13.2
	IM:AFC	0.51	0.54	0.59	0.6	0.6	0.67	0.66
Total buffalo population		6054	6340 -4.7	7775 -22.6	9756 -25.5	10414 -6.7	11092 -6.5	12976 -17
Total livestrock		49650	40916 (-17.6)	48445 -18.4	54348 -12.2	49136 (-9.6)	56663 -15.3	57732 -1.9
Small ruminants		28611	22506 (-22.6)	27849 -23.7	31556 -13.3	26863 (-14.9)	32693 -21.7	30746 (-6.0)
Sheep		13431	9913 (-26.2)	12497 -26.1	14585 -16.7	10054 (-31.1)	11190 -11.3	9080 (-18.9)
Goat		15480	12593 (-18.6)	15352 -21.9	16971 -10.5	16809 (-1.0)	21503 -27.9	21666 -0.8
Camels		756	721 (-4.6)	744 -3.2	669 (-10.1)	498 (-25.6)	422 (-15.3)	326 (-22.7)

*AFC, Adult Female Cattle comprised of population of in-milk, dry, not yet calved and other breedable female animals; **IM, population of in milk animals; Figures in parenthesis denote percentage change over previous census.

(Kanwalet al., 2020)

Flood

Around 55% of India's buffaloes, 38% of its cattle, 41% of its goats and 47% of its pigs are vulnerable to floods, which regularly devastate farmlands. Every year nearly one million cattle are lost to floods through heavy rains. Over the previous 20 to 30 years, the disaster-prone hill state has been hit by a series of natural disasters. Between June 14 and 18, 2013, Uttarakhand experienced one of the biggest natural calamities in its history, when widespread heavy rains caused floods across the state, killing thousands and causing billions of dollars in damage. According to government records, around 6,000 individuals were killed, missing, or were assumed dead, 4,200 communities were affected, 9,200 cattle/livestock were lost, and 3,320 homes were completely destroyed during this flood.

Because animals can swim, they can avoid drowning if they are not chained or imprisoned. In flooded locations, livestock may be unable to eat forages due to contamination by waste water or a lack of supply. Therefore, alternate source of fodder/ feed should be arranged until the fresh fodders are available. Hay/ dry fodder are the preferred feed, as digestion of such feed generates heat that will help to keep the animals warm during flood/ winter.

Rasool *et al.* (2020) conducted a study in three flood-affected districts of Kashmir Division (Pulwama, Srinagar and Bandipora) based on maximum inundation levels and found that each household lost 1-3 cattle/buffalo during the floods of 2014. In PulwamaDistrict highest herd loss of cattle/buffalo (42-82%) was reported. The average loss of two sheep/goats per family was observed for small ruminants, with the maximum flock loss reported from Bandipora District (>92%). In the case of backyard poultry, 39.16% people reported a loss of more than 81% and in Pulwama District reporting the largest loss (>81%).

According to the report of Animal Husbandry Department Kashmir, 7944 cattle died in the floods of 2014, including 4336 Milch animals, 3591 Draught animals and 17 calves. During the floods of 2014, the sheep husbandry department of Jammu and Kashmir, India, reported a loss of 79,855 sheep/goats. The overall number of sheep/goats affected was 446120 and there were 360 animal barns damaged. The findings on economic losses in these three districts are more or less consistent with the statistics provided by the department of animal/sheep husbandry on losses.

According to the report of Uttrakhand principal secretary (agriculture), about 18,228 cattle were killed and 20,000 hectares of agricultural land was severely damaged in the deluge that struck in Rudrapryag, Chamoli and Uttarkashi districts on 16 and 17 June 2013.

Year-wise damage caused due to floods, cyclonic storms, landslides etc. in India

Year	Live Lost human (in No.)	Cattle Lost (in No.)	Houses damaged (in No.)	Cropped areas affected (in Lakh hectares)
2001-02	834	21,269	3,46,878	18.72
2002-03	898	3,729	4,62,700	21.00
2003-04	1,992	25,393	6,82,209	31.98
2004-05	1,995	12,389	16,03,300	32.53
2005-06	2,698	1,10,997	21,20,012	35.52
2006-07	2,402	4,55,619	19,34,680	70.87
2007-08	3,764	1,19,218	35,27,041	85.13
2008-09	3,405	53,833	16,46,905	35.56
2009-10	1,677	1,28,452	13,59,726	47.13
2010-11	2,310	48,778	13,38,619	46.25

Ministry of Home Affairs (MHA)

STRATEGY FOR DISASTER RISK REDUCTION

As yet, there are no specific systems within India that measure and assess a disaster's impact on animals and their losses. Such measures would help to fulfill the requirement of the Sendai Framework to quantify the 'number of people whose livelihoods were disrupted or destroyed attributed to disasters'.Although animals are included in the national disaster management plans, making them work for animals is challenging. This is because there are no dedicated resources – people, funds, equipment and infrastructure – to meet front-line animal protection requirements.

Animal Disaster Management and Livestock Emergency Guidelines and Standards(LEGS) have been adopted by India's National Institute of Disaster Management. This is expected to lead to more human resources being dedicated to protecting animals in disasters. These standard draws on evidence-based good practice in protecting livestock affected by disasters from around the world. World Animal Protection (WAP) trained 50 government veterinary officers in Bihar and Andhra Pradesh states in LEGS. NIDM also trained 150 government veterinary officers from four states – Himachal Pradesh, Assam, Tamil Nadu, Haryana –in the management of animals in emergencies.

Since 2008, India's national and state governments, academic institutions and NGOs have worked with NIDM, simulation exercises and mock drills to better prepare to protect animals from disasters. The main focus is onthe frequently affected areas of Bihar, Andhra Pradesh, Tamil Nadu, Gujarat.

Veterinary Emergency Response Units (VERU) has been established in six zones (North, South, East, West and Central India with the support of NDMA and World Animal Protection. They are based in veterinary institutions to train and build capacities of veterinary and disaster management workers to protect animals from disasters. India's first VERU was founded in Bihar Veterinary College in 2009 after the success of other VERUs World Animal Protection helped develop in Thailand, Mexico, and other Latin American countries. Around one million animals have benefitted from the VERUs since 2009. Total 850 veterinary students have been trained on veterinary emergency response operations in India.

ANIMAL PROTECTION LAW (SECTION 51 A)

Animals have a strong place in Indian law but none specifically requiring their protection before, during and after disasters. They are protected in the country's constitution

1. The Prevention of Cruelty to Animals Act of 1960
2. The Wildlife Protection Act of 1972.

The national policy on disaster management has a dedicated section on animal care in chapter 7: Response. It mentions as follows: "Animals both domestic and wild are exposed to the effects of natural and man-made disasters. It is necessary to devise appropriate measures to protect animals and find means to shelter and feed them during disasters and their aftermath, through a community effort, to the extent possible".

PLAN TO SAVE ANIMALS

The Indian government is one of the first countries in the world to integrate animals into its national disaster management plans and has worked closely with us to do so. Such plans were issued by its National Disaster Management Authority (NDMA) and the Department of Animal Husbandry, Dairying and Fisheries (DAHDF) in 2016.

The NDMA plan gives framework and direction to all the government agencies covering all sectors during all phases of the disaster management cycle. World Animal Protection provided recommendations to NDMA on integrating animal related components into this plan.

The DAHDF national disaster management plan specifically spells out how to protect animals before, during and after disasters. DAHDF is responsible for farm animals/ livestock, poultry and fisheries and worked closely with our technical experts to prepare the plan.

To support the plans, we trained the National Disaster Response Force (NDRF), a dedicated search and rescue force for disaster response operations normally dedicated to rescuing people. More than 250 trainers were trained in all 12 battalions nationwide. Training was organized in six states – North (Himachal Pradesh), South (Tamil Nadu), East (Assam), West (Gujarat) and Central (Bihar and Madhya Pradesh).

Countering Climate Change to Revitalise Livestock Productivity

It would be beneficial to practice mixed farming and employ bio-fertilizer to integrate crops and livestock. Traditionally farmers are aware how to manage their livestock in accordance with climate variations. Practices for preserving water and soil can help to maintain production of food, feed, fodder, fruits and vegetables and simultaneously reducing the effects of climate change. Faster weather forecasts and meteorological information could help the farmers for preparedness in time. The effects of climate change on livestock can be controlled through physical environment modification, genetic creation of heat-resistant breeds, and nutritional management.

The impact of high temperatures and/or humidity can be reduced by forced ventilation and air circulation. Hormonal treatments are also used to enhance the animal reproduction during the heat stress. Use of timed AI, embryo transfer and other latest reproductive techniques are also helpful. Modification of the feed composition, feeding times and feeding frequencies will help in managing effects of heat stress. It would be possible to meet the challenges of climate change to meet with the needs of improving livestock productivity and the food and nutritional security, with farmer-centric policies and significant investment by the government and private sector in agriculture and technology. Further research on climate resilient animal agriculture is the need of the hour for sustainability in livestock farming system, especially in hot tropical countries.

Contingency Plan for Tackling the Extreme Events

Common measures should be planned for preparedness to tackle the any type of extreme weather events are as follows and specific plan for specific weather events are given in the tabular form:

- Weather forecasting and early warning systems
- Prepare contingency plan for local needs
- Constituting efficient team of workers to act as a Rapid Action Force during emergencies.
- Collaboration of the district veterinary officials to handle endemic animal diseases.
- Mass awareness programme on management of animals during extreme weather events.
- Popularizing livestock insurance and its implementation

Extreme weather events		Contingency measures to be Taken
1. Drought	Before	• Sell the unproductive, weak and sick animals for efficient utilization of available resources. • Conservation of water at community level for adequate water supply. • Veterinary preparedness: Vaccination against endemic diseases and timely deworming. • Provision for balanced feeding of productive animals.
	During	• Arrangement of good quality feed. • Use of stored and non-conventional source of feed for livestock. • Judicious use of available water. • Animal health camps for treatment of the sick animals. • Cleaning of animal sheds to minimize disease incidences. • Restriction of free movement of individuals in the animal farm and use of foot baths at the farm entrance to minimize disease transmission. • Use of netting in sheds to prevent arthropod borne diseases.

Extreme weather events		Contingency measures to be Taken
	After	• Culling of unproductive animals. • Providing of good quality feed to obtain optimum growth • Availing insurance wherever required. • Maintenance of proper hygiene and sanitation in the sheds and timely vaccination of all the animals. • Disposal of dead animals by burning or by deep burial with lime powder in pits.
Flood	Before	• Shift the animals to safer and higher place which has to be identified before. • Procurement and storage of sufficient good quality feed ingredients • Preserve the clean water in tank. • Add antibiotic powder in drinking water to prevent disease outbreak • Vaccination against prevalent diseases. • Stocking of emergency medicine for prevalent diseases.
	During	• Arrangement of safe drinking/ medicated water. • Shifting of animals and feed to raised sheds/ places. • Conducting animal health camps. • Isolation of diseased affected and suspicious animals. • Prevent water logging surrounding the sheds. • Assure supply of electricity. • Dust lime powder to prevent ammonia accumulation due to dampness.
	After	• Compensation and re-establishment of normal managemental conditions. • Culling unproductive animals. • Use of good quality feed to obtain optimum growth. • Treating drinking water. • Disposal of manure to prevent protozoal problem. • Maintenance of proper hygiene and sanitation in the shed • Disposal of dead animals by burning or by deep burial with lime in pits at proper depth.

Extreme weather events		Contingency measures to be Taken
Cold/ Heat wave/ Frost	Before	• Arrangement of adequate feed and water. • Construct the shed at community/ individual level. • Measures for modification of micro environment comfortable. • Nutritional manipulation like use of fats/edible oil in the ration, extra supplementation of methionine, biotin, choline chloride and vitamin C etc.
	During	• Organize health camp. • Modulate energy content and increase protein content in feed, add antioxidants, provide drinking water as per the ambient conditions.
	After	• Prepare scientific housing with locally available materials. • Organize health camp. • Re-establishment of normal managemental conditions.
Hailstorm	Before	• Ensure enough water quantity in the water bodies • Efficient team of workers to act as a Rapid Action Force during emergencies. • Procurement and storage of enough good quality feed ingredients and storing of house hold feeds like broken rice, pulse, oil seeds, etc
	During	• Use of unconventional and locally available feed ingredients for feeding of animals. • Avoid soaked and mould infected feeds. • Provide clean drinking water. • Treatment of diseased animals, proper litter management and spraying of fly repellents in the sheds.
	After	• Follow up surveillance and monitoring. • Repair of sheds and restocking. • Cleaning and disinfection of the shed. • Disposal of manure to prevent protozoal problem.

CONCLUSION

The weather stress is main challenge induced by global warming and climate change is also influencing fertility, productivity and welfare of livestock. Therefore, there is an urgent need to develop efficient and effective extension services, sufficient feeds and fodder, effective animal health services etc. Further we need efficient policy support and infrastructure through effective collaborations between different agencies involved in livestock development. Adequate policy support for all livestock species with regional livestock development priorities, and building capacities of livestock extension functionaries to handle the emerging challenges (especially climate change and extreme weather events) will provide ample impetus for the development of the livestock sector. It is likely that newer science tools will enhance animal productivity and make the sector more profitable occupation.

REFERENCES

ADB-WB (2005), "Preliminary Damage and Needs Assessment –Pakistan 2005 Earthquake", prepared by Asian Development Bank and World Bank, Islamabad, Pakistan.

Birthal, P. S., Jha, A. K., Tiongco, M. and Narrod, C. (2008). Improving farm-to-market linkages through contract farming: A case study of small holder dairying in India. IFPRI Discussion Papers814. International Food Policy Research Institute (IFPRI), Washington DC, USA.

Chand, R. (2017). Doubling Farmer's Income: Rationale, Strategy, Prospects and Action Plan,NITI Policy Paper No. 01/2017

Choudhary, B.B. and Sirohi, S. (2019). How sensitive are buffaloes (Bubalusbubalis) to heatstress? Journal of Dairy Research. 86:399-405.

Choudhary, B.B. (2017). Climate sensitivity of agricultural production system in trans and upper Gangatic plains of India: potential economic impact and vulnerability. Ph.D. thesis, National Dairy Research Institute, Karnal, India.

Cruden, D.M. and Varnes, D.J. (1996) "Landslide types and processes," in A.K. Turner and R.L. Schuster (eds.), Landslides: Investigation and Mitigation, Nat'l. Res. Council, Wash., D.C., Transp. Res. Bd. Spec. Rept. 247: 36-75.

Cohen, J.E. (2001) World population in 2050: assessing the projections Conference Series-Federal Reserve Bank of Boston, 46, pp. 83-113

Das,V.K. and Kumar,A.G.(2017).Drivers of farmers' income: The role off arm size and diversification, working paper 013, Indira Gandhi Institute of Development Research, Mumbai.

FAO. (2015)The impact of Natural Hazards and disasters on agriculture and food security and Nutrition security.1:54. www.fao.org/3/a-i5128e.

IPCC (2007) adaptation and vulnerability. Summary for policy makers. See http://www.ipcc.ch/publications_and_data/ar4/wg2/en/spm.html.

Joshi, P .K. and Kumar, P. (2016). Food demand and supply projections for India. Brower F, Joshi PK(Eds.).International trade and food security-the future of Indian agriculture. CABI International, Wallingford, UK.

Kanwal, V. (2018). Analysis of risk and vulnerability of rural farm households to natural disasters in Rajasthan. Ph.D. Thesis, National Dairy Research Institute, Karnal

Kanwal,V.,Sirohi, S. and Chandra, P.(2020).Effect of drought on livestock enterprise: Evidence from Rajasthan. Indian Journal of Animal Sciences**90** (1): 94–98

Kumar,A.,Thapa, G., Roy, D. and Joshi, P. K. (2017). Adoption of food safety measures on milk production in Nepal: Impact on small holders'farm-gate prices and profitability. Food Policy 70: 13–26.

Lacetera, N. (1998) Influence of high air temperatures on colostrum composition of dairy cows and passive immunization of calves. Zoot. Nutr. Anim. 6: 239–246

Lacetera, N., Bernabucci, U., Ronchi, B., Nardone, A. (1996) Body condition score, metabolic status and milk production of early lactating dairy cows exposed to warm environment. Riv. Agric. Subtrop. Trop. 90, 43–55.

Lal, S.N., Verma, D.N. and Husain, K.Q. (1987) Effect of air temperature and humidity on the feed consumption, cardio respiratory response and milk production in Haryana cows. Indian Veterinary Journal 64(2):115–121.

Mandal, D.K., Rao, A.V.M.S., Singh, K. and Singh, S.P. (2002a) Effects of macro-climatic factors on milk production in a Frieswal herd. Indian Journal Dairy Science 55(3):166–170.

Mandal, D.K., Rao, A.V.M.S., Singh, K. and Singh, S.P. (2002b) Comfortable macro-climatic conditions for optimum milk production in Sahiwal cows. Journal of Applied Zoolohical Research 13(2/3):228–230.

Martin, S.W., Schwabe, C.W., Franti, C.E., (1975) Dairy calf mortality rate: characteristics of calf mortality rates in Tulare County,California. Am. J. Vet. Res. 36: 1099–1104.

Moore, C.E., Kay, J.K., Van Baale, M.J., Collier, R.J., Baumgard, L.H. (2005) Effect of conjugated linoleic acid on heat stressed Brown Swiss and Holstein cattle. J. Dairy Sci. 88:1732–1740.

Nardone, A., Lacetera, N., Bernabucci, U., Ronchi, B. (1997) Composition of colostrum from dairy heifers exposed to high air temperatures during late pregnancy and the early postpartum period. J. Dairy Sci. 80: 838–844

Nardone, A., Ronchi, B., Lacetera, N., Ranieri, M.S. and Bernabucci, U. (2010). Effects of climate changes on animal production and sustainability of livestock systems. Livestock Science. 130:57-69.

Rathore, J. S. (2004). Drought and household coping strategies: A case of Rajasthan. Indian Journal of Agricultural Economics 59(4): 689–708.

Sanober, R.,Hamdani, S.A., Abdul, H., Fayaz A. and Akand, A.H. (2020) A study of economic losses suffered by livestock farmers during the floods of 2014 in Jammu and Kashmir (India). Journal of Entomology and Zoology Studies; **8**(2): 1091-1094.

Saxena, R., Singh, N.P., Choudhary, B.B., Balaji, S.J.,Paul, R.K., Ahuja,U., Joshi, D., Kumar, R. and Khan, A.(2017). Can Livestock Sector be the Game Changer in Enhancing the Farmers' Income? Reinvesting Thrust with Special Focus on Dairy Sector. Agricultural Economics Research Review. 30:59-76.

Singh, O.P., Alikhan, T.M. and Rahman, M.S. (2000). Changes in the frequency of tropical cyclones over the north Indian ocean, Meteorol. Atmos. Phys. 75: 11-20.

Sobia, N., Ahmad and Abid, Q. S.(2008) State of Livelihood Assets in the Earthquake Affected Areas:A Way Forward.Working Paper Series # 109 September 2008.

Tailor, S.P. and Nagda, R.K. (2005) Conception rate in buffaloes maintained under subhumid climate of Rajasthan. Indian Journal of Dairy Science; **58**(1):69–70

Thornton, P.K., Van de, S.J., Notenbaert, A. and Herrero, M. (2009). The impacts of climate change on livestock and livestock systems in developing countries: A review of what we know and what we need to know. Agricultural Systems. 101: 113-127.

Bhat, W.A., Lone, F.A., Ahsan, S. and Bhat, S.R. (2019) Impacts of Cloud Bursts on Horticultural Production in Kashmir Valley. Journal of Agro-ecology and Natural Resource Management; **6**(3):134-137

Wason, H.R. and Sharma, M.L. (2000) Source parameters study of local earthquakes in the Garhwal Himalaya based on the digital broadband data. In: Proceedings of 12th World Conference on Earthquake Engineering pp 1–6

Chapter 21

Impact of Climate Change on Animal Production and Health

Gyanendra Singh, Anamika Pandey, VP Maurya, Amit Kumar and Anjali

Physiology & Climatology Division

ICAR-Indian Veterinary Research Institute

Izatnagar-243122

INTRODUCTION

Population expansion, economic reform, environmental degradation, and increasing demand for food all contribute to climate change, and it is one of the critical issues faced in the last few decades. The climate prediction model also indicates that the temperature of the globe will further rise rapidly. Shifts in weather patterns can endanger food production and increase the possibility of catastrophe, flooding is some of the climate change effects. A rising human population and escalating needs severely deteriorate the climate and environment. In developing nations, rapid urbanization is anticipated to continue, and in the ensuing decades, there will be a significant increase in the demand for animal products globally *(Delgado et al., 1999)*. Substantial changes in physical and biological systems have already occurred on all continents and in most oceans. Most of these changes are going in the direction expected with warmer temperatures *(Rosenzweig et al., 2008)*. Climate change has become a serious concern due to the continuous increase in concentrations of greenhouse gases in the atmosphere. In India, 59% of the population relies directly on climate-sensitive industries like agriculture, forestry, and fisheries. Our nation's economy and food security are set to suffer significantly due to the projected global increase in surface temperature due to climate change. Agriculture and animal output, input resources, and other elements of the agricultural system are all impacted by climate change and variability. The three main contributors to the rise in greenhouse gases seen during the previous 250 years, according to the Intergovernmental Panel on Climate Change (IPCC), are the use of fossil fuels, land use pattern, and agriculture. The livestock industry is thought to be the most susceptible because it is a significant source of greenhouse gases and suffers badly due to climate change's direct and indirect effects. Due to its impact on the quality of feed crops and forage, water availability, milk production, livestock illnesses, animal reproduction, and biodiversity, climate change threatens the livestock production system, particularly for smallholders.

The potential effects of climate change on animal health and production are highly variable. Diseases that are vector-borne, soil-associated, water- or flood-associated, rodent-associated, air temperature/humidity-associated, and climate air-temperature likely have the most pronounced direct consequences. Furthermore, Climate change influences the emergence and proliferation of disease hosts or vectors and pathogens and their breeding, development, and disease transmission.

Farmers and pastoralists with limited resources are particularly exposed to the effects of climate change on livestock productivity and health. Early warning systems, improvised shelters, and improved healthcare services should be strengthened to lessen the adverse effects of climate change. If the demands of vulnerable livestock keepers are to be adequately served in the ensuing decades, research and development organizations' priorities need to be redefined.

CLIMATE CHANGE EFFECTS ON LIVESTOCK

The changes in meteorological variables such as temperature, humidity, rainfall, and the frequency and severity of extreme events like droughts directly affected livestock yields *(Adams et al., 1998)*. Climatic variables or seasonal changes significantly influence the behavior of animals due to neuroendocrine response to climatic elements, consequently affecting the production and health of animals *(Shelton, 2000; Sejian et al., 2010a; Baumgard et al., 2012)*. Climate change is a significant threat to the viability and sustainability of livestock production systems in many world regions *(Gaughan et al., 2009)*. High-production animals are substantially influenced by climatic factors, particularly those that are under tropical conditions *(Gaughan et al., 2008; Martello et al., 2010)*. Parons et al. (2001) have demonstrated that heat stress may reduce feed intake, lower milk production, and lead to energy deficits that may lower cow fertility, fitness, and longevity. Chase (2006), using the Cornell Net Carbohydrate and Protein System model, suggested that the maintenance energy requirements of a dairy cow weighing 635kg yielding 36kg of milk per day may be increased by 22% at 32°C compared with the energy requirements at 16°C. For the same temperature rise, Thornton et al. (2008) predicted a decrease in dry matter intake by 18% and a milk decrease by 32%.

Depending on the area and length of the growing season, the climate change effects can be seen in fodder quantity and quality *(Polley et al., 2013, Thornton et al., 2009)*.In arid and semi-arid environments, an increase of 2 °C will have a detrimental effect on pasture and cattle productivity. Because it affects the length and timing of the forage's availability, the length of the growing season is also a crucial element in determining the quality and amount of forage. Methane emissions can rise in proportion to the amount of gross energy consumed as forage quality declines *(Benchaar et al., 2001)*.To minimize the methane emissions by animals, it may be necessary to reduce forage consumption and replace it with grain if forage quality diminishes *(Polley et al., 2013)*.

Water availability is one of the crucial factors that will be severely impacted due to the climate change scenario *(Thornton et al., 2009)*. A temperature rise may result in a two to three-times increase in animal water consumption, which accounts for around 8% of all human water consumption worldwide *(Nardone et al., 2010)*.To solve this problem, it is necessary to grow crops and rear cattle in livestock systems that use less water or in areas where water is abundant *(Nardone et al., 2010)*. However, research on the effects of decreased water availability for land-based livestock systems owing to climate change is lacking *(Thornton et al., 2009)*. Therefore, in the framework of sustainable livestock production, it is crucial to consider water availability and appropriate mitigating measures.

ANIMAL PRODUCTION & REPRODUCTION

Due to the sensitivity of dairy cattle to excessive temperature, heat stress is one of the main reasons for lower productivity in the dairy and cattle industries *(Nardone et al., 2010)*, and there have been significant monetary losses. When the temperature rises above the thermo-neutral zone, there are physiological and behavioral changes in the livestock and metabolic expenses in maintaining the body temperature and cooling the body. Also, feed or dry matter intake decreases, and water intake increases. Thus, a decrease in energy production and an increase in energy expenditure, together with heat stress, cause a reduction in milk production *(Berman, 2005)*. Dairy cattle with high milk production levels produce more metabolic heat and are thus more susceptible to heat stress than the low producers. Long-term increased temperatures can have an impact on several different physiological processes, including metabolic rate, endocrine status, oxidative status *(Bernabucci et al., 2002)*, glucose, protein, and lipid metabolism, liver function, and non-esterified fatty acids (NEFA). Additionally, more enormous energy deficits impact animal longevity and fitness *(King et al., 2006)*.

Heat stress also impacts in similar ways to the milk production of sheep, goats, and buffalo *(Finocchiaro et al., 2005)*. In lactating goats, during hot summer water loss mechanism helps reduce the urine water loss and supports milk production *(Olsson and Dahlborn, 1989)*; thus, goat milk composition and production are impacted. Sheep are more sensitive to the combined effects of temperature and relative humidity (the temperature humidity index); however, different breed types have different index values that cause heat stress in sheep *(Finocchiaro et al., 2005)*. Howden et al. (2010) reported that a temperature increase between 1 and 5 °C may cause substantial mortality in grazing cattle. High temperatures also lead buffalo to produce less milk since they impact their physiological processes like heart rate, respiration rate, and rectal temperature *(Seerapu et al., 2015)*. However, these animals have received less attention due to their capacity to adapt to hotter environments *(Nardone et al., 2010)*.

The consequences of heat stress can be noticed in the meat of pigs and beef cattle. Heat stress can increase the risks of pale-soft-exudative meat in pigs, dark-cutting beef in cattle, and dehydration in most species. Regarding meat production, beef cattle with heavy weights, thick coats, and darker colors are more susceptible to warmth *(Nardone et al., 2010)*. Ruminant body size, carcass weight, and fat thickness may decrease due to global warming *(Mitloehner et al., 2001)*. In pig production, the same is true, with larger pigs experiencing higher reductions in growth, carcass weight, and feed intake *(Nardone et al., 2010)*. The likelihood of piglets surviving may be decreased if sows consume less feed when nursing at temperatures above 25 °C, which also lowers the sow's milk production.

Heat stress may impact the effectiveness of both male and female reproduction. Heat stress and increasing energy shortages may impair cow reproduction *(King et al., 2006)*. It impairs embryo development, pregnancy rate *(Nardone et al., 2010)*, and oocyte growth and quality in cows and pigs *(Barati et al., 2008)*. In bulls, pigs, and poultry, heat stress has also been linked to reduced sperm concentration and quality.

LIVESTOCK DISEASES

Climate change will affect the geographical region, land use, disease characteristics, and animal disease susceptibility *(Thornton et al., 2009)*. Climate change, particularly rising temperatures, can impact animal health directly or indirectly *(Nardone et al., 2010)*. The consequences of climate change on microbial communities (pathogens or parasites), the expansion of vector-borne and food-borne illnesses, host resistance, and the scarcity of feed and water are considered the indirect effects *(Nardone et al., 2010, Thornton et al., 2009, Tubiello et al., 2008)*.

The growth of viruses and/or parasites that spend part of their life cycle outside of their host could be accelerated by temperature changes, which would be detrimental to livestock *(Karl et al., 2009)*. Climate change could lead to changes in diseases pattern, disease outbreaks, or even the introduction of new diseases that could damage livestock that isn't typically exposed to these kinds of illnesses *(Thornton et al., 2009)*. Therefore, livestock must be evaluated for disease dynamics and response to preserve their resilience. Variations in precipitation and global warming impact the amount and spread of pests carried by vectors like flies, ticks, and mosquitoes *(Thornton et al., 2009)*. Additionally, warmer temperatures will increase the likelihood of disease transmission between hosts *(Thornton et al., 2009)*. There is a strong likelihood that the advent of new diseases will serve as a mixing bowl for humans and livestock, allowing for the blending of new genetic material and facilitating its transmissibility. Because diseases depend on animal exposure and other circumstances, it is challenging to evaluate the real disease risk *(Randolph, 2008)*.

According to Nardone et al. (2010), several climate change-related livestock health issues exist. After prolonged exposure to UV radiation, mammalian cellular immunity may be reduced, and T helper lymphocytes, implicated in the immunological response to intracellular infections, also decrease in number. Successful adaptations may therefore be demonstrated as a more effective means of coping with the detrimental effects of climate change on animal health.

The nature and extent of how heat stress impacts feed nutrient absorption and utilization, animal production, reproduction, and health need to be explored further, involving genomics and proteomics. With more understanding of heat stress's metabolic and nutritional consequences, management approaches could be modified to improve animal performance under climate change scenarios.

REFERENCES

Barati, F., Agung, B., Wongsrikeao, P., Taniguchi, M., Nagai, T. and Otoi, T., 2008. Meiotic competence and DNA damage of porcine oocytes exposed to an elevated temperature. *Theriogenology*, 69(6), pp.767-772.

Benchaar, C., Pomar, C. and Chiquette, J., 2001. Evaluation of dietary strategies to reduce methane production in ruminants: a modelling approach. *Canadian Journal of Animal Science*, 81(4), pp.563-574.

Berman, A., 2005. Estimates of heat stress relief need for Holstein dairy cows. *Journal of animal science*, 83(6), pp.1377-1384.

Bernabucci, U., Ronchi, B., Lacetera, N. and Nardone, A., 2002. Markers of oxidative status in plasma and erythrocytes of transition dairy cows during hot season. *Journal of dairy science*, 85(9), pp.2173-2179.

Delgado, C.L., Rosegrant, M.W., Steinfeld, H., Ehui, S.K. and Courbois, C.B., 1999. The coming livestock revolution. *Choices*, 14(316-2016-7248).

Finocchiaro, R., Van Kaam, J.B.C.H.M., Portolano, B. and Misztal, I., 2005. Effect of heat stress on production of Mediterranean dairy sheep. *Journal of Dairy Science*, 88(5), pp.1855-1864.

Howden, N.J.K., Burt, T.P., Worrall, F., Whelan, M.J. and Bieroza, M., 2010.Nitrate concentrations and fluxes in the River Thames over 140 years (1868–2008): are increases irreversible? Hydrological Processes, 24(18), pp.2657-2662.

Karl, T.R., Melillo, J.M., Peterson, T.C. and Hassol, S.J. eds., 2009. *Global climate change impacts in the United States*.Cambridge University Press.

King, J.M., Parsons, D.J., Turnpenny, J.R., Nyangaga, J., Bakari, P. and Wathes, C.M., 2006.Modelling energy metabolism of Friesians in Kenya smallholdings shows how heat stress and energy deficit constrain milk yield and cow replacement rate. *Animal Science*, 82(5), pp.705-716.

Nardone, A., Ronchi, B., Lacetera, N., Ranieri, M.S. and Bernabucci, U., 2010. Effects of climate changes on animal production and sustainability of livestock systems. Livestock Science, 130(1-3), pp.57-69.

Olsson, K. and Dahlborn, K., 1989. Fluid balance during heat stress in lactating goats. *Quarterly Journal of Experimental Physiology: Translation and Integration*, 74(5), pp.645-659.

Polley, H.W., Briske, D.D., Morgan, J.A., Wolter, K., Bailey, D.W. and Brown, J.R., 2013.Climate change and North American rangelands: trends, projections, and implications. *Rangeland Ecology & Management*, 66(5), pp.493-511.

Randolph, S.E., 2008.Tick-borne disease systems. *Rev sci tech Off int Epiz*, 27(2), pp.1-15.

Rosenzweig, C., Karoly, D., Vicarelli, M., Neofotis, P., Wu, Q., Casassa, G., Menzel, A., Root, T.L., Estrella, N., Seguin, B. and Tryjanowski, P., 2008. Attributing physical and biological impacts to anthropogenic climate change. *Nature*, 453(7193), pp.353-357.

Seerapu, S.R., Kancharana, A.R., Chappidi, V.S. and Bandi, E.R., 2015.Effect of microclimate alteration on milk production and composition in Murrah buffaloes. *Veterinary World*, 8(12), p.1444.

Thornton, P.K., van de Steeg, J., Notenbaert, A. and Herrero, M., 2009. The impacts of climate change on livestock and livestock systems in developing countries: A review of what we know and what we need to know. *Agricultural systems*, 101(3), pp.113-127.

Thornton, P.K., van de Steeg, J., Notenbaert, A. and Herrero, M., 2009. The impacts of climate change on livestock and livestock systems in developing countries: A review of what we know and what we need to know. *Agricultural systems*, 101(3), pp.113-127.

Tubiello, F., Schmidhuber, J., Howden, M., Neofotis, P.G., Park, S., Fernandes, E. and Thapa, D., 2008. Climate change response strategies for agriculture: challenges and opportunities for the 21st century. *Agriculture And Rural Development Discussion Paper*, 42.

Chapter 22

Gender and Circadian Bias in Immune Responses Coupled with Hormones

Aasif A. Sheikh, Z. A. Pampori, D. Hasin, O. Aarif, Fozia Shah, M. R. Dar, Sumeira Shafi, Nowsheen Amin and Uroos Ali

Division of Veterinary Physiology, Faculty of Veterinary Sciences and Animal Husbandry, Sher-e-Kashmir University of Agricultural Sciences and Technology of Kashmir, Srinagar, Jammu & Kashmir

ABSTRACT

The biological process referred as immunity protects an organism from diseases or provides resistance to noxious agents. The immune system is highly time-of-day dependent. Hormones on the other hand are long being associated with homeostasis, metabolism and reproduction. However, the effects of hormones extend beyond these functions and are now recognized as important candidates involved in immune modulation. The role of sex steroids particularly estrogen and progesterone have been demonstrated to work contrarily with respect to immune competence. Estrogen has long been associated with heightened immunity and a higher life expectancy in females than males. Progesterone and androgens, on the other hand have been demonstrated to compromise immunity thus preventing embryo rejection and favour pregnancy. Besides gender bias in immunity associated with sex hormones, diurnal bias is also revealed in immune competence in correlation with various hormones. Immune competence is demonstrated to augment during the mid-day when compared to morning and evening. Hormones like melatonin, growth hormone & thyroxin promote immunity whereas, cortisol causes immune suppression. The current chapter focuses on different perspectives of gender and circadian specific hormones on immune function.

INTRODUCTION

Immune system is considered as an effector mechanism with defensive responses to any obnoxious or antigenic challenge designed to eliminate 'foreign' material and return to a surveillance mode. However, the substantial evidence now suggests that immunity is not effector biased but is a sensory organ that forms part of an integrated homeostatic network. The bidirectional flow of information between the neuroendocrine and immune system functions to maintain homeostasis of the organism. Scientists have delimited the immune, endocrine, and neural systems to study physiology and disease (Figure 1). Neuroendocrine, immune and even metabolic systems are interconnected by a profuse network of mediators (Perez et al., 2021). The constant monitoring role of the neuroendocrine system to control and regulate the function of the immune system is vital for the homeostatic integrity of the host. Any impedance in this two-way communication may result into autoimmune disorders, septic shock, or chronic infection.

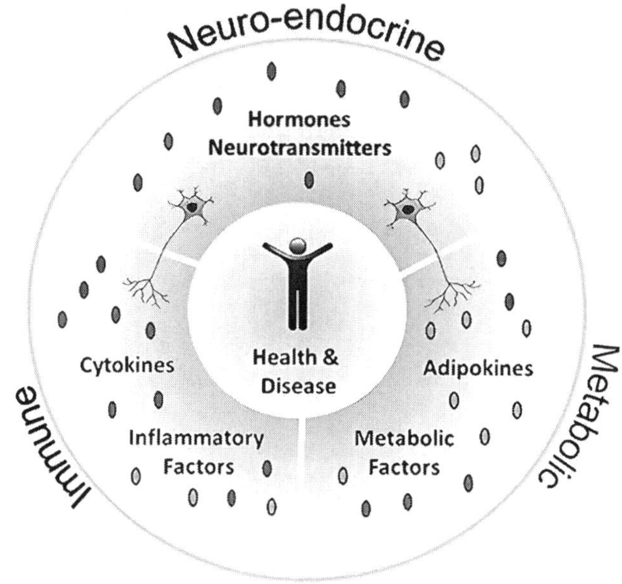

Figure 1: Neuro-endocrine, Metabolic and Immune pathways determine health and disease

Sex steroids are in use for last more than a millennium to correct reproductive disorders and augment reproductive efficiency in animals. However, it has been increasingly apparent that the effects of sex hormones extend far beyond their predominant role in sexual differentiation and reproduction and are now being realised as integral signalling modulators of mammalian immune system. Sexual dimorphism in disease incidence and host response in wide range of animal species provides an indirect evidence of role of sexual hormones in immune modulation (Ahmed et al., 1985; Ramzan et al., 2009). Immunological evidence suggests that female sex hormones play a role in the aetiology and course of chronic inflammatory diseases (Cutolo & Wilder, 2000). The number and activity of immune cells in reproductive tract of animals and humans vary throughout the phases of the reproductive cycle and are believed to be controlled by changes in the levels of estradiol and progesterone hormones (Kaushic et al., 2000; White et al., 1997) Ramadan et al. (1997) in sheep and Wulster-Radcliffe et al (2003) in gilts have reported a higher resistance to uterine infections at oestrus and least during luteal phase. Lymphocyte proliferation response, a promising marker of host immunity has been reported to exhibit variability during various physiological and reproductive phases in different animal species in dairy cattle (Kashiwazaki et al., 1985) and hamsters (Bilbo & Randy, 2001) that has been attributed to sex hormones. Use of sex steroids or sex steroid blockers or ovariectomy or castration in animal models has provided insight for their role in immune modulation (Olsen & Kovacs, 2001; Roden et al., 2004).

Over the past fifteen years, evidence for circadian oscillations of various components of the immune system has emerged as an integral regulator that has the potential to impact disease onset and therapies (Arjona et al., 2012; Lange et al., 2010). Way back in 1969, Feigin and coworkers highlighted the circadian variation in combating bacteria (*Diplococcus pneumoniae*) inoculated in mice. The mice inoculated with at 4 am showed higher survival rate than the mice infected at 8 am, 12 noon and 8 pm. Bellet et al (2013) demonstrated that mice infected during the resting phase exhibited severe signs of inflammation than mice infected during the active phase. It coincided with higher expression of TNFα, CXCL-1, LCN-2 genes. Studies in human and rodents have shown circadian rhythm in most of the biological functions viz., blood cellular components, hormones and cytokines (Haus and Smolensky, 1999).

Several studies have revealed two-way connections between the immune and the neuroendocrine systems (Mocchegiani et al., 1990; Fabris et al., 1995). This link is illustrated by a bidirectional communication circuit in which the endogenous substances of the neuroendocrine system act on the immune system and vice versa. Blalock et al (1985) demonstrated that immune-endocrine network shares a common language via compounds (acetylcholine, adrenocorticotropic hormone (ACTH), endorphin, vasoactive intestinal peptide (VIP), somatostatin and growth hormones) synthesized in both the systems. The knowledge of immune status at different stages of life in different sexes at different time intervals and physiological states can be of great importance in management of livestock, by exercising extra care during the periods of compromised immunity to improve the animal health, production and reproduction.

SEXUAL DIMORPHISM AND IMMUNE RESPONSE

Females and males differ in the energy consumption, nutritional requirements and immune modulation which are based on the interactions between environmental factors and sex hormones (Wu and O'Sullivan, 2011). The severity of host response to some diseases differs between sexes and this dimorphism has been attributed to immunomodulating effects of steroid hormones. Sex hormones can also control the immune response via circadian rhythm. Many hormones like cortisol, regulating T cell mediated inflammation show a circadian rhythm with a maximum peak at 8:00 a.m. and progressively lower levels as the day progresses (Sherman et al., 1985). In humans, sexual dimorphism exists with females having higher Ig levels, high antibody response and higher incidence of autoimmune diseases and strong cell mediated immune responses as evidenced by more efficient rejection of allograft (Butterworth et al., 1967). However, the heightened immune response in females is advantageous to respond to infection and sepsis but unfavourable against self, making females more prone to autoimmune diseases. Human females are more commonly affected with autoimmune diseases, with a female to male ratio varying widely; 2-4:1 in Rheumatoid arthritis, 5-13:1 in Systemic lupus erythematosus (SLE), 3:1 in Scleroderma, 4-8:1 in Grave's disease (Ahmed et al., 1985; Masi, 1989). Sex hormones interact with genetic and environmental factors and determine immunity in an individual (Figure 2). Gut microbial composition is influenced by many factors including genetic, diet and sex hormones (Marietta et al., 2015). The gut microbiota can impact systemic levels of testosterone via 17 β reduction of androgen consequently changing the intestinal metabolic landscape (Ridlon et al., 2013).

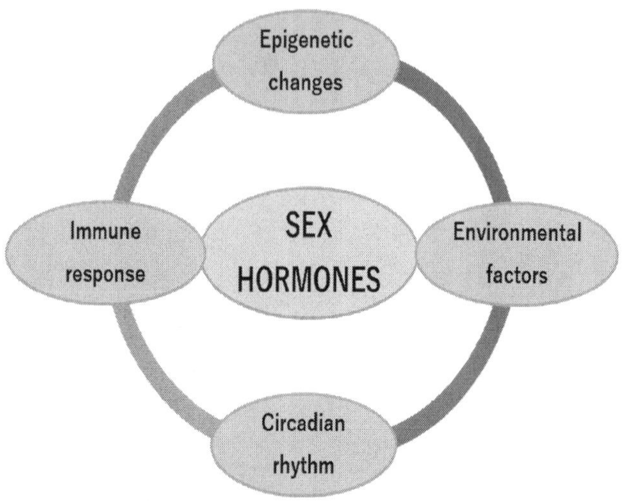

Figure 2: Environmental factors like smoking and gut microbiome gives rise to sex-hormones dependent immunity leading to variation in circadian rhythm, innate and adaptive immune response and epigenetic changes between males and females

In general, females have stronger innate and adaptive (humoral and cellular) immune responses in comparison to males. Bereshchenko et al (2018) pointed to a possible interaction between glucocorticoid and sex steroid receptors that could unravel the sexual disparity of autoimmune diseases. Raju and Chaudry (2008) reported that females in the proestrus cycle (with high estrogen) tolerate traumatic hemorrhage and sepsis far better than males either in human or animal models. There is emerging evidence that sex hormones impact microbial composition and the resulting immune response via secondary metabolites binding with receptors like estrogen receptors (ERs), peroxisome proliferator-activated receptors (PPARs) etc. (Park and Choi, 2017). Estrogen influences physiological functions via ERs which are expressed in brain, gut epithelial cells, lymphoid tissue cells as well as immune cells (Klein, 2004).

Females from different species show greater and more sustained production of antibodies after immunization and infection (Brick et al., 1985; Sperry and Minei, 2008). Immunoglobulins are higher in the pubertal girls than the boys of the same age and these levels are lower than the levels determined in adults of both sexes (Cotuna, 2005). Pampori and Pandita (2013) reported a positive correlation of plasma IgG levels with age and demonstrated significantly higher levels of IgG in post pubertal buffaloes than pre-pubertal group. A higher plasma IgG level was reported during diestrus than estrus phase of reproductive cycle in buffaloes. A notably lower lymphocyte proliferation index (LPI) was registered in post-pubertal buffaloes when compared to pre-pubertal buffaloes. The cyclic females registered higher LPI during estrus than at diestrus, but statistically the difference was non- significant (Pampori and Pandita, 2013). Females rejected allografts more efficiently because of stronger cell mediated immune response in them (Graff et al., 1969). Rebecca et al (2006) reported that after the onset of puberty, female mice had higher expression of adaptive immune response genes, while males had a higher expression of innate immune genes, which suggested a gender dimorphic immune response. Immune responses to environmental factors like infections and vaccinations are also sex-biased (Ruggieri et al., 2016).

The pro-inflammatory cytokine, TNF-α is one of the most important pro-inflammatory mediator, which induces a plethora of biological effects in various cells, initiating and regulating the immune responses (Bemelmans et al., 1996, Cavaillon et al., 2003). There is evidence that the outcome of some infections may be aligned with and may perhaps be predicted by plasma levels of cytokines, particularly TNF-α (Cavaillon et al., 2003). Pampori and Pandita (2013) reported the age and sex bias in TNF-α secretion in buffaloes. The levels were high in young pre-pubertal buffaloes as compared to post-pubertal counterparts. Females had lower levels as compared to males irrespective of age that might probably be responsible for augmented pathophysiological changes in males after sepsis as compared to females. Kahl and Elsasser (2004) reported that testosterone increases TNF-α and amyloid precursor protein (APP) which may be responsible for a differential presentation of disease symptoms between sexes or between steers and bulls. Epidemiological studies reveal that females of all ages experience lower rates of infection and resultant mortality as compared to men. Immunological evidence suggests that female sex hormones govern the aetiology and course of chronic inflammatory diseases because menstrual cycle, pregnancy and menopausal status are important influencing factors (Olsen & Kovacs, 2001; Cutolo & Wilder, 2000). Lately, immune response has been found to differ between phases of oestrus cycle in bovine which is attributed to the diversity in sex steroids during different phases of cycle (kahl et al., 2009; Pampori and Pandita, 2013). However, the mechanism by which the sex steroids modulate immunity is poorly understood. It may be due to their effect on production of immune mediators like cytokines and nitric oxide or indirectly through pituitary hormones. The immune response to the antigenic challenge in different sexes with respect to the primary immune mediators like TNF-α, nitric oxide and superoxide can provide a satisfactory tool to anticipate the immune reactions in animals to infections.

The males on other hand suffer with infectious diseases, ascribed to the androgens that are generally accepted as immunosuppressive. Immune suppression following traumatic haemorrhage has been reported the major cause of subsequent sepsis resulting into high mortality in males, attributed to the androgens as castration or administration of androgen receptor blockers prevented immunodepression following traumatic haemorrhage (Martin et al., 1998). The deprivation of androgens in male mice exacerbates the severity of various autoimmune like disorders whereas exogenous administration in female mice reverses gender based predilection to autoimmune diseases (Roden et al., 2004).

The homeostatic response to infection involves coordinated changes in both neuroendocrine and immune systems which communicate with one another and is supported by the demonstration of shared molecular network of ligands and receptors. Leukocytes express receptors for hormones and modulate diverse biological activities such as growth, proliferation and differentiation. Further, hormones share intracellular signalling substrate and biological activities with cytokines; thus neuroendocrine and immune cells share a common molecular language. The intercommunication between these homeostatic systems modulates pituitary growth hormone as well as other CNS controlled behavioural and metabolic events in response to endotoxin elicited pro-inflammatory cytokine cascade from leukocytes. Cytokine response to provocative stress challenges modelled by endotoxin administration has received great attention as biomarkers and mediators of both homeostatic and pathophysiological processes *in vivo*.

ROLE OF SEX HORMONES IN IMMUNITY

Sex hormones exert a broad range modulation of immune cell functions, and a dichotomy exists in the immune response between the sexes. Many studies have revealed that there is sex bias in the occurrence and incidence of diseases in humans as well as animals and suggested the variation because of different hormonal milieu in males and females particularly steroids. Nathan and Chaudhuri (1997) ascribed the disorders frequently affecting women after menopause, such as cardiovascular disease, osteoporosis, or neurodegenerative disorders to the loss of sex hormone-dependent regulation of physiological and immunological functions. In humans, epidemiological, laboratory and clinical studies have shown variations between gender in parasitic diseases including Schistosomiasis, Filariasis, Leishmaniasis and Onchocerciasis, as well as other infections such as Rubella, Measles, Hepatitis-B and Tuberculosis (Goble and Konopka, 1973). Similarly Ramzan et al (2009) reported toxoplasmosis among sheep and goat with higher prevalence in the females than in the males. The immune component of sex hormones is summed up in Table 1.

There is growing evidence that immune cells have sex hormone receptors and can respond directly to the presence, absence or changes in the concentrations of sex steroid hormones. Androgens (including testosterone), oestrogens (including 17β-oestradiol), and progesterone can have distinct and overlapping effects on the recruitment and activity of diverse immune cell populations in humans, rodents and primary cell culture systems. Generally, testosterone and progesterone are anti-inflammatory, suppressing several of the immune responses necessary for inflammation. Oestradiol has bipotential effects: low concentrations of oestradiol (for example, during the follicular stage of the reproductive cycle) can be pro-inflammatory, whereas high concentrations of oestradiol (for example, during the luteal phase of the reproductive cycle or during pregnancy) can be anti-inflammatory.

Table 1: Effects of sex steroid hormones on innate and adaptive immunity*

Immune Component	Effect of Sex Hormones		
	Oestradiol	Progesterone	Androgens
TLRs	↑TLR4, TLR7 & TLR9	↓TLR3 & TLR7	↓TLR4
Macrophages	↑TLR4	↓iNOS & NO, ↑FIZZ1 & YM1	↓iNOS & NO, ↓TNF
NF-kB	↓Activity	↓Activity	↓Activity
DCs	↑Activation, ↑TLR7 & TLR9, ↑CCL2 ↓CXCL10, ↓IFNα	↓CD40, CD80, CD86 & ↑CD11c, ↑IL-18 & IL-10	ND
Neutrophils	↑Numbers, ↑ Degranulation, ↑Elastase release	ND	↑Numbers, ↓Kinases & leukotriene formation
NK cells	↑IFNγ, ↑Granzyme B, ↓FASL	↑Numbers, ↑Apoptosis (caspase dependent)	ND
Eosinophils	↓Numbers, ↓Mobilization	↑Numbers	ND
Inflammatroy cytokines	Low oestrogen: ↑IL-1β, IL-6, & TNF High oestrogen: ↓L-1β, IL-6 & TNF	↓TNF & IFNγ ↑IL-6	↑IL-1β & IL-2 ↓TNF
Suppressive cytokines	↑IL-4, IL-10 & TGFβ	↑IL-4, IL-5 & TGFβ	↑IL-10 & TGFβ
Chemokines	↓CCL2, ↑CXCL1	↓CXCL2	↓CCL3
T_H1 cells	Low oestradiol: ↑Activity	↓Activity	↓IFNγ
T_H2 cells	High oestradiol: ↑Activity	↑Activity	↓IL-4 & IL-5, ↓GATA3
T_H17 cells	↓Numbers, ↓IL-17	↓Percentages	↑IL-17
T_{reg} cells	↑Numbers	↑Percentages	↑Numbers
$CD8^+$ T cells	↑Response	↓Response	↓Numbers, ↓Activity
B cells	↑IgG & IgM	↓CD80 & CD86	ND
Antibody response	↑Response	↑Total antibody↓Autoantibodies	↓Response

*CCL - CC-chemokine ligand; CXCL - CXC-chemokine ligand; DCs - dendritic cells; FASL - FAS ligand; IFN - interferon; IL - interleukin; iNOS - inducible nitric oxide synthase; ND - not defined; NF-κB -nuclear factor-κB; NK - natural killer; NO - nitric oxide; TGF β- transforming growth factor-β; TH -helper; TLR - Toll-like receptor; TNF - tumour necrosis factor; Treg - regulatory T

Sex hormones appear to be involved in regulating the immune response, which is evident from a striking difference between a male and female immune response and disease prevalence. The removal of ovaries in female rats did not produce any effect on the intensity of the parasitism (Roberts and Horsnell, 2015). Conversely, the administration of testosterone or removal of the testis in male rats altered the response to parasitic infection (Nakazawa et al., 1997). The hormonal diversity exists between sexes, which becomes evident around puberty and remains throughout reproductive life of the animal. Sex steroids have been demonstrated to have significant effect on lymphocyte proliferation and secretion of proinflammatory cytokines.

Pampori and Pandita (2012) reported that estrogen stimulated whereas, progesterone inhibited lymphocyte proliferation and testosterone did not have any serious effect on lymphocyte proliferation. The buffalo lymphocytes produced appreciable amounts of NO *in vitro* after treatment with estradiol and NO in culture supernatant was high at the lowest dose of progesterone which was proportional to the lymphocyte proliferation. Pampori and Pandita (2013) revealed a reproductive stage bias in physiological and immune responses to endotoxin challenge in buffaloes. Higher plasma TNF-α , nitric oxide, xanthine oxidase, cortisol and glucose was reported during estrous as compared to the diestrous stage of the cycle after endotoxin challenge. Sex steroids have been shown to play definitive role in lymphocyte maturation, activation, immunoglobulin and cytokine production.

Estrogen is generally believed to stimulate immunologic processes driven by $CD4^+$ Th2 cells. Th2 cells drive certain antibody mediated responses, particularly those involved in allergy with cytokines allocated IL-4, IL-5 and IL-10 (Olsen and Kovacs, 1996; Beagley et al., 2003; Tanriverdi et al., 2003). Estrogen reduces the number of immature thymic lymphocytes ($CD4^+/CD8^-$) and dampens lymphocyte development in thymus whereas encourages hepatic T cell lymphopoiesis. Ovariectomy or testosterone treatment causes shift favouring $CD4^-/CD8^+$ cell phenotype (Konya et al., 2009). Paavonen et al (1981) reported that pregnancy and late follicular levels of estrogen enhanced immunoglobins which is mediated through T cell mediated suppression of B cells. Estrogen enhanced IgG and IgM production without altering cell viability or proliferation, probably through the increased B cell stimulating cytokine IL-10 from monocytes and that is likely the reason why diseases like SL, Myasthenia gravis (MG) and thyroiditis appear in women in reproductive years predominantly (Kanda et al., 1999). Montoya et al (2002) reported that pregnancy levels of estrogen in women inhibited important proinflammatory cytokines IL-6, IL-8 and TNF-α . Estrogen has been shown to be protective following shock like states in males.

Estrogen reduced neutrophil accumulation, attenuated ICAM, cytokine induced chemo-attractants in rats after traumatic haemorrhage (Yu et al., 2006). Estrogen treatment in case of burn injury patients has shown improved immunity, reduced mortality & morbidity, restored immune suppression, T cell proliferation and reduced IL-6 production that otherwise causes depression of lymphocyte proliferation (Gatson et al., 2009).

Progesterone is reported to compromise immunity and potentiate the disease severity and occurrence. Although progesterone has been recognized as essential for the establishment and maintenance of pregnancy, this steroid hormone has been implicated to have a functional role in immune response. Progesterone inhibited the immune response to lipopolysaccharide (LPS) and CpG oligodeoxynucleotides (CpG ODNs) through modulation of Toll-like receptor (TLR) signalling (Su et al., 2009). Large number of Chlamydia were found in the vaginal secretions of progesterone-treated animals, while estradiol-treated animals had none, indicating that progesterone increases and estradiol decreases susceptibility to intrauterine chlamydial infection (Kaushic et al., 2000). In gilts, the progesterone was reported to increase the susceptibility to uterine infections after intra-uterine challenge.

Androgen administration exogenously in female mice reversed gender based predilection of female to autoimmune diseases, whereas as removal of androgen in male mice exacerbates severity of various autoimmune like disorders (Fox et al., 1992 and Fitzpatrick *et al.*, 1991). Androgen administration in female mice can abrogate immune responses to pathogen, allograft or traumatized host tissue (Martin et al., 1998). Androgen deprivation has shown to stimulate B cell lymphopoiesis in post-pubertal male animals (Olsen and Kovacs, 2001). Marketon and Glaser (2008) reported that stress hormones (cortisol and catecholamines), have detrimental effects on immune function, including reduced NK cell activity, lymphocyte proliferation, antibody production and reactivation of latent viral infections. Such effects on the immune system have severe consequences on health which include delayed wound healing, impaired responses to vaccination and development and progression of cancer.

CIRCADIAN BIAS AND IMMUNITY

A circadian rhythm or circadian cycle is a natural, internal process that regulates the sleep-wake cycle and repeats roughly every 24 hours. Land animals coordinate their behavior and physiological events according to circadian rhythms and species differences too exist with regard to the precise schedules of such rhythms. The animals have been classified as nocturnal or diurnal on the basis of their activity in 24 hr circadian cycle. Most biological processes in the body fluctuate with such daily rhythms. Hormone levels, body temperature, blood flow, urine production, hair growth, and metabolic rate fluctuate during circadian cycle. Melatonin is regarded a modulator of haemopoiesis and immune cell production and function, both *in vivo* and *in vitro* (Miller et al., 2006). The circadian nature of immune function is demonstrated in Figure 3. Singh et al (2020) reported increased monocyte, eosinophil, and basophil counts in response to melatonin in fresh water snakes. Interestingly, the phagocytic response of neutrophils was inhibited when treated with melatonin.

Nitrite release and superoxide production by leukocytes were higher in snakes receiving melatonin injections. Sleep seems to have much in common between the mammals. It occurs regularly each day, largely under the influence of the 24-hour circadian cycle.

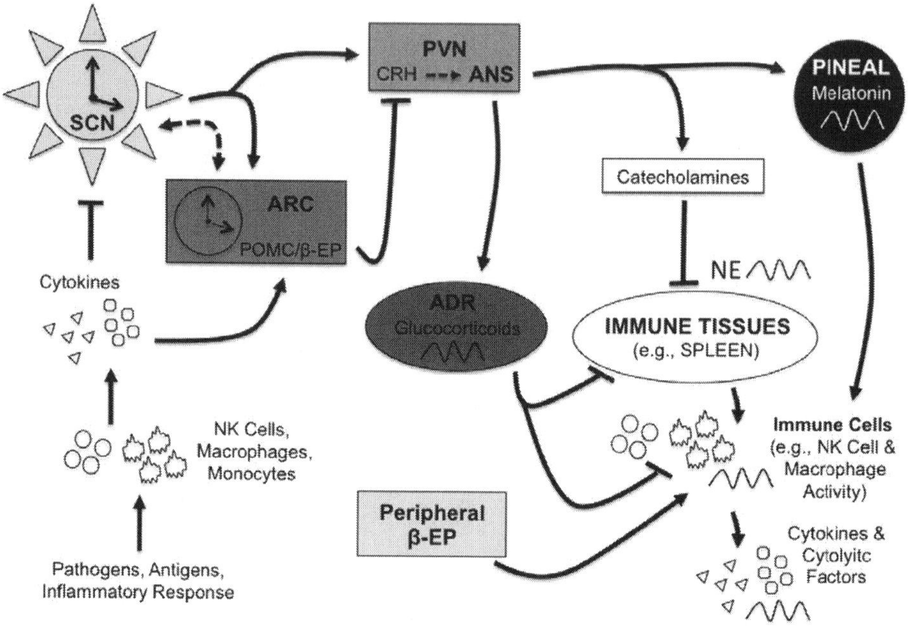

Figure 3: Circadian nature of Immune Function

The reciprocal relationship between the circadian rhythm (sleep-wake cycle) and the immune response has been the subject of extensive research. Changes in the immune system can cause changes in sleep, and conversely, sleep has an important role in maintaining the immune system. Sleep-deprived animals have a severely shortened lifespan and a compromised immune system (Ruiz et al., 2007). Since the endocrine and immune systems are intricately linked, as such any disruption may contribute to decreased resistance to infectious disease (Everson & Crowley, 2004). Pampori and coworkers (2023) have reported circadian rhythmicity in growth hormone, cortisol, prolactin, melatonin with higher secretions of growth hormone, melatonin during darkness and more cortisol during morning in cattle. They also reported higher lymphocyte proliferation index and neutrophil phagocytic activity during the mid day as compared to morning & evening (data unpublished).

CIRCADIAN BIAS IN HORMONE SECRETION AND IMMUNE COMPETENCE

It is established that many important hormones viz. growth hormone, adrenal corticoids, thyroid hormones, catecholamines and melatonin have temporal secretion in humans as well as animals (Czeisler and Klerman, 1999). Hormones have been implicated in the immune system giving birth to immune-endocrine physiology. Gnocchi and Bruscalupi (2017) strongly highlighted the existence of circadian rhythms in many physiological parameters including hormone secretion in most living organisms. Scheiermann et al (2013) reported the existence of clocks in immune system in different hematopoietic cell lineages, including macrophages and lymphocytes.

Arjona and Sarkar (2005) reported an increased expression of components of the innate immune system, such as the pattern recognition receptor (PPR), Toll-like receptor 9 (TLR9), as well as enhanced phagocytic and cytotoxic ability of leukocytes during the active phase in mice. Similarly, Petrovsky and Harrison (1998) reported the diurnal variation in immununo-inflammatory disorders like rheumatoid arthritis and asthma in humans. They also reported an inverse relation between cytokine secretion and plasma cortisol. Siopes and Underwood (2008) reported a melatonin dependent diurnal variation in both cellular and humoral immune response in quail.

A diurnal rhythm was found in the total number of lymphocytes, T cells, inducer/ helper cells, suppressor/cytotoxic cells and B cells. The lowest levels of all subsets were seen at 09:00 hours and the highest levels at 21:00 hours (Bertouch et al., 1983). Diurnal rhythmicity of pro-inflammatory cytokine production, viz. IFN-, TNF-α, IL-1 and IL-12 production was inversely related to the rhythm of plasma cortisol and were related to the diseases. Borghetti et al (2009) reported that growth hormone and insulin like growth factor I (IGF-I) are part of a neuroendocrine immune axis that stimulates cellular proliferation of primary lymphoid organs (bone marrow, thymus) as well as stimulates activation of peripheral lymphocytes and macrophages to enhance specific immune responses.

HORMONE RECEPTORS ON IMMUNE CELLS

Neifeld et al (1977) investigated steroid hormone receptors in human lymphocytes and reported the presence of glucocorticoid binding sites in these cells. Phytohemagglutinin stimulated lymphocytes had 2 to 3-fold increase in receptor activity than non-stimulated cells. Melatonin receptors in human lymphocytes were reported by Lardone et al (2009). The MT1 receptor expressed in the thymus and the spleen, as well as in CD4, CD8, and B cells. Slominski et al (2012) reported the presence of the MT2 receptor in the thymus, as well as confirmed the MT1 receptor expression in the thymus, spleen, and lymphocytes. Figure 4 illustrates the sex hormone receptor expression in the immune system. Borghetti et al (2009) reported the presence of both GH and IGF-I receptors in lymphocytes. Thellin and coworkers (1998) demonstrated expression of hGH-N-R on activated T cells. They also found B-cell population displaying similar levels of hGH-N-R expression.

CONCLUSION

Emerging intersectional research on circadian rhythms, sexual dimorphism and immunity presents exciting opportunities for using scientific understanding to augment the immune resilience. Gender and circadian rhythm interact at several levels to determine the entity and effectiveness of the immune response. Overall, the topic highlights the great complexity that there are secondary mechanisms that need to be analyzed and deepened to unravel such biological networks.

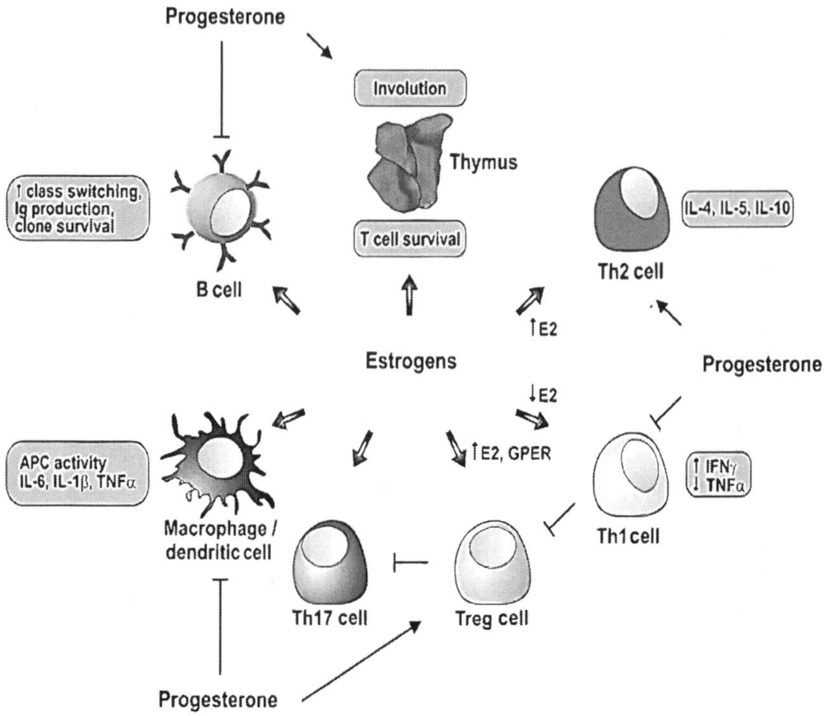

Figure 4: Generally accepted hormone effects on the immune system

REFERENCES

Ahmed SA, Penhale WJ, Talal N. 1985. Sex hormones, immune responses, and autoimmune diseases. Mechanisms of sex hormone action. The American Journal of Pathology. 121(3):531-551.

Arjona A, Sarkar DK. 2005. Circadian oscillations of clock genes, cytolytic factors, and cytokines in rat NK cells. *The Journal of Immunology*. **174(12)**:7618-7624.

Arjona A, Silver AC, Walker WE, Fikrig E. 2012. Immunity's fourth dimension: approaching the circadian–immune connection. *Trends in immunology*. **33(12)**:607-612.

Asai K, Hiki N, Mimura Y, Ogawa T, Unou K, Kaminishi M. 2001. Gender differences in cytokine secretion by human peripheral blood mononuclear cells: role of estrogen in modulating LPS-induced cytokine secretion in an *ex vivo* septic model. *Shock*. **16(5)**:340-343.

Bauer H, Jung T, Tsikas D, Stichtenoth DO, Frölich C, Neumann C. 1997. Nitric oxide inhibits the secretion of T-helper 1-and T-helper 2-associated cytokines in activated human T cells. *Immunology*. **90(2)**:205-211.

Beagley KW, Gockel CM. 2003. Regulation of innate and adaptive immunity by the female sex hormones oestradiol and progesterone. *FEMS Immunology & Medical Microbiology*. **38(1)**:13-22.

Bellet MM, Deriu E, Liu JZ, Grimaldi B, Blaschitz C, Zeller M, Edwards RA, Sahar S, Dandekar S, Baldi P, George MD. 2013. Circadian clock regulates the host response to Salmonella. *Proceedings of the National Academy of Sciences.* **110(24)**:9897-9902.

Bemelmans MH, Van Tits LJ, Buurman WA. 1996. Tumor necrosis factor: function, release and clearance. *Critical Reviews in Immunology.* **16(1)**.

Bereshchenko O, Bruscoli S, Riccardi C. 2018. Glucocorticoids, sex hormones, and immunity. *Frontiers in Immunology.* **9**:1332.

Bertouch JV, Roberts-Thomson PJ, Bradley J. 1983. Diurnal variation of lymphocyte subsets identified by monoclonal antibodies. *British Medical Journal (Clin Res Ed).* **286(6372)**:1171-1172.

Bilbo SD, Nelson RJ. 2001. Sex steroid hormones enhance immune function in male and female Siberian hamsters. *American Journal of Physiology-Regulatory, Integrative and Comparative Physiology.* **280(1)**:R207-213.

Blalock JE, Bost KL, Smith EM. 1985. Neuroendocrine peptide hormones and their receptors in the immune system: production, processing and action. *Journal of Neuroimmunology.* **10(1)**:31-40.

Bogdan C, Röllinghoff M, Diefenbach A. 2000. The role of nitric oxide in innate immunity. *Immunological Reviews.* **173**:17-26.

Borghetti P, Saleri R, Mocchegiani E, Corradi A, Martelli P. 2009. Infection, immunity and the neuroendocrine response. *Veterinary Immunology and Immunopathology.* **130(3-4)**:141-162.

Bouman A, Schipper M, Heineman MJ, Faas MM. 2004. Gender difference in the non-specific and specific immune response in humans. *American Journal of Reproductive Immunology.* **52(1)**:19-26.

Brick JE, Wilson DA, Walker SE. 1985. Hormonal modulation of responses to thymus-independent and thymus-dependent antigens in autoimmune NZB/W mice. *Journal of Immunology.* **134(6)**:3693-3698.

Butterworth M, McClellan B, Allansmith M. 1967. Influence of sex in immunoglobulin levels. *Nature.***214**:1224-1225.

Carson RL, Wolfe DF, Klesius PH, Kemppainen RJ, Scanlan CM. 1988. The effects of ovarian hormones and ACTH on uterine defense to *Corynebacterium pyogenes* in cows. *Theriogenology.* **30(1)**:91-97.

Castro JE. 1974. Orchidectomy and the immune response II. Response of orchidectomized mice to antigens. *Proceedings of the Royal Society of London. Series B. Biological Sciences.* **185(1081)**:437-451.

Cavaillon JM, Adib-Conquy M, Fitting C, Adrie C, Payen D. 2003. Cytokine cascade in sepsis. *Scandinavian Journal of Infectious Diseases.* **35(9)**:535-544.

Cotuna D, Hefco V, Neacsu I. 2005. Variations of immunoglobulins in the serum of adolescents of puberty age. *Journal of Experimental and Molecular Biology.* **6**.

Cutolo M, Wilder RL. 2000. Different roles for androgens and estrogens in the susceptibility to autoimmune rheumatic diseases. *Rheumatic Disease Clinics of North America*. **26(4)**:825-839.

Czeisler CA, Klerman EB. 1999. Circadian and sleep-dependent regulation of hormone release in humans. *Recent Progress in Hormone Research*. **54**:97-130.

Druckmann R, Druckmann MA. 2005. Progesterone and the immunology of pregnancy. *The Journal of Steroid Biochemistry and Molecular Biology*. 97(5):389-396.

Ebru K, Fenaux JB, Phillips RA, Lengi AJ, Elvinger F, Ansar Ahmed S. 2006. Estrogen up-regulates inducible nitric oxide synthase, nitric oxide, and cyclooxygenase-2 in splenocytes activated with T cell stimulants: role of interferon-. *Endocrinology*. **147(2)**:662-671.

Everson CA, Crowley WR. 2004. Reductions in circulating anabolic hormones induced by sustained sleep deprivation in rats. *American Journal of Physiology-Endocrinology and Metabolism*. **286(6)**:E1060-1070.

Fabris N, Mocchegiani E, Provinciali M. 1995. Pituitary-Thyroid Axis and Immune System: A Reciprocal Neuroendocrine-lmmune Interaction. *Hormone Research in Paediatrics*. **43(1-3)**:29-38.

Fitzpatrick F, Lepault F, Homo-Delarche FR, Bach JF, Dardenne M. 1991. Influence of castration, alone or combined with thymectomy, on the development of diabetes in the nonobese diabetic mouse. *Endocrinology*. **129(3)**:1382-1390.

Fox HS. 1992. Androgen treatment prevents diabetes in nonobese diabetic mice. The Journal of Experimental Medicine. **175(5)**:1409-1412.

Gatson JW, Maass DL, Simpkins JW, Idris AH, Minei JP, Wigginton JG. 2009. Estrogen treatment following severe burn injury reduces brain inflammation and apoptotic signaling. *Journal of Neuroinflammation*. **6(1)**:1-10.

Gnocchi D, Bruscalupi G. 2017. Circadian rhythms and hormonal homeostasis: pathophysiological implications. *Biology*. **6(1)**:10.

Goble FC, Konopka EA. 1973. Sex as a factor in infectious disease. *Transactions of the New York Academy of Sciences*. (Series II):325-346.

Graff RJ, Lappé MA, Snell GD. 1969. The influence of the gonads and adrenal glands on the immune response to skin grafts. *Transplantation*. **7(2)**:105-111.

Greenstein BD, Fitzpatrick FT, Adcock IM, Kendall MD, Wheeler MJ. 1986. Reappearance of the thymus in old rats after orchidectomy: inhibition of regeneration by testosterone. *Journal of Endocrinology*. **110(3)**:417.

Haider A, Siddique M, Abubakar M, Arshad MJ, Hussain M. 2008. Prevalence and distribution of peste des petits ruminants virus infection in small ruminants. *Small Ruminant Research*. **79(2-3)**:152-157.

Haitao L, Samouilov A, Liu X, Zweier JL. 2004. Characterization of the effects of oxygen on xanthine oxidase-mediated nitric oxide formation. *Journal of Biological Chemistry*. **279(17)**:16939-16946.

Haus E, Smolensky MH. 1999. Biologic rhythms in the immune system. *Chronobiology International*. **16(5)**:581-622.

Janeway C, Walport M, Capra J. 1999. Immunobiology. *The Immune System in Health and Disease*. New York, N.Y. Garland Publishers.

Kahl S, Elsasser TH, Li CJ. 2009. Variability in tumor necrosis factor- , nitric oxide, and xanthine oxidase responses to endotoxin challenge in heifers: Effect of estrous cycle stage. *Domestic Animal Endocrinology*. **36(2)**:82-88.

Kahl S, Elsasser TH. 2004. Endotoxin challenge increases xanthine oxidase activity in cattle: effect of growth hormone and vitamin E treatment. *Domestic Animal Endocrinology*. **26(4)**:315-328.

Kanda N, Tamaki K. 1999. Estrogen enhances immunoglobulin production by human PBMCs. *Journal of Allergy and Clinical Immunology*. **103(2)**:282-288.

Kashiwazaki Y, Maede Y, Namioka S. 1985. Transformation of bovine peripheral blood lymphocytes in the perinatal period. *The Japanese Journal of Veterinary Science*. **47(2)**:337-339.

Kaushic C, Zhou F, Murdin AD, Wira CR. 2000. Effects of estradiol and progesterone on susceptibility and early immune responses to *Chlamydia trachomatis* infection in the female reproductive tract. *Infection and Immunity*. **68(7)**:4207-4216.

Khan MN, Iqbal Z, Sajid MS, Anwar M, Needham GR, Hassan M. 2006. Bovine hypodermosis: Prevalence and economic significance in southern Punjab, Pakistan. *Veterinary Parasitology*. **141(3-4)**:386-390.

Klein SL. 2004. Hormonal and immunological mechanisms mediating sex differences in parasite infection. *Parasite Immunology*. **26(6-7)**:247-264.

Konya C, Goronzy JJ, Weyand CM. 2009. Treating autoimmune disease by targeting CD8+ T suppressor cells. *Expert Opinion on Biological Therapy*. **9(8)**:951-965.

Kumar S, Khurana R, Rakha NK, Khokhar RS. 2006. Epidemiological pattern of various skin disorders in dogs. *The Indian Journal of Veterinary Research*. **15(1)**:1-4.

Kurtis JD, Mtalib R, Onyango FK, Duffy PE. 2001. Human resistance to *Plasmodium falciparum* increases during puberty and is predicted by dehydroepiandrosterone sulfate levels. *Infection and Immunity*. **69(1)**:123-128.

Lacetera N, Bernabucci U, Ronchi B, Scalia D, Nardone A. 2002. Moderate summer heat stress does not modify immunological parameters of Holstein dairy cows. *International Journal of Biometeorology*. **46**:33-37.

Lange T, Dimitrov S, Born J. 2010. Effects of sleep and circadian rhythm on the human immune system. *Annals of the New York Academy of Sciences*. **1193(1)**:48-59.

Lardone PJ, Carrillo-Vico A, Molinero P, Rubio A, Guerrero JM. 2009. A novel interplay between membrane and nuclear melatonin receptors in human lymphocytes: significance in IL-2 production. *Cellular and Molecular Life Sciences*. **66**:516-525.

Marietta E, Rishi A, Taneja V. 2015. Immunogenetic control of the intestinal microbiota. *Immunology*. 145:313–322.

Marketon JI, Glaser R. 2008. Stress hormones and immune function. *Cellular Immunology*. **252(1-2)**:16-26.

Martin KA, Robert AC, Alfred A, William GCB, Irshad HC. 1998. Dehydroepiandrosterone an inexpensive steroid hormone that decreases the mortality due to sepsis following trauma-induced hemorrhage. *The Archives of Surgery*. **133**:1281-1288.

Masi AT. 1989. Epidemiology of the rheumatic diseases. *Arthritis and Allied Conditions*. 16-54.

Miller SC, Pandi PS, Esquifino AI, Cardinali DP, Maestroni GJ. 2006. The role of melatonin in immuno-enhancement: potential application in cancer. *International Journal of Experimental Pathology*. **87(2)**:81-87.

Mocchegiani E, Amadio L, Fabris N. Neuroendocrine-thymus interactions. I. 1990. *In vitro* modulation of thymic factor secretion by thyroid hormones. *Journal of Endocrinological Investigation*. **13**:139-147.

Montoya MC, Sancho D, Bonello G, Collette Y, Langlet C, He HT, Aparicio P, Alcover A, Olive D, Sánchez-Madrid F. 2002. Role of ICAM-3 in the initial interaction of T lymphocytes and APCs. *Nature Immunology*. **3(2)**:159-168.

Münzel T, Feil R, Mülsch A, Lohmann SM, Hofmann F, Walter U. 2003. Physiology and pathophysiology of vascular signaling controlled by cyclic guanosine 3 , 5-cyclic monophosphate–dependent protein kinase. *Circulation*. **108(18)**:2172-2183.

Murray J, Barbara JA, Dunkley SA, Lopez AF, Van Ostade X, Condliffe AM, Dransfield I, Haslett C, Chilvers ER. 1997. Regulation of neutrophil apoptosis by tumor necrosis factor- : requirement for TNFR55 and TNFR75 for induction of apoptosis *in vitro*. Blood, *The Journal of the American Society of Hematology*. **90(7)**:2772-2783.

Nakazawa M, Fantappie MR, Freeman GL, Eloi Santos S, Olsen NJ, Kovacs WJ, Secor WE, Colley DG. 1997. *Schistosoma mansoni*: susceptibility differences between male and female mice can be mediated by testosterone during early infection. *Experimental Parasitology*. **85**:233-240.

Nathan and L, Chaudhuri G. 1997. Estrogens and atherosclerosis. *Annual Review of Pharmacology and Toxicology*. **37(1)**:477-515.

Neifeld JP, Lippman ME, Tormey DC. 1977. Steroid hormone receptors in normal human lymphocytes. Induction of glucocorticoid receptor activity by phytohemagglutinin stimulation. *Journal of Biological Chemistry*. **252(9)**:2972-2977.

Olsen NJ, Kovacs WJ. 1996. Gonadal steroids and immunity. *Endocrine Reviews*. 17(4):369-384.

Olsen NJ, Kovacs WJ. 2001. Effects of androgens on T and B lymphocyte development. *Immunologic Research*. **23**:281-288.

Paavonen TI, Andersson LC, Adlercreutz HE. 1981. Sex hormone regulation of *in vitro* immune response. Estradiol enhances human B cell maturation via inhibition of suppressor T cells in pokeweed mitogen-stimulated cultures. The Journal of Experimental Medicine. **154(6)**:1935-1945.

Pampori ZA, Pandita S. 2012. Analysis of *In Vitro* Effects of Sex Steroids on Lymphocyte Responsiveness in Murrah Buffaloes (*Bubalus bubalis*). *Veterinary Medicine International*. 2012.

Pampori ZA, Pandita S. 2013. Gender and age bias in immune competence and oxidative stress markers in Murrah buffaloes. *Indian Journal of Animal Sciences*. **83(7)**:717-724.

Pampori ZA, Pandita S. 2013. Reproductive cycle stage bias in physiological and immune responses to endotoxin challenge in Murrah buffaloes. *Buffalo Bulletin*. **32(4)**:270-283

Pampori ZA, Pandita S. 2014. Age- and sex-related variability in physiological and immune responses to endotoxin challenge in Murrah buffaloes (*Bubalus bubalis*). *Journal of Applied Animal Research*. **34(1)**:1-9

Park HJ, Choi JM. 2017. Sex-specific regulation of immune responses by PPARs. *Experimental & Molecular Medicine*. **49(8)**:e364.

Perez AR, Maya-Monteiro CM, Carvalho VF. 2021. Neuroendocrine-Immunological Interactions in Health and Disease. *Frontiers in Endocrinology*. **12**:718893.

Petrovsky N, Harrison LC. 1998. The chronobiology of human cytokine production. *International Reviews of Immunology*. **16(5-6)**:635-649.

Raju R, Chaudry IH. 2008. Sex steroids/receptor antagonist: their use as adjuncts after trauma-hemorrhage for improving immune/cardiovascular responses and for decreasing mortality from sepsis. *Anesthesia & Analgesia*. **107(1)**:159-166.

Ramadan AA, Johnson GL, Lewis GS. 1997. Regulation of uterine immune function during the estrous cycle and in response to infectious bacteria in sheep. *Journal of Animal Science*. **75(6)**:1621-1632.

Ramzan M, Akhtar M, Muhammad F, Hussain I, Hiszczy ska-Sawicka E, Haq AU, Mahmood MS, Hafeez MA. 2009. Seroprevalence of *Toxoplasma gondii* in sheep and goats in Rahim Yar Khan (Punjab), Pakistan. *Tropical Animal Health and Production*. **41**:1225-1229.

Rebecca L, Zhao P, Rawat R, Davis A, Hall JC, Chae JJ, Agarwal R, Cohen P, Rosen A, Hoffman EP, Nagaraju K. 2006. Sexual dimorphism in immune response genes as a function of puberty. *BMC Immunology*. **7(1)**:1-4.

Ridlon JM, Ikegawa S, Alves JM, Zhou B, Kobayashi A, Iida T, et al. 2013. Clostridium scindens: a human gut microbe with a high potential to convert glucocorticoids into androgens. *The Journal of Lipid Research*. **54**:2437-2449.

Roberts CW, Horsnell WG. 2015. Effects of sex and maternal immunity on protozoan and helminth infections. *Sex and Gender Differences in Infection and Treatments for Infectious Diseases*. 361-88.

Roden AC, Moser MT, Tri SD, Mercader M, Kuntz SM, Dong H, Hurwitz AA, McKean DJ, Celis E, Leibovich BC, Allison JP. 2004. Augmentation of T cell levels and responses induced by androgen deprivation. *The Journal of Immunology*. **173(10)**:6098-6108.

Rosselli M, Keller RJ, Dubey RK. 1998. Role of nitric oxide in the biology, physiology and pathophysiology of reproduction. *Human Reproduction Update*. **4(1)**:3-24.

Roth JA, Kaeberle ML, Appell LH, Nachreiner RF. 1983. Association of increased estradiol and progesterone blood values with altered bovine polymorphonuclear leukocyte function. American journal of veterinary research. **44(2)**:247-253.

Ruggieri A, Anticoli S, D'Ambrosio A, Giordani L, Viora M. 2016. The influence of sex and gender on immunity, infection and vaccination. *Annali Dell'istituto Superiore Di Sanita*. **52(2)**:198-204.

Ruiz FS, Andersen ML, Zager A, Martins RC, Tufik S. 2007. Sleep deprivation reduces the lymphocyte count in a non-obese mouse model of type 1 diabetes mellitus. *Brazilian Journal of Medical and Biological Research*. **40**:633-637.

Sartin JL, Elsasser TH, Kahl S, Baker J, Daniel JA, Schwartz DD, Steele B, Whitlock BK. 2003. Estradiol plus progesterone treatment modulates select elements of the proinflammatory cytokine cascade in steers: attenuated nitric oxide and thromboxane B2 production in endotoxemia. *Journal of Animal Science*. **81(6)**:1546-1551.

Scheiermann C, Kunisaki Y, Frenette PS. 2013. Circadian control of the immune system. *Nature Reviews Immunology*. **13(3)**:190-198.

Schwarz E, Schäfer C, Bode JC, Bode C. 2000. Influence of the menstrual cycle on the LPS-induced cytokine response of monocytes. *Cytokine*. **12(4)**:413-416.

Sherman B,Wysham C, Pfohl B. 1985. Age-related changes in the circadian rhythm of plasma cortisol in man. *The Journal of Clinical Endocrinology and Metabolism*. **61**:439–443.

Singh A, Tripathi MK, Singh R. 2016. Melatonin modulates leucocytes immune responses in freshwater snakes, Natrix piscator. *Journal of Herpetology*. **50(1)**:130–137.

Sinha BS, Verma SP, Mallick KP, Samantaray S, Kumar B, Kumar RP. 2006. Study on epidemiological aspects of bovine trypanosomosis in some districts of Bihar. *Journal of Veterinary Parasitology*. **20(1)**:69-71.

Siopes TD, Underwood HA. 2008. Diurnal variation in the cellular and humoral immune responses of Japanese quail: role of melatonin. *General and Comparative Endocrinology*. **158(3)**:245-249.

Skarzynski DJ, Bah MM, Deptula KM, Woclawek-Potocka I, Korzekwa A, Shibaya M, Pilawski W, Okuda K. 2003. Roles of tumor necrosis factor- of the estrous cycle in cattle: an *in vivo* study. *Biology of Reproduction*. **69(6)**:1907-1913.

Slominski RM, Reiter RJ, Schlabritz-Loutsevitch N, Ostrom RS, Slominski AT. 2012. Melatonin membrane receptors in peripheral tissues: distribution and functions. *Molecular and Cellular Endocrinology*. **351(2)**:152-166.

Sperry JL, Minei JP. 2008. Gender dimorphism following injury: making the connection from bench to bedside. *Journal of Leukocyte Biology*. **83(3)**:499-506.

Su L, Sun Y, Ma F, Lü P, Huang H, Zhou J. 2009. Progesterone inhibits Toll-like receptor 4-mediated innate immune response in macrophages by suppressing NF-B activation and enhancing SOCS1 expression. *Immunology Letters*. **125(2)**:151-155.

Tajpara MM. 2003. Epidemiological study on canine parvoviral diarrhea in dogs by Polymerase Chain Reaction and its comparative efficacy with other diagnostic assays (Doctoral dissertation).

Tanriverdi F, Silveira LF, MacColl GS, Bouloux PM. 2003. The hypothalamic-pituitary-gonadal axis: immune function and autoimmunity. *Journal of Endocrinology*. **176(3)**:293-304.

Thellin O, Coumans B, Zorzi W, Barnard R, Hennen G, Heinen E, Igout A. 1998. Expression of growth hormone receptors by lymphocyte subpopulations in the human tonsil. *Developmental Immunology*. **6(3-4)**:295-304.

Upadhyay SR, Singh R, Chandra D, Singh KP, Rathore BS. 2007. Seroprevalence of bovine brucellosis in Uttar Pradesh. *Journal of Immunology and Immunopathology*. **9(1-2)**:58-60.

Viselli SM, Reese KR, Fan J, Kovacs WJ, Olsen NJ. 1997. Androgens alter B cell development in normal male mice. *Cellular Immunology*. **182(2)**:99-104.

Washburn SM, Klesius PH, Ganjam VK, Brown BG. 1982. Effect of estrogen and progesterone on the phagocytic response of ovariectomized mares infected in utero with beta-hemolytic streptococci. *American Journal of Veterinary Research*. **43(8)**:1367-1370.

Weber M, Lauer N, Mülsch A, Kojda G. 2001. The effect of peroxynitrite on the catalytic activity of soluble guanylyl cyclase. *Free Radical Biology and Medicine*. **31(11)**:1360-1367.

White HD, Crassi KM, Givan AL, Stern JE, Gonzalez JL, Memoli VA, Green WR, Wira CR. 1997. CD3+ CD8+ CTL activity within the human female reproductive tract: influence of stage of the menstrual cycle and menopause. *Journal of Immunology*. **158(6)**:3017-3027.

Wu BN, O'Sullivan AJ. 2011. Sex differences in energy metabolism need to be considered with lifestyle modifications in humans. *Journal of Nutrition and Metabolism*. **2011**:391809.

Wulster-Radcliffe MC, Seals RC, Lewis GS. 2003. Progesterone increases susceptibility of gilts to uterine infections after intrauterine inoculation with infectious bacteria. *Journal of Animal Science*. **81(5)**:1242-1252.

Yu HP, Shimizu T, Hsieh YC, Suzuki T, Choudhry MA, Schwacha MG, Chaudry IH. 2006. Tissue-specific expression of estrogen receptors and their role in the regulation of neutrophil infiltration in various organs following trauma-hemorrhage. *Journal of Leukocyte Biology*. **79(5)**:963-970.

Zweier JL, Kuppusamy P, Lutty GA. 1988. Measurement of endothelial cell free radical generation: evidence for a central mechanism of free radical injury in postischemic tissues. *Proceedings of the National Academy of Sciences*. **85(11)**:4046-4050.

Chapter 23

Sustainable Livestock Production in North Western Himalayan Region with Special Reference to Climate Change

[1]Jonali Devi, [2]Kamal Sarma, [3]Zahoor A. Pampori, [3]Dilruba Hasin and [1]Kawardeep Kour

[1]Division of Veterinary Physiology & Biochemistry, [2] Division of Veterinary Anatomy-Faculty of Veterinary Sciences & Animal Husbandry, SKUAST-Jammu, R. S. Pura (UT of J & K) [3]Division of Veterinary Physiology, SKUAST-K (UT of J & K)

Livestock plays a major role in Indian economy. Approximately 20.5 million people depend upon livestock for their livelihood in India. Livestock contributed 16% to the income of small farm households against an average of 14% for all rural households. Again, livestock provides livelihood to two-third of rural community and it provides employment to about 8.8 % of the population in India. The vast Livestock sector of India contributes 4.11% of GDP and 25.6% of total Agriculture GDP. The livestock sector of India is one of the largest in the world with 11.6 percent of the world's total livestock population (BAHS-Basic Animal Husbandry Statistics, 2014). In recent years, the livestock sector has emerged as a significant segment of an expanding agricultural sector in the Indian economy (Tisdell and Gali, 2000). It is well known that the livestock farming is a very important socio-economic activity in Indian agriculture, as milk is the second largest agricultural commodity contributing to GNP (Gross National Products), next to rice.

Climate change is one of the most important environmental, social and economic issue facing the world today and has become an important area of concern for India to ensure food and nutritional security for growing population. Climate change will affect livestock production through competition for natural resources, quality and quantity of feeds, livestock diseases, heat stress and biodiversity loss while the demand for livestock products is expected to double by 2050. Therefore, challenge is to maintain a balance between livestock productivity, food security and animal welfare. Predicting the response of livestock to climate change is the need of the hour and it has to become an extremely active field of research. India ranks first in the world's total milk production. More than 2/3 of the milk production comes from the unorganized sectors (small farmers) as a part of integrated farming system comprising the crop production and animal husbandry. Extreme weather conditions cause severe production losses, especially during critical phases of growth, lactation and reproduction causes severe economic losses to individual farmers and to the national economy.

Reports have indicated that developing countries like India are more vulnerable to the effects of climate change due to their high reliance on natural resources, very limited capacity to adapt institutionally and financially and high poverty levels. A commendable share of the population of Jammu and Kashmir is dependent on agriculture for their livelihood. Goat and sheep rearing plays a vital role in socio-economic upliftment of weaker sections of the society of this state i.e., Gujjars and Backcrawls (Kuchay *et al.*, 2011). Sustainable growth of these animals for nutritional security and economic prosperity of Jammu and Kashmir is important. Meteorological data during last 25 years indicated that the environmental temperature of the Jammu region is ranged between 2°C in winter to 48 at summer season with relative humidity ranging from 18 to 91%. Wide ranges of environmental temperature may alter the physiological status of the animals and may lead to stress condition. It is known that different animal breeds show different degrees of heat tolerance because of varied genetic makeup which is due to long time interaction between gene and exposed environmental conditions. Being the original habitats, the local breeds of sheep and goat are highly adapted to the climatic condition and can withstand the extreme hot and cold climate of Jammu region of J&K.

CONTRIBUTION OF LIVESTOCK SECTOR IN INDIAN ECONOMY

The livestock sector of India is one of the largest in the world. The total milk production in our country grew at 6.50 percent and it reached 187.75 million tonnes in the year 2018-19, which was estimated as more than double the growth of world milk production. This record production of milk improved the per capita availability of milk to 394 gm per day per person, which was considerably higher than recommended rate of availability by Indian Council of Medical Research (ICMR) *i.e.*, 280 gm per day per person. Uttar Pradesh, Rajasthan, Madhya Pradesh, Andhra Pradesh and Gujarat are among the top five milk producing states, constituting 53.10 percent of the total milk production of the whole country. Nearly 35 percent of the milk production of India is contributed by indigenous buffalos followed by 26 percent by crossbred cattle. On the other hand, the total meat production reached 8.11 million tonnes in the year 2018-19 with a growth rate of 6 percent. Out of the total meat production in India, contribution of poultry meat is 50 percent (4.06 million tonnes) followed by buffalo meat (19.50 percent). The poultry meat production showed a growth rate of 7.80 percent. Uttar Pradesh, Maharashtra, West Bengal, Andhra Pradesh and Telangana are among the top five meat producing states in the country, constituting 56.90 percent of the total meat production. In 2018-19, egg production reached 103.32 billion with an annual growth rate of 8.50 percent. Presently, the per capita availability of eggs is approximately 79 eggs per person per year, which is much less than the recommended level i.e., 180 eggs per person per year by ICMR. The states like Andhra Pradesh, Tamil Nadu, Telangana, West Bengal and Haryana altogether contributed 65 percent of the total egg production of India and are recognised as the top five eggs producing states. The total egg production from commercial poultry farms is 84.91 billion (82.20 percent) and from backyard poultry is 18.41 billion (17.80 percent). The total wool production in the year 2018-19 was 40.42 million kgs. Telangana, Karnataka and Gujarat are the top five wool producing states of the country and altogether contributed 78.50 percent of the total wool production.

MAJOR CHALLENGES OF LIVESTOCK SECTOR

1. Climate Change

Livestock undergo various kinds of stress such as physical, nutritional, chemical, psychological and thermal stress. Among all, thermal stress is most concerning now a day in the ever-changing climatic scenario. Thermal stress redistributes the body resources including protein and energy at the cost of decreased growth, reproduction, production and health. Thermal stress stimulates complex responses which are fundamental in the preservation of cell survival. Exposure to thermal stress has been related to morphological and physiological modifications. At the molecular and cellular levels, cold stress reduces rates of enzymatic reactions, diffusion and membrane transport where the heat stress accelerates these processes. Thermal stress (both heat and cold) induces denaturation and mis-aggregation of protein slowing of progression through the cell cycle, inhibit translation and transcription, disrupt cellular cyto-skeleton elements and change membrane permeability.

2. Low Productivity

Although India possesses highest livestock population and it ranks number one in milk production in the globe, the productivity, particularly of ruminants has been extremely low, turning this precious asset of the poor people into a liability. It is worthy to mention here that, over 60 percent of the rural households rear large ruminants, mostly for milk and partly for bullock power, although the average milk yield is significantly low.

3. High Economic Losses Due to Animal Diseases

The diseases in livestock cause major economic loss to the farmers. With the improvement in the quality of livestock through cross-breeding program, the susceptibility of these livestock to various diseases including exotic diseases has been increased. The insufficient coverage of vaccination is continuously resulting into economic losses due to various animal diseases. Estimations of losses due to different diseases are not easy because it is very difficult to report all diseases at all places. The direct losses estimation is based on reported diseases and it indicated that average annual economic losses due to diseases like Haemorrhagic Septicaemia (HS), Foot and Mouth Disease (FMD), Brucellosis, Peste des Petits Ruminants (PPR),

Classical Swine Fever were in around Rs. 5255 crores in the year 2014, Rs. 20000 crores in 2016, Rs. 20400 crores in 2015, Rs. 2417 crores in 2016 and Rs. 429 crores in the year 2016, respectively. It indicated that farmers in India faces a direct loss of almost Rs. 50,000 crores every year due to the five fully preventable (with vaccination) diseases although the government of India along with state governments spend equally good amount of funds on vaccination against these five diseases that costs approximately every year. But adequate results are not achieved due to substandard vaccines, inefficient vaccination, ill-education of livestock farmers etc.

4. Inadequate Infrastructure and Human Resources for Support Services

Indian livestock sector is facing the problem of poor infrastructure and human resources. As on 31 March 2017, the number of veterinary institutions stood at 65242. As per the recommendation of the National Commission on Agriculture (NCA)-1976, One Veterinary Institution is to be provided for every 5,000 cattle units (one cattle unit =1 cow or 1 buffalo or 10 sheep or 10 goats or 5 pigs or 100 poultry) to ensure proper and adequate veterinary health care. On the same line, the Veterinary Council of India (VCI) has recommended that for every 5000 livestock population there is need of one veterinarian for effective delivery of veterinary services to the farmers. It is reported that there are a total of 67651 veterinarians in India, whereas estimated requirement by VCI is around 1.1-1.2 lakh (Damodaran, 2015) in the whole country. This highly inadequate human resources resulted in poor and insufficient veterinary services to the farmers. For the purpose of improvement of cattle breed and in turn milk production, Artificial Insemination (AI) technology was adopted in India in 1970 onwards. However, in the last 50 years, due to several such constraints, the average conception rate through AI is not going more than 30-40 percent at field level and the share of milk from crossbred cows to total milk production is not exceeding beyond 26 percent.

5. Shortage of Feed and Fodder

India has only 2.29 percent of land area of the world, but is maintaining nearly 17 percent of world human population and 10.70 percent of livestock (more than 535.82 million) which posing a huge pressure on land, water and other resources. India is having only 5 percent of its cultivable land under fodder production. Again, area under permanent pastures and grazing lands comprises a mere 3.30 percent of the total area, and it has also been declining steadily. Among different resources of livestock fodder, crop residues are major one and these feeding resources are major ingredient meeting more than 50 percent of the livestock sector demand in the country. At prevailing livestock productivity and production, livestock sector is facing severe feed and fodder shortage in the country. In a report titled "Revisiting National Forage Demand and Availability Scenario", released during August 2019 by the ICAR-Indian Grassland and Fodder Research Institute (IGFRI) has reported that there is a deficit of 23.40 percent in the availability of dry fodder, 11.24 percent in green fodder and 28.90 percent for concentrates in India (Roy *et al.*, 2019). There are already proven high yielding varieties of fodder and technologies such as silage making, hay making and urea- molasses treatment for crop residue is in practice.

However, adoption of such technologies is very poor in many of the states, especially in rural areas. According to the Indian Ministry of New and Renewable Energy (MNRE) report, India generates on an average 500 million tons of crop residue per year and a majority of this crop residue is in fact used as fodder and fuel for other domestic and industrial purposes. But there is still a surplus of 140 million tons, out of which 92 million tons is burned each year, which can be effectively used for animal fodder (Bhuvaneshwari *et al.*, 2019).

6. Inadequate Public Institution Support

In India, the livestock sector did not receive the policy and adequate financial attention as it deserved. The sector is granted with only about 12 per cent of the total public expenditure on agriculture and allied sectors, which is disproportionately lesser than its contribution to agricultural GDP. The sector has been also neglected by financial institutions. The share of livestock in the total agricultural credit has not ever exceeded four percent in the total credit. The government mechanisms to protect animals against various risk are not strong enough. At present, only 6 percent of the animal heads (excluding poultry) are provided insurance cover. Livestock extension machinery has remained grossly neglected in the past. However, in May 2019, Government of India has constituted separate ministry *i.e.,* Ministry of Fisheries, Animal Husbandry and Dairying at central level to address various challenges of livestock sector, which is definitely going to boost the livestock sector.

7. Inadequate Processing and Value Addition

Processing and value addition of livestock product is being regarded as the potential tool for sustainability of livestock production. In India, the milk processing industry has expanded at a Compound Annual Growth Rate (CAGR) of 14.80 percent as of 2018 (Laura Wood, 2019). Moreover, the meat industry is one of the most important part of food processing industry. The processing rate of kara beef (buffalo meat) and poultry meat are approximately 21% and 6 %, respectively. The major reason for inadequate processing and value addition in meat product chiefly lack of necessary infrastructure. As on 2019, in the country, there are only 1377 slaughter houses, 68 abattoirs with proper meat processing facilities approved by Agricultural and Processed Food Products Export Development Authority (APEDA), 32 APEDA registered meat processing plants, 11 APEDA registered stand-alone abattoirs, 9 carcass utilization centres, and 25000 small scale meat retail shops apart from a few private companies. There is a forecast in the report of FAO (2011) entitled "Mapping Supply and Demand for Animal-Source Foods to 2030" that the demand for various livestock products will increase by 80-100 percent by the year 2030 and out of the total increase, nearly 60 percent of demand will be due to change in consumption pattern and frequency of intake of the people and remaining 40 percent demand increase will be due to population growth. It clearly indicates the importance of value addition and processing of livestock products (Robinson and Pozzi, 2011).

8. Issues in Marketing of Livestock and Livestock Products

Paving the way to the markets is critical to speed up the commercialization of livestock production. Lack of access to markets may act as a disincentive to farmers for adopting latest technologies and quality inputs. The change in the present market is not uniform. The changes are either species specific or products. But there are phenomenal changes from informal to formal market system seen currently in dairy and poultry sectors. However, nearly 60 percent of milk in the country is sold by the unorganized sector. On the other hand, sheep, goat and beef remains in the informal sector without much investment from private firms. If it is to be expressed concisely, the Indian livestock and livestock product market are mostly underdeveloped, irregular, uncertain, and lack transparency and often dominated by informal market intermediaries who exploit the producers.

9. Lack of Attention of Small Ruminates

The small ruminants (sheep and goats) are generally reared by small, marginal and landless farmers, who cannot afford to own large ruminants. However, most of these small ruminants which are dependent on free grazing without any investment on supplementary feeding and health care, do not make significant contribution to the income due to low productivity. As the demand for meat is expected to grow high during the next two decades, the present system of unsustainable husbandry practices, which highlights the status of these species getting deprived of technological and managerial support services, needs to be addressed.

10. Inadequate Attention Towards Extension Services

The delivery system of livestock services has chiefly three components viz. providing technical services to the animals, giving technical inputs and educating the livestock farmers. Providing various services to animals includes vaccination, deworming, breeding and disease management for which technical inputs such as vaccines, medicines, semen, AI guns, syringes and needles, etc. needs to be supplied. The livestock farmers have no option but to depend on vets or para-vets for all the above-mentioned services and, to some extent, supply of technical inputs. Unfortunately, the third component, *i.e.*, educating livestock farmers on various aspects of livestock management, (feeding, vaccination, disease management, breeding etc.) is totally neglected. Often, supply of inputs and providing services are considered as an extension service ignoring the fact that "education of farmers is the core of livestock extension service" (Rao, 2013). The main focus of any extension services requires building the capabilities or capacities of the farmers so that they can take care of their animals and crop in addition to offering knowledge on transfer of technology and strengthening of various infrastructure and support services. Earlier, the State Departments of Animal Husbandry (SDAH) were part of State Department of Agriculture but with the changing times, this department got bifurcated and now every state of India has independent department for Animal Husbandry. However, since beginning, the orientation of the SDAH remained confined towards giving healthcare and breeding services rather than focus on production. Again, in most of the states, the designation of veterinarians is Veterinary Officer (VO), Veterinary Assistant Surgeon (VAS) rather than Livestock Development Officer (LDO) which normally psychologically restricts their role on livestock development and building farmer's capacities. The veterinarians are supposed to educate the farmers on scientific management practices, sustainability of livestock farming, ways to meet paucity of animal feed and fodder, marketing of livestock, processing of livestock products, environmental issues, etc. Thus, the development role of veterinarians on livestock production aspect is not adequately explored in India. In spite of above challenges, the Indian livestock sector is performing well, however in view of fulfilling the increasing demand of livestock products, these needs to be addressed.

MITIGATION STRATEGIES TO IMPROVE PRODUCTION

1. **Smart Livestock Farming:** To mitigate all the above-mentioned challenges and drawbacks of the livestock sector, it is the need of hour to shift towards the smart livestock farming. The objective of Smart livestock farming is to achieve more productive, efficient and sustainable farm operations with the effective use of available digital technologies. The largest potential of it lies in individual animal monitoring and analysis, which is called the Precision Livestock Farming (PLF). The smart livestock farming consists of the following components - Artificial Intelligence, Cyber-Physical Systems (CPS) and Internet of Things (IoT), Platforms, Information and Communication Technologies (ICT), Cloud Computing, Crowdsourcing, Transparent supply chains, Flexible production systems etc.
2. **Development of genetically fewer sensitive breeds:** selective crossbreeding is most preferable. For example, the exotic breeds of cattle which are more tolerant due to more sweat gland density (Jersey) should be given more preference over less heat tolerant breeds (Holstein Friesian).
3. **Physical modification of the environment:** it includes the methods for modification of microenvironment like shades, ventilation, wetting, combination of ventilation and wetting etc. Shades may either natural or artificial. Tree shades are proved to be more efficient (Hahn, 1985). Shades are effective in reducing heat stress and the physiological responses in the dairy animals (Upadhyay et al., 2009). Singh and Upadhyay (2009) found that animals in shade show lower physiological responses in terms of respiratory rate, pulse rate, rectal temperature and skin temperature during afternoon and milk production from these animals were more with more protein percentage. Forced ventilation provided by the fans or cooler is a very effective method for lowering the temperature (Kumar et al., 2013). Another effective cooling system during hot days is using water spray. Several cooling devises like mist, foggers, sprinkling systems can be adopted. However, the single use of sprinkling and fan system for 30 minutes before milking has proved to be useful to relief from heat stress. Different roofing materials have been suggested by different workers in different agro-climatic conditions.
4. **Improves nutritional and managemental practices:** For evolving ameliorative strategies of adverse effect of thermal stress, several studies have been carried out. Properly balanced and palatable ration along with continuous availability of fresh water is inevitable for wellbeing of livestock, reared under all types of climatic conditions. Also, the feeding of vitamin E showed a positive impact by lowering the levels of thermal stress mark-

ers like Heat shock protein expression in lymphocytes and antioxidant enzyme (SOD and CAT) levels. Likewise, vitamin C also plays a role in lowering the heat stress in livestock. Ganaie *et al.* (2013) and Kour (2018) showed the beneficial effect of vitamin C feeding in buffaloes and goats during environmental stress conditions. Some studies conducted on supplementation of chromium during summer and winter seasons (Kumar, 2013) stressed about the beneficial effects of its supplementation over the control group by improving the immunity and growth performance.

5. **Global best practice roll-out:** best practices are regarded as the methods or techniques that have consistently shown results superior to those achieved by other means. Large yield and productivity gaps exist across the livestock sector, especially between the industrialized advanced and developing countries. Digitalization can make a roll-out in to an easier, faster, and less expensive by leveraging transparent supply chains, cloud computing, improved networks and global knowledge platforms.
6. **Precision feeding:** Precision feeding can be a highly effective tool in enabling a reduction of feed intake per animal at the same time maximizing individual growth rates in livestock. It enables the intake of the right amount of feed, in the right nutrient composition, at the right time and for each animal individually.
7. **Smart waste management:** About 20% of all meat goes to waste every year. Although most waste is generated at the consumer end, the root causes lie across the whole supply chain, e.g., poor packaging or bad meat quality. Smart waste management offers high efficiency to first identify such root causes and second, to improve existing processes and thereby decrease waste amounts. The intelligent collection and use of data are the key for understanding what is produced and what is thrown away. Through this, players along the supply chain can make focused adjustments to reduce waste at their end as far as possible.
8. **Animal health and welfare monitoring:** Various health issues and diseases can decrease production efficiency of livestock by up to 33%. The trend towards more and more intensification of livestock farming systems in one hand increases productivity, but on the other hand can also have adverse effects on animal health and welfare, and also increases the risk of rapid and far-reaching disease outbreaks within stocks. Through ICT and the IoT, comparatively more performance-related data can be collected from the animals than the traditional methods by the use of cameras and image recognition software's, wearables, as well as weight or sound monitoring, etc. Additionally, data from livestock facilities can also help to improve animal health, for example through climate, air quality and ventilation monitoring and by using drones.

Vision

- To provide information regarding effect of individual/combined elements of weather (solar radiation, temperature, precipitation, humidity and wind) on physiology and production parameters of animals.

- There is a need of develop strategies to adopt and mitigate the expected increase in temperature due to climate change which will help to adopt and protect the productive animals against extreme weather conditions.
- To gather knowledge on weather-livestock relationship in different agro-climatic zone of Jammu region to identify weather sensitive critical stages on livestock rearing.
- Development of species and breed specific farming system models for different agro-climatic zones.
- Establishment of weather-based advisories for animal husbandry sector including a) timely dissemination of mobile based weather information to the registered farmer, b) information dissemination to farmers through training and c) brainstorming session on awareness regarding adverse effect of climatic stress on livestock and strategies to mitigate the stress.

REFERENCES

Bhuvaneshwari, S, Hettiarachchi, H. and Meegoda, J. N. (2019). Crop Residue Burning in India: Policy Challenges and Potential Solutions. International Journal of Environment Research and Public Health 6(5), 832; https://doi.org/10.3390/ijerph16050832

FAO (2011) FAOSTAT. Food and Agriculture Organization of the United Nations

Ganaie, A.H., Hooda, O.K., Singh, S.V., Ashutosh, Upadhyay, R.C. (2013). Effect of vitamin C supplementation on immune status and oxidative stress in pregnant murrah buffaloes during thermal stress. Indian Journal of Animal Sciences. 83(6): 649-655.

Hahn, G.L. (1985). Management and housing of farm animals in hot environment, In : M.Yousef (Ed.) Stress physiology in Livestock. 2: 151-174.

Kour, S. (2018). Effects of vitamin C on physio-biochemical parameters in water deprived goats. PhD thesis submitted to SKUAST-Jammu, R.S.Pura, J&K.

Kuchay, J.A.; Chishti, M.Z.; Zaki, M.M. and Javid, A. (2011). Prevalance of nematode parasites in Ladakh-India. *Journal of Agricultural Extension and Rural development*, **3** (13): 229-231.

Kumar, S. (2013). Thermal stress alleviation and immune modulation in Sahiwal calves supplemented with chromium propionate. MVSc thesis submitted to NDRI, Karnal, Haryana.

Laura Wood (2019). The Dairy & Milk Processing Market in India, 2018- 2019 & 2023. Business Wire.Retrievedfromhttps://www.businesswire.com/news/home/20190322005336/en/Dairy-MilkProcessing-Market-India-2018-2019-2023.

Rao, S.V.N. (2013). Why Collaboration Matters for Livestock Development?, AESA Blog 06, Livestock Extension. Retrieved from https://www.aesanetwork.org/wp-content/uploads/2013/08/AESA-BLOG-6.pdf

Robinson, T.P. and Pozzi, F. (2011). Mapping supply and demand for animal-source foods to 2030. Animal Production and Health Working Paper. No. 2. Rome. pp.10, 48. Retrieved from http://www.fao.org/3/i2425e/i2425e00.pdf

Roy, A. K., Agrawal, R. K., Bhardwaj, N. R., Mishra, A. K. & Mahanta, S. K. (2019). Revisiting National Forage Demand and Availability Scenario. Retrieved fromhttps://www.researchgate.net/publication/336230799_Revisiting_National_For age_Demand_and_Availability_Scenario.

Singh, S.V. and Upadhyay, R.C. (2009). Impact of temperature rise on physiological function, thermal balance and milk production of lactating Karan fries and Sahiwal cows. Indian Vet J. 86(2): 141-144.

Tisdell, C. and Gali, J. (2000). Trends and developments in India's livestock industry. Econ. Ecol. and Env. Working paper 43 (Aug).

Upadhyay, R.C., Ashotosh, Raina, V.S. and Singh, S.V. (2009). Impact of climate change on reproductive functions of cattle and buffaloes. In: Global Climate Change and Indian Agriculture (Edited by P.K. Aggarwal). Published by ICAR, New Delhi. Pp. 107-110.

Chapter 24

Antibiotic Resistance in India: An Update After the National Action Policy for Antimicrobial Resistance

Varshetha Muthukumar[1], Nukula Ramesh[2], Chandrasekhar B.[3], Pavan Kumar Pesingi[4] and Thulasiraman Parkunan[5*]

[1]*Department of Public Health, School of Health, Bioscience and Sport, University of East London, UK*

[2]*Department of Veterinary Extension, College of Veterinary Science, Rajendranagar, Hyderabad, P. V. Narasimha Rao Telangana Veterinary University, Telangana, India*

3Dairy Microbiology Department, Warner College of Dairy Technology, SHUAT, Prayagraj, Uttar Pradesh, India

[4]*Department of Veterinary Public Health and Epidemiology, Faculty of Veterinary and Animal Sciences, Institute of Agricultural Sciences, Rajiv Gandhi South Campus, Banaras Hindu University, Barkachha, Mirzapur, Uttar Pradesh, India*

[5]*Department of Veterinary Physiology and Biochemistry, Faculty of Veterinary and Animal Sciences, Institute of Agricultural Sciences, Rajiv Gandhi South Campus, Banaras Hindu*

ABSTRACT

Background: Antimicrobial drugs are needed to treat the growing number of infectious diseases worldwide. With overuse and abuse of Antimicrobial drugs, resistant strains of pathogenic microflora have emerged, thereby placing a dire need for regulations on consumption. India becomes the antibiotic capital in the global arena. A policy to curb this practice of antibiotic abuse requires a holistic approach towards controlling the emergence of Antimicrobial Resistance (AMR).

Objective: Here we aim to present the problems of antimicrobial usage at various stakeholders -level contributing towards emergence and spread of AMR in India, review mitigation strategies and discuss alternate tackling initiatives which can be adopted in place of antimicrobial drugs.

Conclusion: (a) This paper outlines that with joint collaboration and political commitment, AMR is a solvable public health issue that if left in inaction could potentially infiltrate our rather weak public health system and create a huge economic burden. (b) This article demonstrates the current scenario and policies implemented since the launch of the mitigation strategies outlined according to the National Action Plan (NAP) in 2017.

INTRODUCTION

Antimicrobials have become a ubiquitous part of any health care system in the world. They have shaped how modern medicine has advanced over the decades. People had ill-fated outcomes in the pre-antibiotic era where elective surgeries, cesarean deliveries and post-operative infections would often become fatal (Adedeji, 2016).With the advent of antibiotics, modern medicine has taken a huge upsurge in better treatment outcomes of infectious diseases and operative surgical procedures. Over the decades, antimicrobials have been made accessible to all the populations in the world. The excruciating gains achieved in public health in the last century will possibly be reversed with the emergence of resistant microorganisms to current antimicrobial drugs.

As with any species, microorganisms too have evolved to develop resistant mechanisms against antibiotics (Tello *et al.*, 2012). The emergence of resistance will render any antibiotic useless and will push us into a global public health threat or the post-antibiotic era where even minor infections and simple treatment procedures would complicate into fatal outcomes resulting in prolonged hospital admission, expensive treatment and high economic burden (Mainous *et al.*, 2011). The so called 'superbugs' are the resistant microbes that are causing a silent pandemic infiltrating all healthcare systems in the world. This resistance to antibiotics is found to be driven by the irrational consumption of antibiotics in all sectors of human development. Infections due to drug-resistant pathogens are estimated to cause 10 million deaths every year by 2050 and economic loss of US $100 trillion (O' Neil *et al.*, 2014). Two million deaths are estimated to occur by the year 2050 in India due to AMR. There has been a strong distinctive correlation demonstrated between antimicrobial usage and the development of resistance (Bronzwaer *et al.*, 2002). Furthermore, India being the second most populated country in the world was one of the largest consumers of antibiotics in 2010 in the world (Van Boeckel *et al.*, 2014). Between the years 2000 and 2015, total antibiotic consumption in India rose alarmingly by 103% (Klein *et al.*, 2018). These figures frighteningly forecast that AMR is not just confined to any particular country but could rise to a global challenge due to widespread travel and trade in the world.

Antimicrobial drugs play a vital role to limit the morbidity and mortality rate of many infectious diseases in the country (Kourtis, Athena, 2016). India faces the top spot of prevalence in tuberculosis which is a chronic bacterial infection that requires appropriate treatment and management with antimicrobials(WHO 2011).Over 1.9 million deaths were reported due to infectious diseases in the Southeast Asian region which accounts to 14% of total deaths occurring every year (WHO, 2016). Development of antimicrobial resistance against infectious diseases will prove to be fatal and skyrocket these numbers to a global level. Hence, tackling this burden of AMR against infectious diseases should be sought as a global mission. Antimicrobial resistance can be postulated as a strain that is resistant against an antibiotic if its minimal inhibitory concentration (MIC) is higher than for the corresponding parental wild-type strain. A resistance gene is a part of genome which in its presence, allows a bacterium to withstand a higher antibiotic concentration or in its absence increases susceptibility of the antibiotic (Bengtsson-Palme, 2018).

In 2014, Jim O'Neill and his team stated that the broader public health issues such as HIV,Tuberculosis and Malaria for which resistance is a concern and the countries having high rates in these diseases will develop drug resistance further exacerbated by regional variations (O' Neil *et al.*, 2014). India being a high burden country in all these diseases will pay a huge price for the debilitating impact of HIV-TB co-morbidity and multi-drug resistant malaria. There has been soaring numbers of resistance to last-resort antibiotics saved to treat life-threatening conditions (Van Boeckel *et al.*, 2014). WHO regards AMR as a 'one health' issue with extended ramifications in not just human health but also animal, plant, and environmental health. One health concept acknowledges that human health is very much interconnected with that of the ecosystem and other species. The presence of antibiotic residues and antimicrobial resistant microbes in other species of food animals and agriculture invariably enters the human food chain and effects of bio-accumulation potentiate the transmission of AMR and poses a wider public health threat to all mankind (Destoumieux-Garzón *et al.*, 2018). Inadequacies in data gathering or lack of wanting to share data of sales and dispensing of antimicrobials by pharmaceutical agencies also surmounts to India being the global antibiotic capital. This data on sales and consumption is regarded key in surveillance studies as proposed in the GLASS report by WHO (WHO Report on Surveillance of Antibiotic Consumption, 2016).

As with tackling any disease, surveillance studies are necessitated for formulating policies and implementation of developed strategies. The lack of substantial data to support any pivotal decision making acts as a loophole in tackling AMR in India. This review highlights the progress made through various policies and regulations that have been implemented in India since the formulation of national action policy AMR in India in 2017. Since 2017 only 3 states have implemented state action policies for addressing AMR. This paper also establishes the challenges faced on the way forward and adds additional research input that might be necessary to reduce antibiotic consumption and adopt alternate products for antimicrobials.

STAKEHOLDERS CONTRIBUTING TO AMR IN DIFFERENT SECTORS

Antimicrobial use in humans: Antimicrobial resistance in human health is largely caused due to irrational prescription and consumption of antibiotics. Antibiotics form a part of the schedule H1 drugs that can only be purchased with a valid prescription by a registered medical practitioner, but access is made available to almost everybody over-the-counter or through prescriptions prescribed by illegitimate medical professionals and/or quacks. Lack of availability of qualified medical practitioners in rural set up constraints people to seek medical advice from quacks. According to a WHO report in 2016, 57.1% of healthcare professionals in India claiming to be allopathic doctors have no medical qualification (Anand and Fan, 2016). The wide disparity in lack of a medical qualification is concentrated in rural areas. Only 18.8% of allopathic doctors had a medical qualification in rural areas as compared to 58.4% of doctors having a medical degree in urban areas (Anand & Fan, 2016). Despite India achieving the WHO recommended norm of 1:1000 doctor population ratios in 2017, the tug of war in urban-rural discrepancies has paved way for the lack of quality healthcare. This disparity exposes the predominant weakness in India's health care system (Kumar & Pal, 2018).In many instances, patients in rural areas requiring emergent help are forced to travel more than 100km to seek treatment which invariably leads to people accessing services offered by private healthcare practitioners in their native villages who are often quacks (Singh & Badaya, 2014).

Seeking healthcare advice from unqualified professionals who are commonly called rural medical practitioners (RMP) or private medical practitioners (PMP) cater to the health needs of the rural population. It is illegal for these practitioners to prescribe allopathic drugs. Despite this law, RMP and PMP prescribe antibiotics illicitly without serious knowledge of potential risks and complications. They also involve in corrupt practices such as parenteral administration of drugs to many people with the same syringe thereby transmitting various infectious diseases. Thus, an increase in number of infectious diseases requires antibiotic drugs for treatment, hospital admissions, loss of work days which have essentially incurred added costs that could have been entirely avoided.

Incentives from pharmaceutical companies to practicing physicians remain another predominant cause of irrational use of antibiotics (Davies *et al.*, 2019). It is reported that promotional practices for drug marketing by pharmaceutical companies involve inducement or bribery, persuasion, emotional appeals, sponsorship for national and international conferences, gift cards and vouchers which are promised if the doctor gives suitable business through their prescriptions (Davies *et al.*, 2019). The Aggressive drug promotion and marketing practices have led to exaggeration of medical benefits and downplaying risks of the drugs ultimately resulting in the creation of superbugs (Gulhati, 2004). AYUSH practitioners are liable to medical negligence if found to have prescribed allopathic drugs. Nevertheless, allopathic drugs are marketed to physicians practicing alternative forms of medicine such as AYUSH and rural medical practitioners (Davies *et al.*, 2019). Unethical and cross practice performing by other medical professionals have led to excessive use of irrational, hazardous, non-indicated high cost antimicrobial drugs and less adherence of doctors to the 5D's - diagnosis, drug, dosage, duration and de-escalation of antibiotics (Gadre & Diwate, 2019). Irrational antibiotic combination largely leads to antibiotic resistance. Out of large sales of medicines in India almost 50% of Fixed Dose Combinations (FDC) are irrational. These irrational FDC are potentially undesirable, hold unnecessary risks and adverse effects, and expose the patient to avoidable expenses (Srinivasan, 2016). Various approaches or conflicts in treatment regimen, incentives to physicians by pharmaceutical companies, practicing empirical treatment practices due to delayed laboratory diagnostic services, prescribing high end antibiotics or reserved drugs by untrained clinicians, compulsion of the need to prescribe drugs to seek validation from patients as opposed to educating the patient on harmful adverse effects of antibiotics comprise contribution of AMR by physicians.

Healthcare facilities in India are not adequately equipped to tackle hospital acquired infections (HAI). Failure in setting up an Antibiotic stewardship team, which regulates the administration of medication to patients admitted for surgical treatment, absence of monitoring of antibiotic susceptibility tests, lack of implementation of infection control (IFC) guidelines stokes fears of AMR in the hospital setting which are potentially multi-drug resistant. Only 25% of health care institutions in India had AMA (Antimicrobial Agents) usage data and only 30% had AMA prescription audit and feedback. Antimicrobial Stewardship Programme teams were actively functioning in only 50% health care institutions (Walia *et al.*, 2015). Lack of appropriate data to identify and substantiate the needs of the population hinders the framing of policies and implementation. Research studies in gauging the ground realities among various stakeholders have impeded surveillance and effective interventions with regards to AMR. There is lack of data in many aspects of drug sales and dispensing or lack of wanting to share data by drug manufacturers to avoid commercial rivalries (WHO, 2016). There is also a dire need for newer generations of antibiotics since no major drug discovery has been made in the last four decades. As newer resistant microbes have emerged against current generations of antibiotics over the years, a constant antibiotic pipeline is not made available. Potential and advanced research is required to reverse or manipulate the genomic sequences of resistant organisms. One of the key causes of administering antibiotics to viral diseases is due to delay in confirming laboratory diagnosis. Despite various breakthroughs and advancements made in medicine, a diagnosis based on bacterial culture takes several hours to few days to conclude. Furthermore, applied research is necessary in developing rapid diagnostic tests for quick confirmatory results for bacterial infections which can prevent incidence of Health Care Acquired Infection (HCAI). Table 1 figures out various causes of AMR in modern human medicine.

Table 1: Potential stakeholders contributing to AMR in the service provider-consumer spectrum of human health

Health care Facilities Tertiary care hospitals)	Registered medical Practitioner/ Private medical Practitioner	Pharmacists	Consumers/ Community people	Research	Quacks	Role of government
No reporting systems for Nosocomial infection in India (Dixit et al., 2019; De & Mukherjee (2018)	Incentives from Pharma companies to prescribe higher generation and expensive antibiotics (Dixit et al., 2019)	Sale of schedule H and schedule H1 drugs without prescription from a registered medical practitioner (Kumar et al., 2013)	Inaccessibility to healthcare and laboratory facilities Taneja & Sharma, 019)	Absence of Research on AMSP about effective intervention, Surveillance, and management of antimicrobial usage data.	Over 57.3% of people claiming themselves to be allopathic doctors did not have a medical qualification (Anand & Fan, 2016)	To formulate laws to curb unequal distribution of healthcare providers in urban and rural settings.
Only 50% of health care institutions had documented antibiotic stewardship team in hospitals but data on implementation and follow-up lacks (Walia et al 2015)	Unlicensed practitioners in the private sector (Kumar et al., 2013)	Inadequate monitoring of prescription audit for OTC drugs (Singh et al., 2019)	Self-medication upon hearsay/ internetc.	Inefficient rapid diagnostic tests for optimal treatment as opposed to empirical diagnosis.	81.2% healthcare providers in rural areas lacked a medical qualification.41.6% of healthcare providers in urban areas lacked a medical qualification (Anand & Fan, 2016)	Lack of rules and regulation to control antibiotic sale (Gulhati, C. M. 2004) No strict implementation of existing policies/laws

Health care Facilities Tertiary care hospitals)	Registered medical Practitioner/ Private medical Practitioner	Pharmacists	Consumers/ Community people	Research	Quacks	Role of government
Only 65% hospitals have Anti-Microbial Agent's(AMA) prescription guidelines (Walia et al., 2015)	Restrictive prescriptive authority which requires approval to use certain restricted antibiotics, except trained clinicians	Product degraded by improper storage and handling	Non-compliance to recommended treatment duration (Kumar et al., 2013)	Bacterial diagnostics have not kept up with medical innovation over the last 70 years.		
Lack of formularies and audit restrictions	Varying approaches while treating infectious diseases.	Unregistered or unregulated manufacturers producing drugs with no active ingredient/ Counterfeit drugs (Glass, 2014)	Prompting pharmacists for purchase of antibiotics for a shorter or a longer treatment duration than the recommended one (Kumar et al 2013)	Extensive Research required to overhaul Vaccines and reduce antibiotic usage.	Corrupt practices and botching surgeries leads to rising cross transmission of infectious diseases posing a public health threat.	

Health care Facilities Tertiary care hospitals)	Registered medical Practitioner/ Private medical Practitioner	Pharmacists	Consumers/ Community people	Research	Quacks	Role of government
Lack of regular Continuing Medical Education Programme for hospital personnel regarding AMR .	Prescription of antibiotics by practitioners of alternative medicine such as homeopathy, Ayurveda, Unani, siddha, etc. (Dixit et al., 2019)	Absence of record keeping for sale of schedule H1 drugs (Dixit et al, 2019)	Poverty, Illiteracy, Overcrowding, poor sanitation facilities and malnutrition becomes the silent barrier (Kumar et al., 2013; Taneja & Sharma, 2019)	Global innovation fund for early stage research and R&D lacking commercial imperative		
Lack of Implementation of Infection Prevention and Control guidelines	Although there is no Indian law banning Registered Medical Practitioner from dispensing and selling drugs in the doctor's office, appropriate records on purchase of antibiotics are lacking which are liable for inspection and audit in the doctor's office according to patient needs without involvement of pharmacists (Math et al., 2019; Kumar et al., 2013)			Lack of rapid Antibiotic Sensitivity Testing methods/kits at rural level		

ANTIMICROBIALS USE IN ANIMAL

Indiscriminate use of antimicrobials as a mode of disease prevention, along with inappropriate therapeutic purpose fuels the burden of AMR in livestock and poultry farms (National policy for containment of antimicrobial resistance, 2011). Knowingly and unknowingly some of the livestock farmers use antibiotics for growth promotion without knowing the consequences (Mahalmani *et al.*, 2019). Considering the recent emergence of colistin-resistant bacterial infections in food animals, colistin is banned in India and China as growth promoters (Bandyopadhyay and Samanta, 2020; Walsh and Wu, 2016). Substitution of hygiene and sanitation in livestock and poultry farms with prophylactic use of antimicrobials in feeds to prevent diseases transcends to emergence of resistance. Lack of strict implementation of legislative framework and regulatory checks by authorities for antibiotic residues in food animals and animal products, fisheries and hatcheries cultured for human consumption leads to the transfer of these antibiotic resistant genes to humans. Greater number of livestock farmers are not aware of the concept of withdrawal period after antibiotic administration and whoever knows fail to follow due to financial burden. In addition it is also believed record keeping is of least importance among many livestock farmers including commercial farms. Illiteracy of livestock farmers, quackery, over the counter (OTC) antibiotic availability, distantly located animal health centers, poor handling and cleanliness in farms, and improper animal waste (liquid and solid) disposal are the crucial factors aggravating the situation of AMR.

ANTIMICROBIAL USE IN ENVIRONMENT

The predominant cause of development of AMR in the environment is poor hygiene, sanitation and lack of implementation of suitable public health measures. It is not uncommon for untreated sewage to be let out in open drains which menacingly burden any public health measures being taken. The general public is not sufficiently made aware of appropriate treatment and disposal of human waste. The emergence of antibiotic resistant bacterial infection with a novel NDM-1 (New Delhi metallo -beta lactamase)gene in the year 2009 stokes fears of exponential versatility of the bacterial genome to develop resistance against antibiotics. An environment point prevalence study carried out in New Delhi after NDM -1 gene, pointed to samples isolated from both drinking water samples and seepage samples .This concludes transmission of resistant genes to different arrays of hosts through the environment.

India is the pharmaceutical hub in manufacturing and dispensing of generic drugs. Holding the top spot in drug production, pharmaceutical industries do not impart adequate infrastructure to treat effluents of drug processing, thereby active compounds of many antibiotic drugs remain unchanged and are emitted into surrounding soil and water bodies. As these drug compounds get diluted in huge water bodies, pathogenic or commensal microflora are constantly exposed to sub-therapeutic doses of antimicrobials causing development of resistance genes and dissemination of resistant genes from the environmental reservoir to human pathogens (Bengtsson-Palme *et al.*, 2014). Many industries do not invest in infrastructure for effluent management.In Spite of infrastructure setup to treat effluents from pharmaceutical factories called ETS (Effluent Treatment System) ,few industries require more energy and money to run the effluent treatment plant than to the drug manufacturing unit (Bhushan *et al.*, 2016).

Veterinary practitioners	Para-clinical Staffs	Veterinary Pharmacists/ Pharmaceutical companies	Farmers/Farm Owners	Public	Research
Imprudent prescription of antibiotics due to lack of diagnostic facilities at dispensary level.	Informal prescription of antimicrobials	Suggesting the drugs to livestock farmers based on experience.	Use of antimicrobials for non-therapeutic purpose (Mahalmani et al., 2019)	Drastic shift from plant based to animal-protein based diets	Lack of surveillance data on antimicrobial resistance in the public domain.
Unable to dedicate time for clinical services due to non-clinical work burden (schemes, etc)	lack of knowledge on antibiotics and AMR	Lack of data on antimicrobial sales by Veterinary Pharma companies/ pharmacy shops	Lack of maintaining antimicrobial usage data.	Shifting from quantity to quality	Lack of diagnostic kits (e.g. ABST) at a cheaper rate.
Shortage of human resource	use of antibiotics, which is beyond their brief. (68)	Direct marketing of drugs to farmers (Mahalmani et al., 2019)	unaware about legislative framework on antimicrobial usage in livestock production	lack of knowledge on antibiotic residues.	lack of regional wise antibiotic resistance pattern.

Veterinary practitioners	Para-clinical Staffs	Veterinary Pharmacists/ Pharmaceutical companies	Farmers/Farm Owners	Public	Research
Choice of antibiotic is less in government supply.	With or without Imitating veterinarians in treatment is unauthorized.	over the counter sale	Antimicrobial drug withdrawal periods rarely observed	Poor availability of ready-made kits to test the quality of product at cheaper rate.	Very few integrated antimicrobials surveillance studies.
Little continuing veterinary education programmes.	easily accessible and low cost to farmers	counterfeit drug sale	Use of antibiotics against non-bacterial infections.		Comparatively less funding availability to curb the AMR in livestock.
	Treatment with higher generation of antibiotics to impress the farmers.	Sale of drugs by seeing used sachets or vials on farmers demand.	Use of antibiotics labelled for humans		Little convergence to combat on AMR.
		lack of stringent legislative rules for veterinary pharmacy shops	lack of doorstep animal health service.		Less significance on one health approach.
			Approaching non-qualified persons for treatment at begining stage of infection.		missing continuity in AMR research.

Pharmaceutical industries also set their own standards of antibiotic residue limits in effluents, violating the proposed standards by MoEFCc. These manufacturing waste are usually disposed off into nearby water bodies and soil which forms the environmental reservoir of AMR causing determinants such as resistant microbes, antibiotic residues and resistance conferring genes that are actively transmitted to other non-resistant microbes (Framework & Resistance, 2019).

ANTIMICROBIAL USE IN AQUACULTURE

The aquaculture industry boomed in the past four decades due to mounting demand for food security and it represents the world's fastest growing food production sector. Food security is a global priority in 2030 according to the UN Agenda of Sustainable Development Goal which focuses on eradicating poverty and sustainable food production without environmental degradation (Reverter *et al.*, 2020). A shift in human dietary consumption for fish and seafood is suggested to supplement the protein needs of the growing global population and aquaculture represents an untapped opportunity to contribute to the global food systems (Froehlich *et al.*, 2018). Despite China holding the top spot in global aquaculture production at 63.2% in 2008, it was seemingly projected to decline to 56.9% in 2030. The rapid expansion of aquaculture production is expected in Southeast Asia and India. In India, aquaculture is termed as the 'sunrise sector'. Mirroring the name as sunrise sector, it is forecasted to expand production from 6.7% to 9.2% from 2010 to 2030 in global shares representing a 121% change in the 2010-30 time frames (FAO, 2020 & Bank, 2013). As this industry with tremendous potential, gains momentum to change into a key food source for India, it puts immense pressure on the need to cultivate productivity wisely and responsibly. Antimicrobials administered to fisheries and hatcheries are administered en-masse which leads to co-resistance. The presence of antibiotic residues in water excreted by aquatic food animals becomes a reservoir containing resistant microbes whose effluents are left untreated and drained into water bodies (Bandyopadhyay and Samanta, 2020). Until 2019 no national policy on Aquaculture and fisheries were existing. In light of this, a national policy called the National Inland Fisheries and Aquaculture policy was drafted (National Inland Fisheries and Aquaculture Policy. 2019).

Aquaculture
Fisheries officers of the Department of Fisheries in concerned states are usually graduates, post-graduates or PHD's who are not authorized to prescribe medicines. Fisheries science professionals are not adequately trained and authorized to prescribe medicines (Bhushan, 2016).
Antimicrobials are prohibited for use in brackish water aquaculture. But they were found to be used and recommended for use as growth promoters and for disease prevention
Pharmacists dispense Schedule H drugs to fish farmers without valid prescription.
Fish farming leads to water contamination and inadequacies in aquaculture wastewater management results in continuous interplay between antibiotics and microbes increases the reservoir of antibiotic resistance in aquatic environments.

Despite guidelines for Effluent Treatment systems(ETS) as mandated by Coastal Aquaculture Authority for shrimp aquaculture, no fisheries or hatcheries were found to have established ETS system.
Intensification of fish farming practices
Species diversification and new growing techniques have paved the way for unanticipated interaction between cultured and wild populations of aquatic animals.
Increased globalization in trade and market opportunities for farmed aquatic animals HAS simultaneously facilitated spread of diseases and pathogens.
Imprudent use of veterinary drugs for aquaculture.

EXISTING POLICIES FOR TACKLING AMR IN INDIA

(A) Policies Framed for Surveillance

1. The National Programme on the Containment of Antimicrobial Resistance was launched under the aegis of the National Centre for Disease Control (NCDC) in 2011 . The objectives of this programme were to – establish a laboratory based AMR surveillance system of 30 network laboratories; generate quality data on AMR for pathogens of public health importance; strengthen infection control guidelines and practices, and promote rational use of antibiotics; and generate awareness about the use of antibiotics in both health care providers and in the community (Kakkar M et al 2017& Srivastava, R. K. 2011).
2. The Antimicrobial Resistance Surveillance Research Network (AMRSN) launched in 2013 established by the ICMR is a national network on surveillance of AMR in laboratories based in academic centres , targeting medically important microbes. AMRSN is currently limited to the human health sector and is planning to notch up surveillance in animal, environmental and food samples.

(B) Policies Framed/Programmes Launched for Awareness and Containment

1. National policy for containment of AMR in India outlined in 2011 (Travasso, 2016).
2. Schedule H1 under the Drugs and Cosmetics Rules, to regulate the sales of antibiotics (NCDC, 2016)
3. Red line campaign (NCDC, 2016)
4. National Treatment Guidelines for Antimicrobial Use in Infectious Diseases, which were released in February 2016 to ensure rational use of antibiotics.
5. ICMR launched the programme on Antimicrobial Stewardship, Prevention of Infection and Control (ASPIC) in 2012

6. National action plan in 2017
7. Chennai declaration launched a 5 year plan to tackle the challenge of AMR in 2014
8. Jaipur declaration

EXISTING STRATEGIES THAT REQUIRE REVIEW

Tackling AMR at the grassroots level requires a One-health approach as proposed by the Tripartite Coalition of World Health Organisation (WHO),World Organisation for Animal Health(OIE) and Food & Agriculture Organisation (FAO). Aligning with the Global Action Plan by WHO released in 2015, A National Action Plan on AMR was released in 2017 directing all states of India to develop state action plans. Given the huge population and vast diversity in food-animal sectors ,public healthcare systems, geographical distribution of Natural Resources and environment , cultural and farming practices; and industrial variance in each state , individual state action plans developed could only sought to tackle this challenge .This approach thus enables each state to take lead and design targeted interventions to tackle local challenges and overcome competing interests according to its feasibility and capabilities. Kerala ,Madhya Pradesh and Delhi have been the only three states that have their respective state action plans developed to combat antimicrobial resistance.

In alignment with the Nation Action Plan on AMR, Kerala Antimicrobial Resistance Strategic Action Plan (KARSAP) involves a multi-sectoral collaboration and multidisciplinary approach involving the department of agricultural development and farmers welfare, animal husbandry, health& family welfare, environment, of strong political commitment by the Government of Kerala and collaborative fraternization among the stakeholders have yielded promising results in tackling and containment of AMR. This model of steering committee and action could be adopted by other states as well. Despite the successful implementation in surveillance and intervention of AMR, Kerala faces local challenges.

With the state being a consumer in pharmaceuticals and antibiotics comprising 20% of the total drugs consumed annually by the state, the National Drug Survey declares that 10%of drugs from government sources and 2% drugs from retail outlets were found to be not of standard quality (NSQ) in Kerala. The local challenges faced by Kerala are as follows: a) Lack of sufficient trained personnel/human resources in inland departments b) Difficulty in traceability of animal food sources to its respective farm of origin). Lack of antibiotic residue control programmes d) OTC sale of antibiotics e) Lack of appropriate treatment of urban sewerage systems leading to antibiotic residues and antibiotic resistant microbes in natural water bodies. As part of increasing surveillance on AMR, microbiology laboratories in Government hospitals proposed, to conduct a community based study to collect baseline AMR burden data in community and expand 'one-health' approach to surveillance in food, animal and environment (Antimicrobial resistance and its containment in Kerala, 2017).

Since the launch of KARSAP in 2018, Kerala has tackled resistance among six bacterial species of which four are gram negative bacillus and two belong to gram positive cocci. There had been significant drop in resistance in *Acinetobacter* species, *Klebsiella* spps , *Pseudomonas aeruginosa, E. coli, Staphylococcus* spps and *Enterococcus* spss. With widespread training and awareness workshops Kerala has managed to reduce the production of ESBL (Extended Spectrum Beta Lactamases) compared to the national average.

Despite the local challenges, key strategies developed to existing challenges include governance, regulatory action,capacity building,community participation and research. State action plans developed for all states could drastically reduce the emergence and transmission of resistant microbes. Following its launch, e-pharmacies selling drugs have been sought as a major threat that would hinder the implementation of KARSAP. Robust tracking of sales and dispensing with periodic inspection and audit would prove to be useful in tackling this challenge. To downsize the role of contribution of AMR by all the stakeholders, the easy accessibility and availability of antibiotics should be made secure and encrypted. The root cause of development of AMR is the easy access and availability of this valuable commodity to various stakeholders without suitable documentation. A digital encrypted portal would break the nexus of imprudent availability to only rationale driven antimicrobial usage.

To combat the unequal distribution of urban-rural health workforce, a recurring roster plan can be implemented wherein physicians and para-clinical staff are posted to rural districts for providing healthcare services. Startups that develop Cloud-based health management platform to connect rural people with doctors for consultation; and supply medicines with the local pharmacist and periodic follow up could bridge many problems in rural -healthcare today. The role of telemedicine and digital healthcare management would be tremendous and rightly feasible to plug the loopholes in the Indian healthcare system. Therefore it is imperative that each state formulate its own action plan to fight antimicrobial resistance by identifying the needs of the respective population and customizing solutions to perilous public health problems.

The medical fraternity has to periodically update the medical education curriculum on promoting medical professionals about generic drug prescription practices (Joshi *et al.*, 2019). With the majority of the qualified health workforce docked in urban areas of the country, Community health workers such as ASHA and Anganwadi workers were intended for providing awareness and care for maternal and child health in rural areas. Given the low number of health workforce in villages and towns of India, ASHA workers advocate education on institutional deliveries, neonatal care and immunizations, providing essential vitamin and mineral supplements, medical provisions such as contraceptives and ORS kits for treating diarrhoea. They are also equipped with administering antibiotics such as oral formulations of Cotrimoxazole and injectable Gentamicin for treating neonatal sepsis and infections. ASHA and Anganwadi workers can be made useful in creating awareness on AMR given their widespread reach and ability to identify and respond to immediate needs of the rural population. All ASHA workers are involved in the Village Health and Sanitation committee by the Gram panchayat and are key advisors in framing the village Health plan. Inductive training for these ASHA and Anganwadi workers on AMR could prove beneficial to the whole community. The ASHA women in liaison with the gram panchayat can bring about regulatory action of incessant usage of antibiotics in animal farms, and agriculture.

The following measures can be implemented to eliminate contribution of AMR in rural villages

a. Antibiotics should not be used in feed as supplements or as growth promoters in farms. Prebiotics, probiotics and phototherapeutics for growth promotion in animals should be encouraged. Use of antibiotics for prophylaxis, therapeutic and metaphylactic purposes should be under strict veterinary supervision.

b. Safe Manure management practices to be adopted. Land application of untreated manure to be discouraged and application of animal waste into biogas generation, development and management of a common biogas generation plant for use by small poultry farmers operating in a cluster.

RESEARCH INPUTS IN ALTERNATE STRATEGIES/TACKLING INITIATIVES FOR REDUCING ANTIBIOTIC CONSUMPTION

(A) Vaccines

A clear distinctive relationship has been demonstrated between antibiotic usage and antimicrobial resistance. Therefore strict enforcement in sales and consumption of Antimicrobials is imperative to tackle this post-antibiotic era. However, consumption of antibiotics can be substantially decreased with use of vaccines. Vaccines exert their potential by effectively killing antibiotic resistant pathogens through antibody -mediated destructive mechanisms and thereby ridding off any risk to infection due to antibiotic-resistant strains. Vaccines also obviate the need for antibiotic usage by decreasing episodes of febrile illnesses and secondary bacterial infections which require antimicrobials for management. The latter form of effect is attributed to antiviral vaccines which as such do not target organisms with antibiotic-resistant strains but result in fewer antibiotic prescriptions due to secondary bacterial infections.

Conclusively, the effect of vaccines are long standing for years together as opposed to antibiotics, which require a constant pipeline for newer class of drugs. Additional research and development in creating vaccines has not been invigorated.

(B) Herbal Alternatives for Antimicrobial Usage

Herbal extracts have been proven to fight infections against methicillin-resistant staphylococcus aureus strains in adjunct to antibiotic therapy, whose synergistic effects will shield the development of wider antibiotic resistant strains. Surprisingly, few phyto-pharmaceuticals have shown exemplary performance in comparison to gentamicin. The high burden on developing new drugs could be eased by adopting a combined treatment combination of antibiotics and phyto-pharmaceuticals taking advantage of the synergistic effects of antibacterial properties of both and reducing adverse effects of multidrug therapy.

(C) Sanitation and Hygiene Measures

Sanitation engineering is one of the very poorly overlooked needs of the Indian society. Adequate equipment or technology is not currently available to maintain public drains and sewers. Considering the crowded population and cramped housing conditions, sanitation and hygiene in houses is imperative to reduce the risk of contagious diseases that are entirely water-borne. The Swachh Bharat mission launched in 2014 has made access to household toilets from 37% in 2014 to 71% in 2018 and a reduction in open defecation practices by 26%. At any given point of time around half of the hospital beds in developing countries are occupied by people with diarrhoeal diseases. The prevention of sanitation and water -related diseases could save $7 billion per year on health system costs and an additional $3.6billion per year in deaths averted. The development of AMR is massively reduced with adopting effective sanitation and hygiene measures thereby preventing imprudent administration of antimicrobials and reducing the number of hospital admissions. Life expectancy of an individual is proved to be longer to those who live under better sanitation and living conditions.

A major policy change in enabling wastewater treatment in individual housing and settlements would drive the change for a hygienic community. Alternative food source for meat: With rising demand for animal protein to sustain the food bowl of the world, food animals are intensively reared and bred with irrational use of antibiotics. By vastly channelizing this demand with alternative sources of protein will prove beneficial economically, ecologically as well as by reducing stress on health care systems. Alternate sources of protein for meat consumers include seafood, fungi (mushrooms) and plant based protein intake. According to agro forest experts, doctors and environmental professionals the general consensus is that fungi could save the world. As more naturalists and conservationists urge people to resort to plant based diet, the burden of demand on animal meat drops which will further deem usage of antimicrobials on animals as unnecessary.

CONCLUSION

A widespread and rapidly evolving AMR calls for invigorating initiatives in policy making and legislative framework with effective enforcement and detection of violation. India being one of the BRICS countries is required to summon political commitment, to tackle these challenges by multidisciplinary approach. Despite AMR being a massive challenge, it is completely worthy of confrontation with tangible action now more than ever to avoid bearing the brunt of collapse of our healthcare delivery systems. The responsibility of the health of the community inevitably lies among all stakeholders of the healthcare sector and this silent pandemic due to AMR calls for a paradigm shift in public health policies and measures.

REFERENCES

Bengtsson-Palme J, Kristiansson E, Larsson DJ. 2018. Environmental factors influencing the development and spread of antibiotic resistance. FEMS Microbiology Reviews. 42(1):fux053.

Bloom DE, Black S, Salisbury D, Rappuoli R. 2018. Antimicrobial resistance and the role of vaccines. Proceedings of the National Academy of Sciences. 115(51):12868-71.

Davidson K. 1994. Double standards. English Today. 10(2):3–13.

Gbinigie O, Allen J, Boylan AM, Hay A, Heneghan C, Moore M, Williams N, Butler C. 2019. Does cranberry extract reduce antibiotic use for symptoms of acute uncomplicated urinary tract infections (CUTI)? Protocol for a feasibility study. Trials. 20(1):1-9.

Kakkar M, Walia K, Vong S, Chatterjee P, Sharma A. 2017. Antibiotic resistance and its containment in India. BMJ. 5:358.

Klugman KP, Black S. 2018. Impact of existing vaccines in reducing antibiotic resistance: Primary and secondary effects. Proceedings of the National Academy of Sciences. 115(51):12896-901.

Kuok CF, Hoi SO, Hoi CF, Chan CH, Fong IH, Ngok CK, Meng LR, Fong P. 2017. Synergistic antibacterial effects of herbal extracts and antibiotics on methicillin-resistant Staphylococcus aureus: A computational and experimental study. Experimental Biology and Medicine. 242(7):731-43.

O'Neil J. Review on Antibiotic resisitance. 2014. Antimicrobial Resistance: Tackling a crisis for the health and wealth of nations. Heal. Wealth Nations. 1-6.

Reverter M, Sarter S, Caruso D, Avarre JC, Combe M, Pepey E, Pouyaud L, Vega-Heredía S, De Verdal H, Gozlan RE. 2020. Aquaculture at the crossroads of global warming and antimicrobial resistance. Nature Communications. 11(1):1870.

Srivastava RK, Chaudhury RR, Bramhachari SK, Singh S, Guleria R, Sinha A, Gupta U, Kakkar M, Rodrigues C, Wattal C, Kotwani A. 2011. National policy for containment of antimicrobial resistance India. Directorate General of Health Services, Ministry of Health and Family Welfare, Nirman Bhawan, New Delhi.

Team CD. 2014. "Chennai Declaration": 5-year plan to tackle the challenge of anti-microbial resistance. Indian Journal of Medical Microbiology. 32(3):221.

Travasso C. 2016. India draws a red line under antibiotic misuse. BMJ. 352:i1202.

Van Boeckel TP, Gandra S, Ashok A, Caudron Q, Grenfell BT, Levin SA, Laxminarayan R. 2014. Global antibiotic consumption 2000 to 2010: an analysis of national pharmaceutical sales data. The Lancet Infectious Diseases. 14(8):742-50.

WHO Report on Surveillance of Antibiotic Consumption. 2016.

World Health Organization (WHO). 2019. Food Agriculture Organization of the United Nations (FAO), & World Organisation for Animal Health (OIE), Global Database for Antimicrobial Resistance Country Self-Assessment - Country progress with development of a national action plan on AMR -2018-2019.

**Rest of the references will be available on request to author

Index

COLOUR PLATES

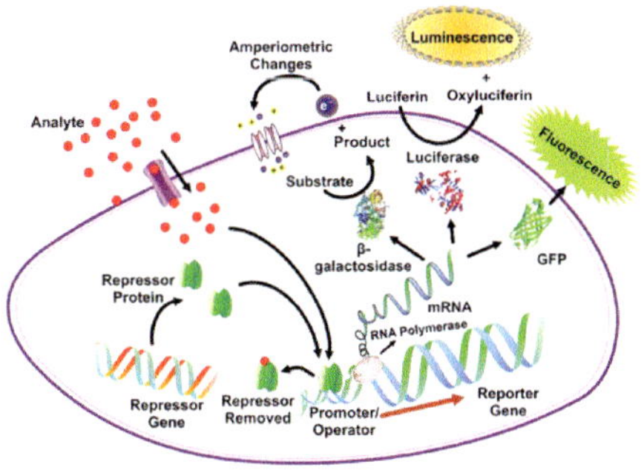

Figure 1a: Whole-cell biosensor: its principle and mechanism.
(p. 2)

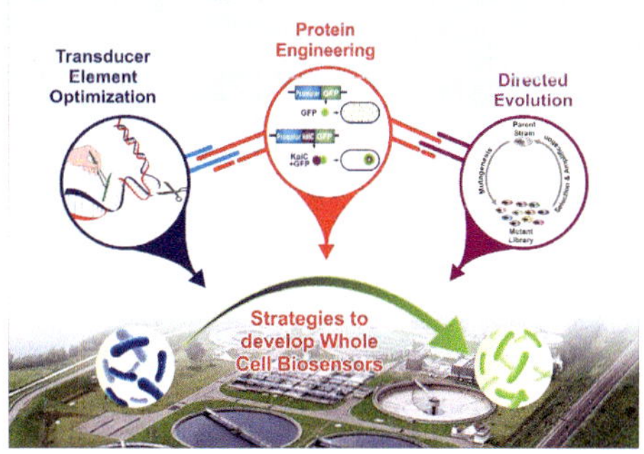

Figure : 1b. Advanced strategies to develop whole-cell biosensors for wider applicability.
(p. 5)

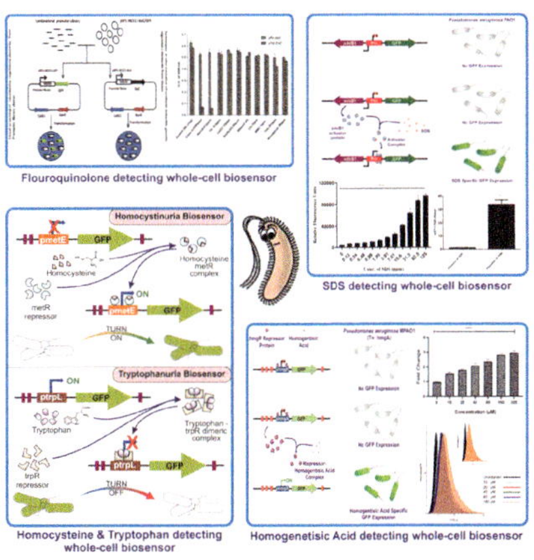

Figure : 1c. Some recently developed whole-cell biosensors for the detection of antibiotics, metabolites, and surfactants 11,12,13,14.
(p. 7)

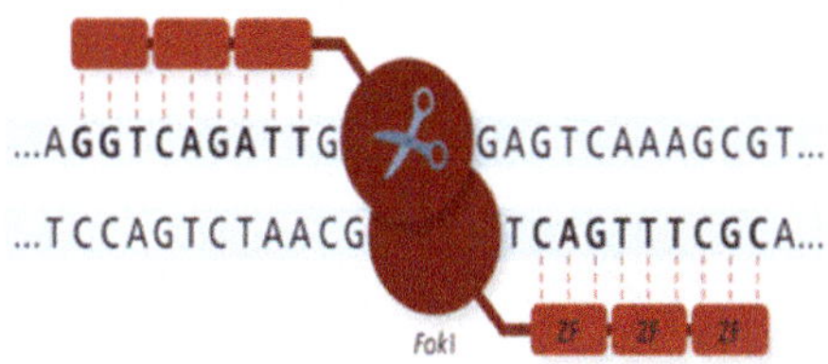

Figure 1: Zinc-finger nucleases (ZFNs)
(p. 10)

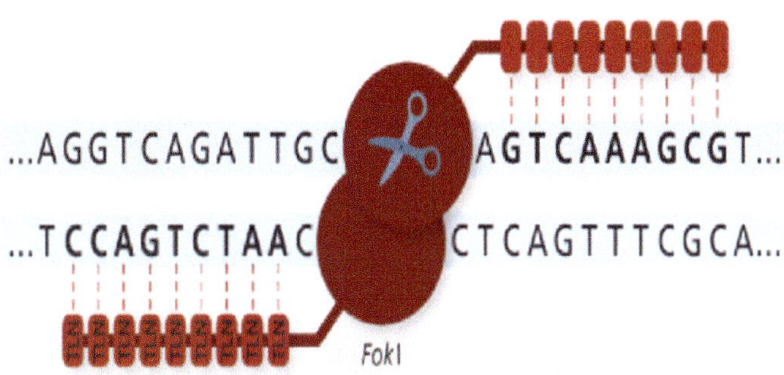

Figure 2: Transcription activator-like effector nucleases (TALENs)
(p. 10)

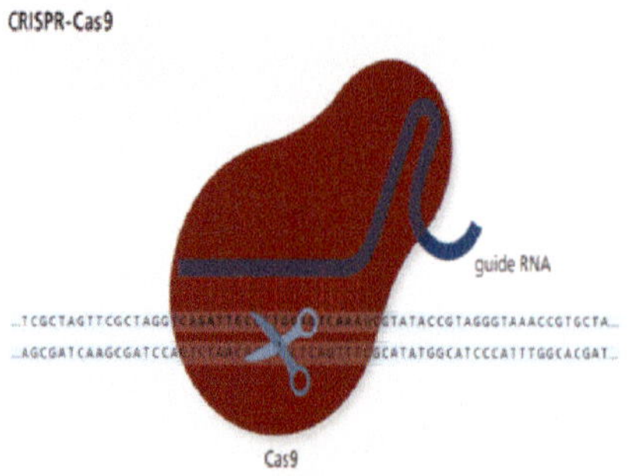

Figure 3
(p. 12)

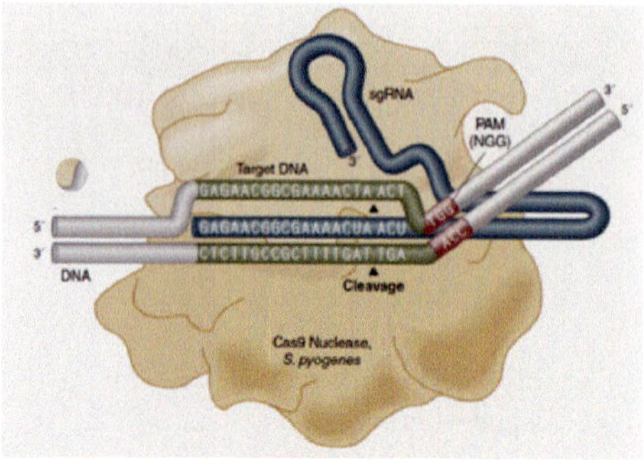

Figure 4
(p. 12)

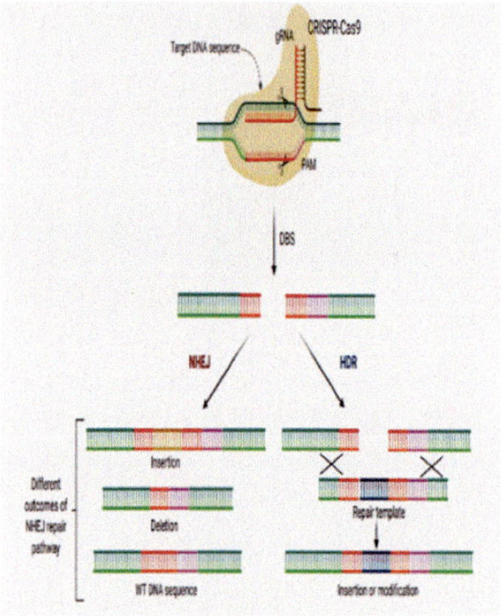

Figure 5
(p. 13)

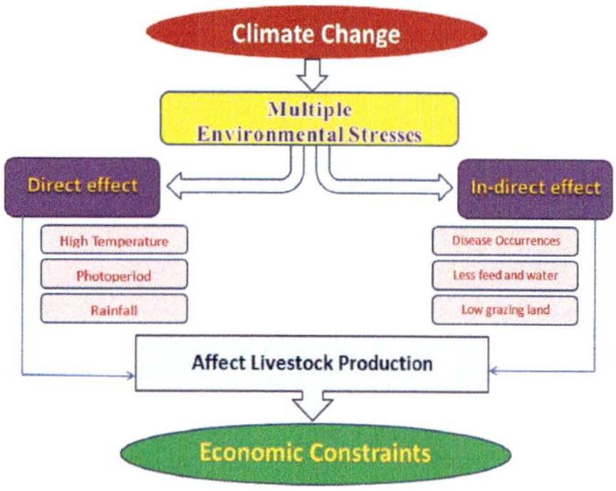

Figure1: Various impacts of climate change livestock production
(p. 26)

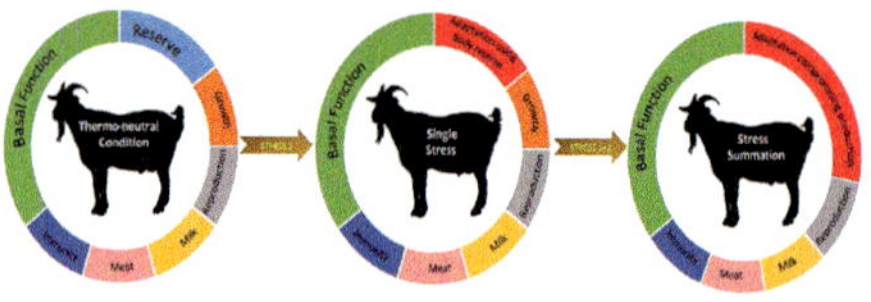

Figure 3: Pictorial representation of concept of multiple stressors on livestock production
(p. 27)

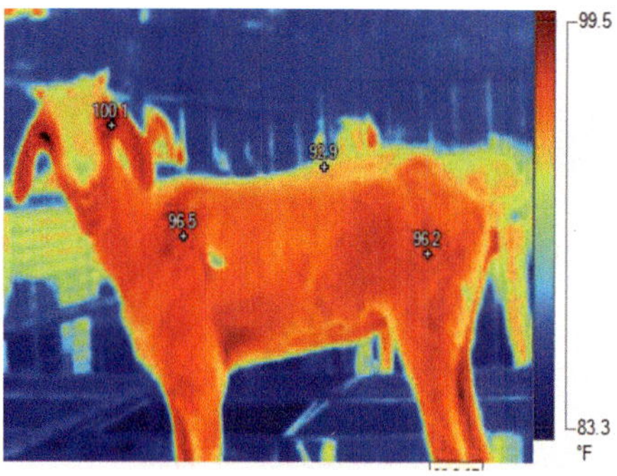

Figure 4: Surface temperature measurement in goat using infrared thermography
(p. 28)

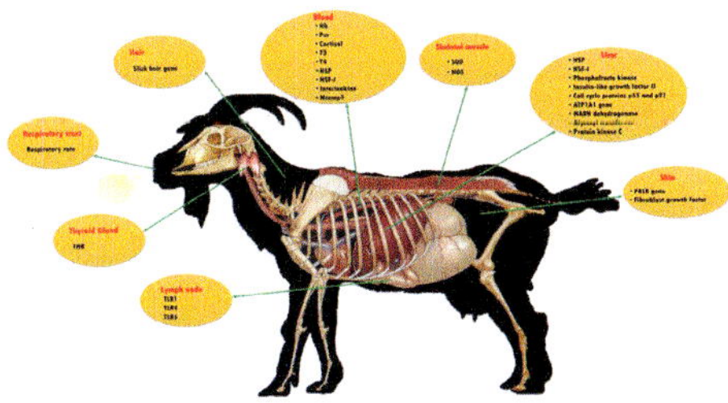

Figure 5: Different biomarkers for heat stress in goats (Source: Sejian et al., 2018)
(p. 29)

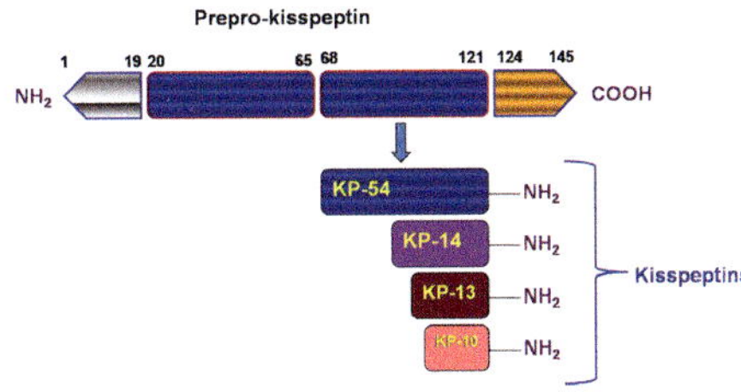

Figure 1: Formation of different types of kisspeptin from its common precursor.
(p. 35)

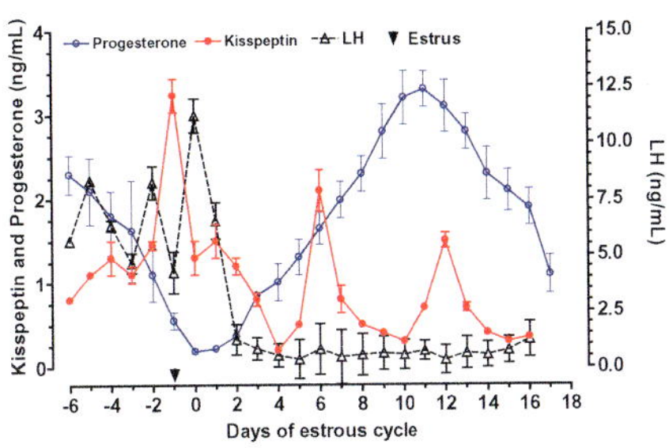

Figure 2: Blood kisspeptin, LH and progesterone profiles (mean±SEM) in cyclic crossbred cows.
(p. 37)

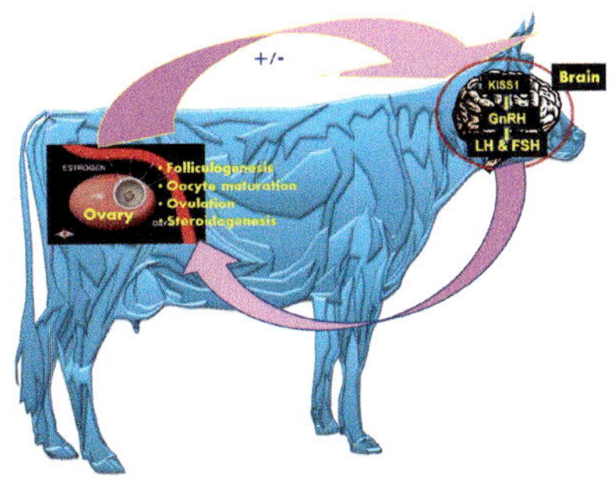

Figure 3: Influence of kisspeptin on ovarian functions and its control through steroid feedback mechanism in bovine species.
(p. 39)

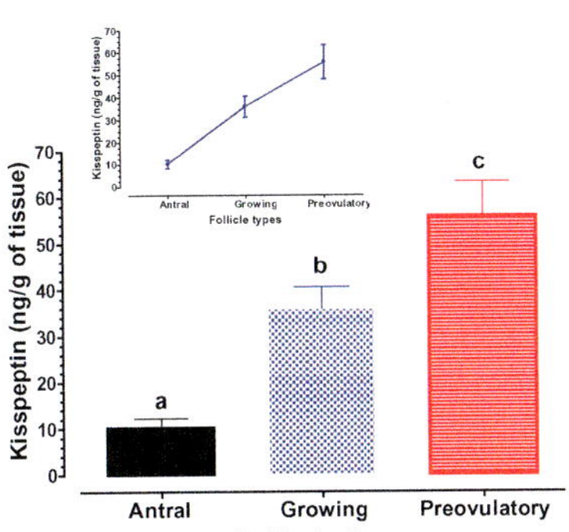

Figure 4: Mean (±SEM) content of kisspeptin in the follicles of different stages of development. A total of 10 grams of antral (5-6 mm), growing (8-10 mm) and preovulatory (15-16 mm) follicles were extracted (n=4). Bars indicated with different letters (a,b,c) differ (P<0.001). [Adopted from Mondal et al., 2015]
(p. 43)

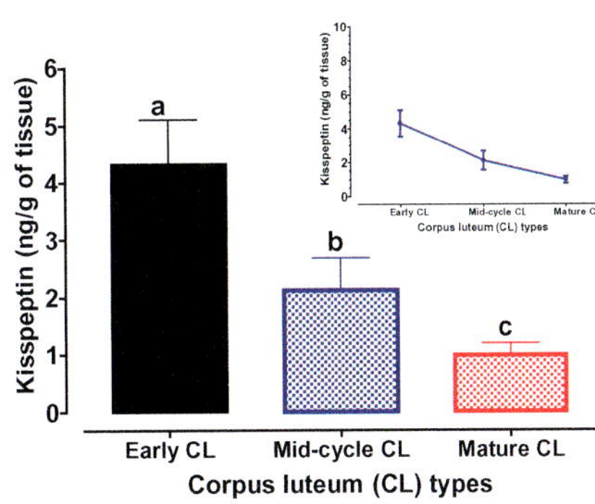

Figure 5: Mean (±SEM) content of kisspeptin in the bovine corpus luteum (CL) during different stages of development. A total of 10 grams of early, mid-cycle and mature CL tissues were extracted (n=4). Bars indicated with different letters (a,b,c) differ (P<0.001).
(p. 43)

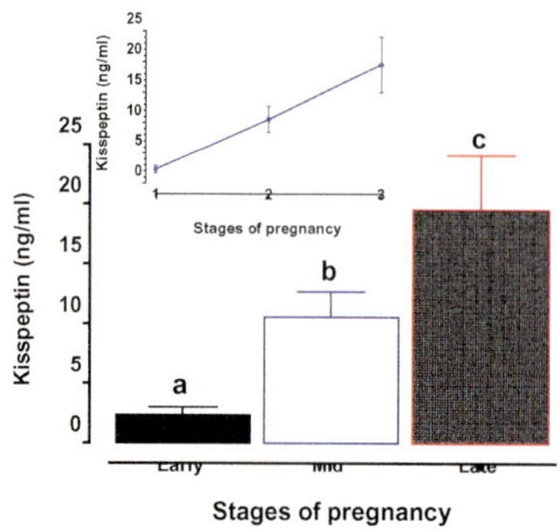

Figure 6: Mean (±SEM) profiles of blood kisspeptin in pregnant cows during different stages of pregnancy viz., early (<10 weeks; n=6), mid (>10 to <20 weeks; n=6) and late (>20 to 36 weeks; n=6) stages of pregnancy. Bars indicated with different letters (a,b,c) differ (P<0.001). [Adopted from Mondal et al., 2015]

(p. 44)

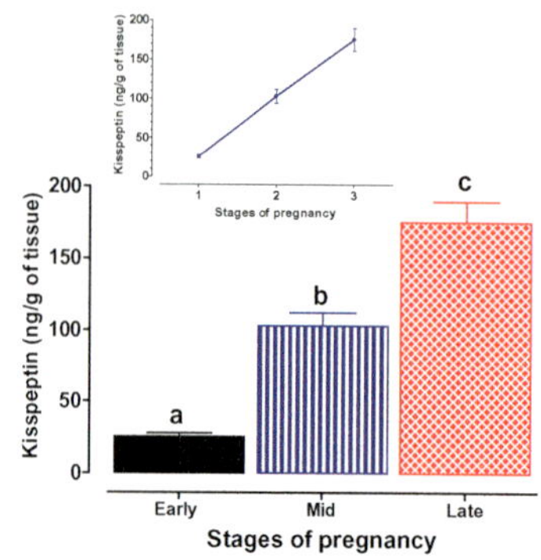

Figure 7: Mean (±SEM) content of kisspeptin in bovine placental tissues collected from animals of different stages of pregnancy. A total of 10 grams of placental tissues were extracted (n=6). Bars indicated with different letters (a,b,c) differ (P<0.001). [Adopted from Mondal et al., 2015]

(p. 45)

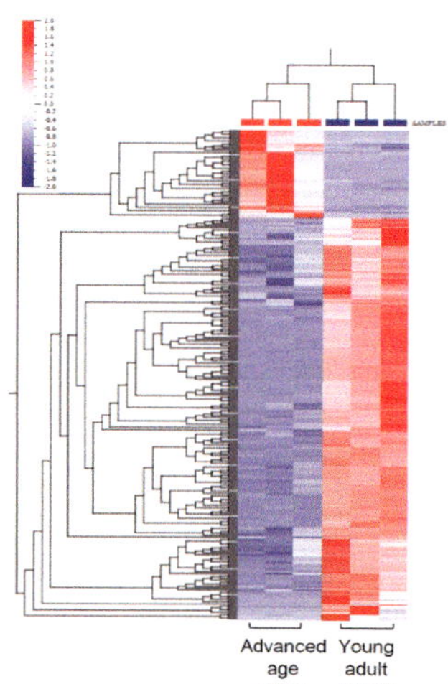

Figure 2. Hierarchical cluster analysis and heat map of 289 differentially expressed proteins of sperms in men for advanced age group (41-51 years; n=5) compared to young adult group (21-30 years: n=6). The 52 upregulated proteins are shown in red color and 237 downregulated proteins are shown in blue color. The criteria for differential expression were probability of P<0.05 and 2-fold change in the protein abundance between two age groups.

(p. 82)

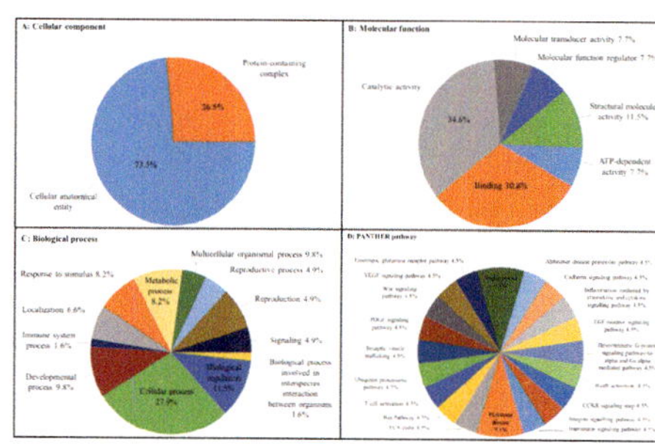

Figure 3. Global proteomic profile of human spermatozoa and aging. Pie diagrams depicting functional classification and spatial distribution of differentially upregulated proteins in the spermatozoa of advanced age group (41-51 years, n=5) compared to young adult group 121-30 years; n=6). PANTHER Classification System was used for functional analysis. Panel A: Cellular component, Panel B: Molecular function, Panel C: Biological process, and Panel D: PANTHER pathway.

(p. 84)

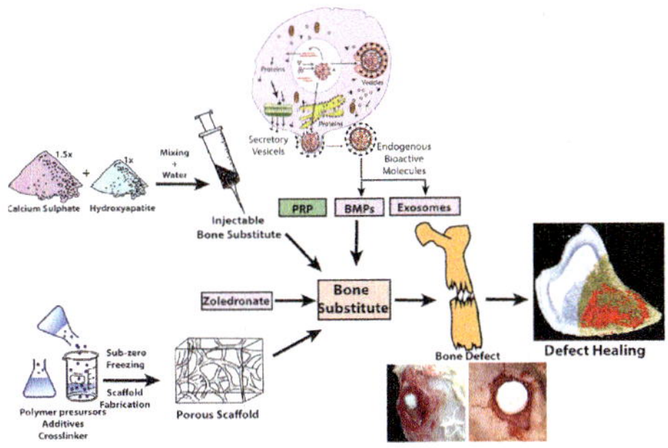

Figure 1: Schematic showing the use of injectable nano cement (NC), bioactive factors and porous scaffolds for bone defect healing [Reproduced with permission from the Ph.D thesis of Dr. Arun Kumar Teotia (Bioinspired functionalized bone substitutes for skeletal regenerative therapies), IIT Kanpur, 2018]..
(p. 92)

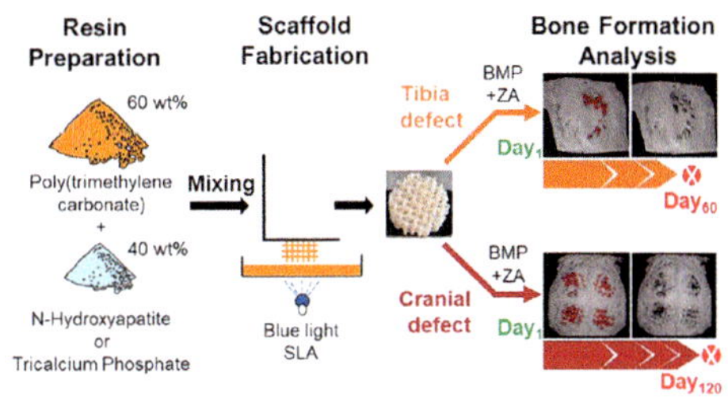

Figure 2: Schematic showing the use of poly (trimethylene carbonate) (PTMC) and nHAP/ TCP for fabrication of 3D printed scaffold and its subsequent effect over bone regeneration. [Reprinted with permission from A.K. Teotia, et al., ACS Appl. Mater. Interfaces. 12 (2020) 48340–48356. Copyright 2020, American Chemical Society]
(p. 93)

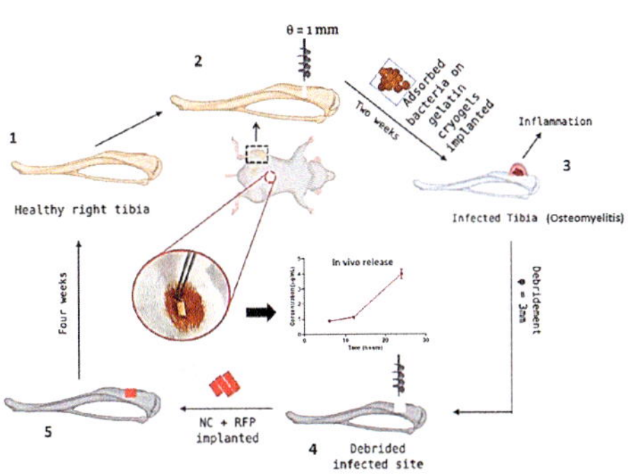

Figure 3: Graphical showing the surgical procedure where the bone defect was created infected with bacteria followed by treatment with nano cement (NC) loaded with rifampicin. [Reprinted with permission from I. Qayoom, et al., ACS Infect. Dis. 6 (2020) 2938–2949. Copyright 2020, American Chemical Society].
(p. 94)

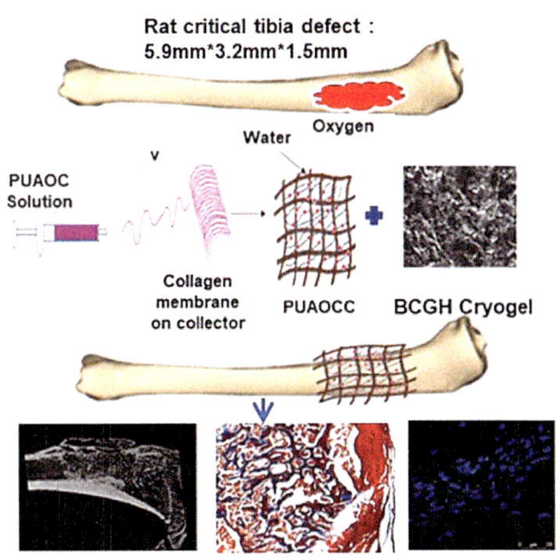

Figure 4: Schematic showing the use of cryogel and membrane for bone defect and periosteum regeneration. [Reprinted with permission from S. Gupta, et al., ACS Appl. Mater. Interfaces. 15 (2023) 8824–8839. Copyright 2023, American Chemical Society].
(p. 95)

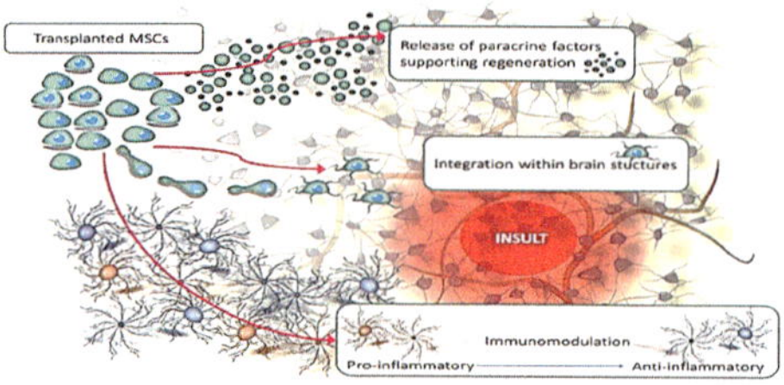

Figure 1
(p. 101)

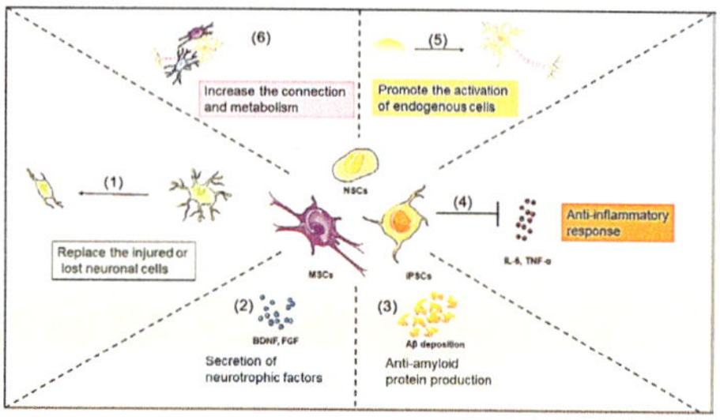

Figure 2
(p. 104)

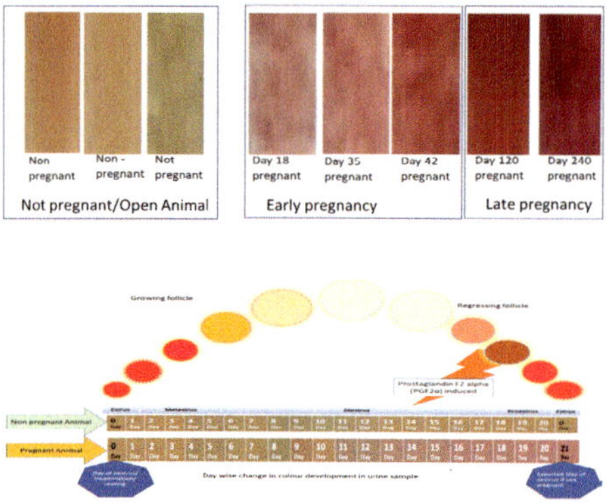

Figure 3: Colour variation with progression of pregnancy
(p. 114)

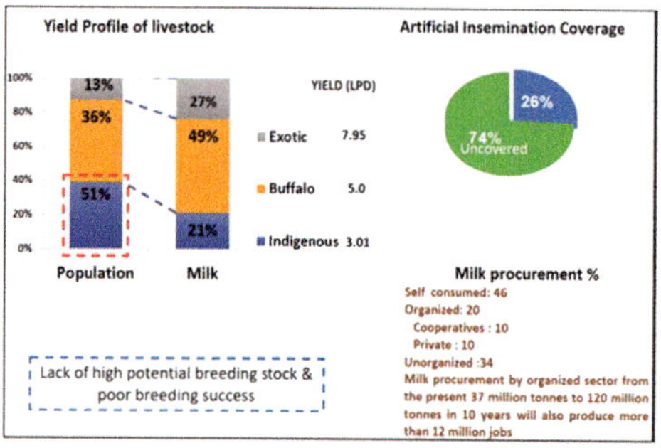

Figure 1
(p. 120)

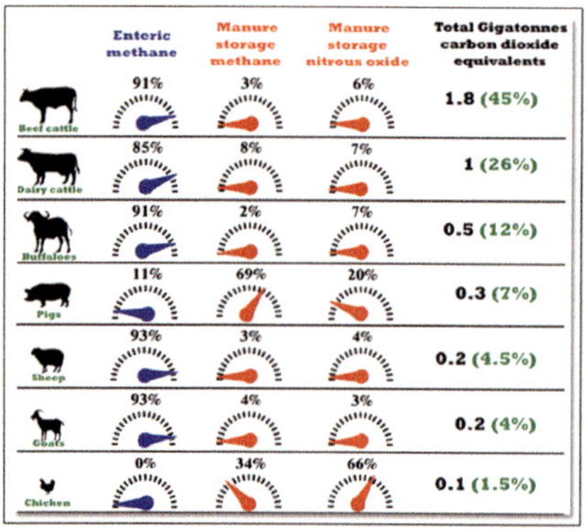

Figure 2
(p. 124)

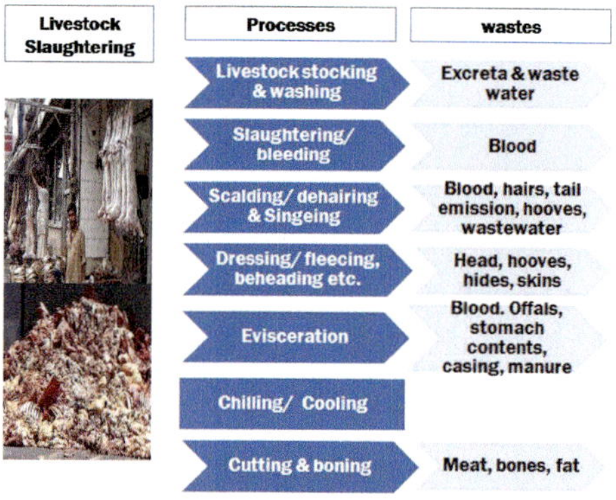

Figure 3: Livestock slaughter processes & waste
(p. 125)

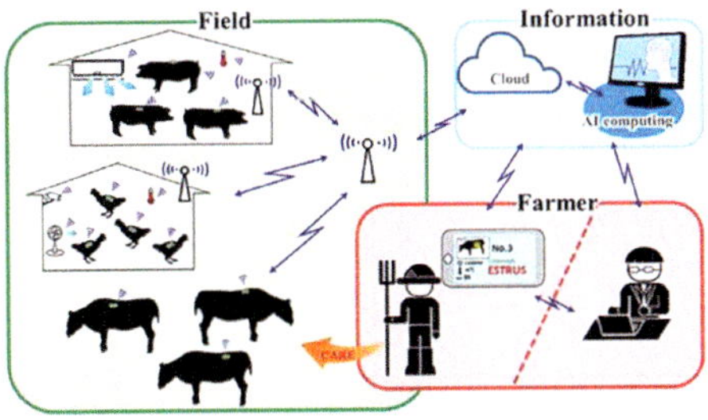

Figure 4: IoT & AI driven livestock farm model
(p. 127)

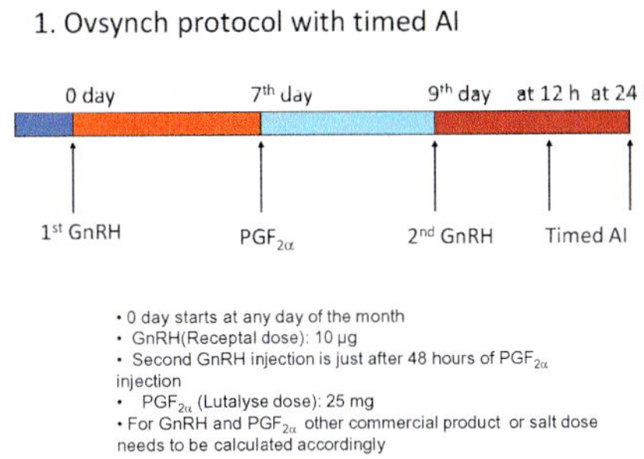

Fig. Different Synchronization Protocol presented in tabular form as ready reckoner:
(p. 137)

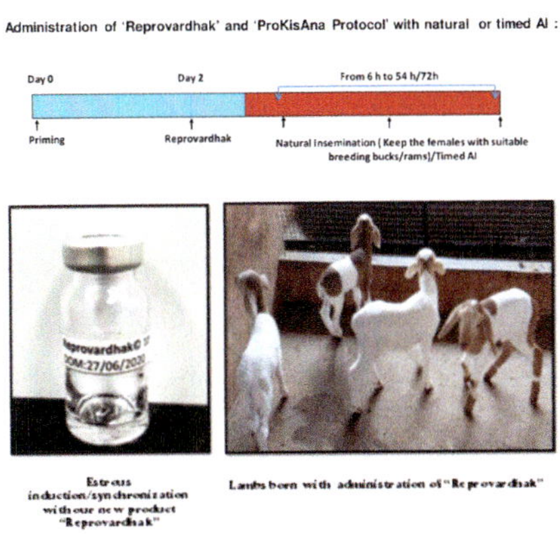

Figure 1
(p. 138)

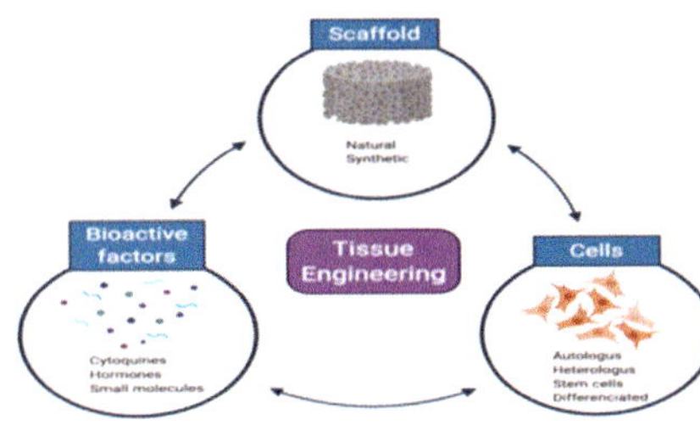

Figure 1: Tissue Engineering Triad
(p. 174)

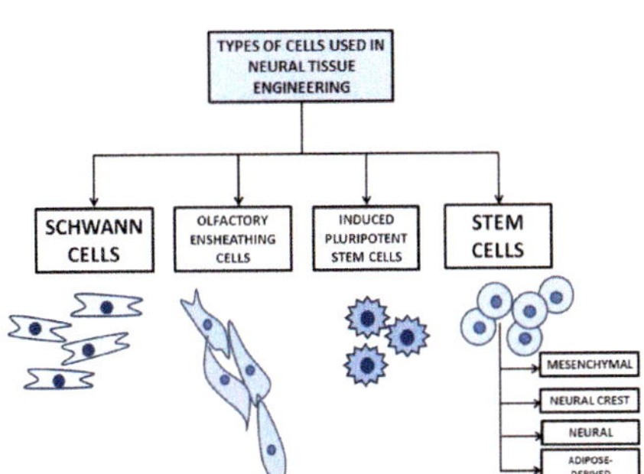

Figure 2: Types of cells used in Neural Tissue Engineering
(p. 175)

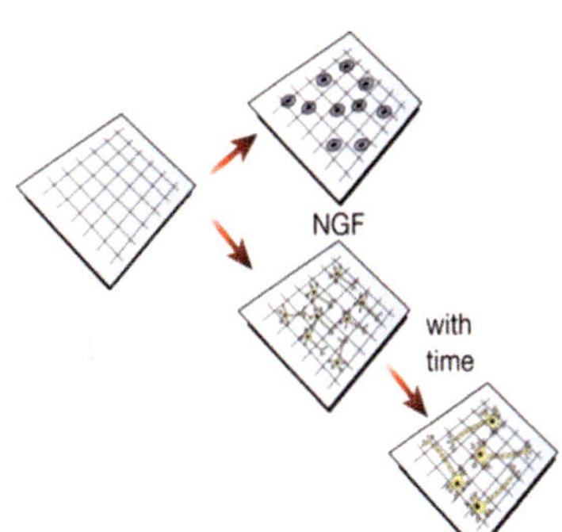

Figure 3: Polymeric structure for neural regeneration
(p. 176)

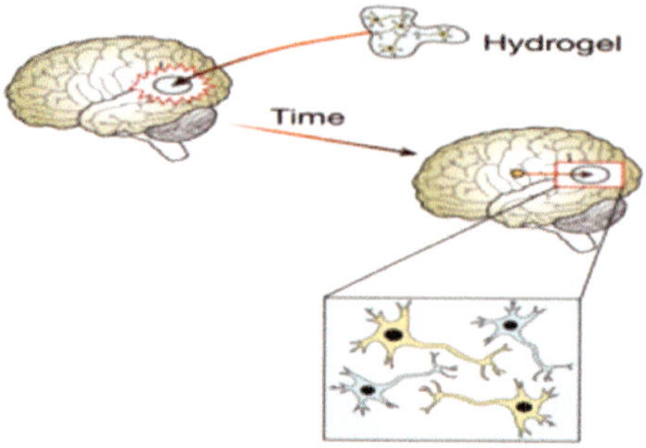

Figure 4: Polymer hydrogel supports the regeneration of the brain tissue
(p. 180)

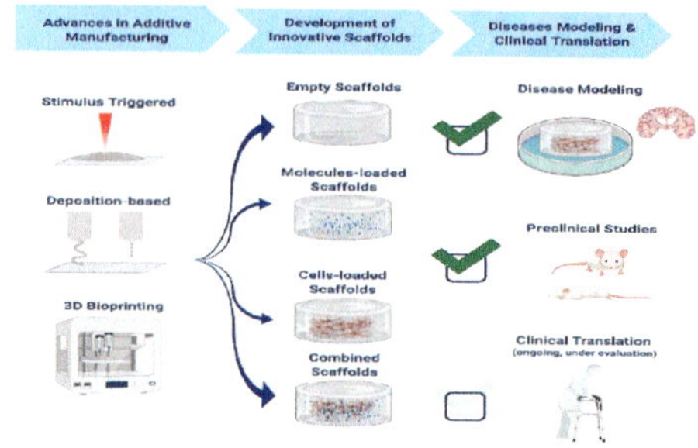

Figure 7: Use of additive manufacturing techniques in neurodegenerative diseases
(p. 181)

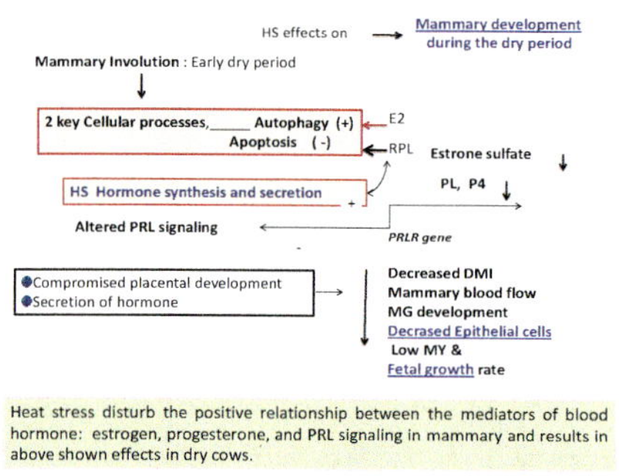

Figure
(p. 190)

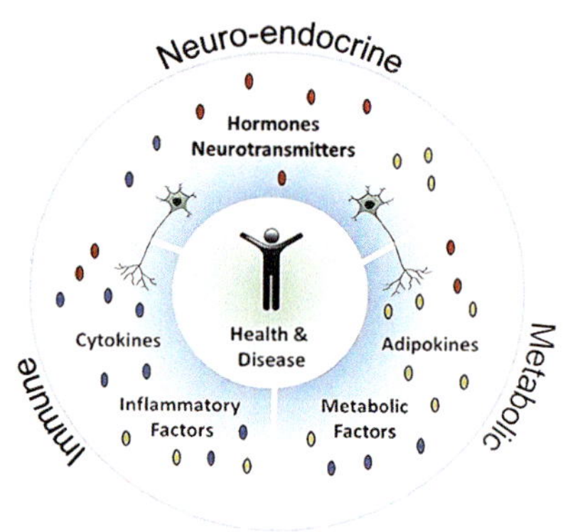

Figure 1: Neuro-endocrine, Metabolic and Immune pathways determine health and disease
(p. 222)

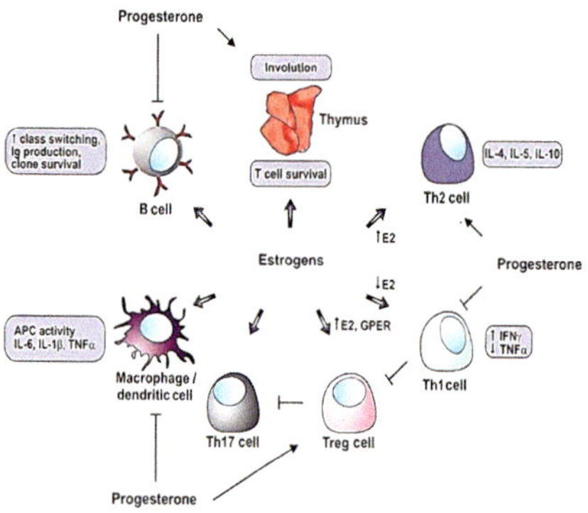

Figure 4: Generally accepted hormone effects on the immune system
(p. 232)